Stay Healthy

by
supplying
what's lacking
in your diet

GW00535878

10th edition
(updated and revised)

Researched by
David Coory

ZEALAND PUBLISHING HOUSE LTD
Private Bag 12029
Tauranga, New Zealand
www.zealandpublishing.co.nz

First published	1988 by Zealand Publishing House as *"NZ Nutrition and Your Health."*
4th Edition	1992 – revised and updated. Retitled *"Stay Healthy by Supplying What's Lacking in Your Diet."*
6th Edition	1996 – revised and updated.
7th Edition	Jan 2001 – revised and updated. New cover.
8th Edition	Sep 2001 – revised and updated. Further revisions 2002, 2003, 2004, 2006, 2007 (latest RDI's).
9th Edition	April 2013 – major rewrite and update. New cover.
10th Edition	Aug 2016 – revised and updated, with both metric and US measurements. New cover.

Further copies of this book can be obtained from Health House (books couriered free within New Zealand and Australia).

Health House
Private Bag 12029, Tauranga 3143, New Zealand.
Internet **www.healthhouse.co.nz**
Free Order Phone (New Zealand) 0800 140 141
Free Order Phone (Australia) **1800 140 141**
International **+64 7 543 0491**

ISBN 978-0-9876619-8-2

All information, advice and figures in this book are provided in good faith and are not intended to replace competent medical advice.

To improve and enhance future editions, researcher David Coory welcomes suggestions, comments or corrections. Please email him at stayhealthybook@zealandpublishing.co.nz

Printed by Brebner Print, New Zealand

"Health is the best wealth" Ancient Greek proverb

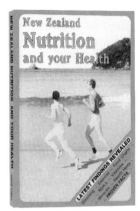

First edition of this book 1988 – re-titled in later editions

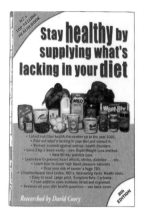

Previous 8th edition

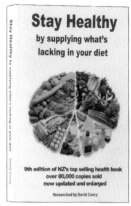

Previous 9th edition

This book is dedicated to researchers worldwide, who painstakingly pursue a better understanding of that most complex and marvellous process – the human digestive system.

Acknowledgments

Special thanks to Robert Dee, John MacKinven, Raymond Mihaere, Raymond Coory, and the staff at Health House for their editing, Caren Glazer for her cartoons and the support of my wife Marie Coory.

Contents

How this book can help you

Types of food

Vitamins

Minerals

Avoiding health disorders

Food additive list – Recipes

Health Hints and articles

More over the page

"Men occasionally stumble over the truth, but most of them pick themselves up and hurry off as if nothing ever happened."

Sir Winston Churchill

Give me the facts

I researched and wrote the first edition of this book 28 years ago. With each new edition (this is the 10th) I try to include updated facts and useful suggestions. Readers like yourself often provide these. The previous 9th edition was a major revision and almost complete rewrite – I also tried to improve readability by adding a little colour.

This book has remained New Zealand's top selling health book since it was first published in 1988 and so far over 88,000 copies have been bought by our modest population of less than 5 million people. I feel this is due to its reasonable price, simple layout, useful feedback from readers, plus my zeal for health and love of research and experimenting.

As this latest 2016 update and revision will also be made available internationally, some New Zealand (abbreviation NZ) terms and measurements have been clarified – such as 100 g (grams) being approx 4 oz. For more on this see page 17.

My passion is that you enjoy optimum health and enjoy good food by following the nutrition and health guidelines outlined in this book. May you have a clear mind and memory, a sound heart, clear arteries, healthy bones, a cheerful, worry-free outlook on life and refreshing sleep. Hopefully you can also be free of diabetes and obesity.

You can avoid or cure many health problems

You'll almost certainly find, by using this book, that your present diet is not giving you enough or the right balance of some important fats, minerals and vitamins. This can mean you're not obtaining all the energy you might otherwise enjoy, or your immune system is not performing as well as it could – also that your memory and mind are not as sharp and clear and relaxed as they should be.

This dietary problem can also be tragic for our children and grandchildren – lack of optimum nutrition is increasingly being linked to learning difficulties, obesity, addictions, ADHD, anti-social behaviour and drug abuse.

Nutritional knowledge is so vitally important – the content and often the taste of our food is steadily being lowered by the modern practice of using NPK (nitrogen-phosphorus-potassium) chemical fertilisers which lack trace minerals. Added to this is on-going genetic selection for higher crop yields and over-processing to extend shelf life.

Sadly, I find with every major update of this book, I have to remove NZ grown crop foods off the book's food tables, as typical daily servings no longer meet the cut-off point of at least 10% of our RDI (Recommended Daily Intake) – the previous 9th edition was no exception.

However, unprocessed meat and fish generally remain consistently nutritious. NZ beef and lamb, which is nearly all grass-fed, have a higher nutritional content than overseas meat. Fish remain nutritious (apart from traces of mercury in some large species) as the mineral content of sea water, unlike soil, remains consistent.

There is brighter news – more and more food growers are beginning to adopt natural soil fertilising methods to enhance the probiotic (healthy bacteria) content of their soil. This is a major step in the right direction.

Mineral and vitamin deficiencies widespread in NZ

In the meantime, as a result of nutrient-poor food, and processing for convenience and long shelf life, nutritional deficiencies are common and widespread. Below is a list of typical mineral and vitamin deficiencies, compared to our Recommended Daily Intake (RDI). These figures are taken from the NZ 2009 Adult Nutrition Survey, with overseas averages for those not tested in the survey.

Iodine	100% deficient (NZ survey)
Vitamin D	84% of elderly deficient (NZ survey)
Chromium	80% deficient (overseas average)
Vitamin B12	80% deficient (overseas average)
Iron	80% women deficient (NZ survey)
Copper	75% deficient (overseas average)
Magnesium	72% deficient (overseas average)
Omega 3 fat	60% deficient (overseas average)
Zinc	52% - 90% deficient (NZ survey)
Calcium	45% - 90% deficient (NZ survey)
Selenium	45% - 78% deficient (NZ survey)

This book will show you how to rectify these deficiencies.

Avoiding serious diseases

I had hoped to limit the size of the previous 9th edition to that of previous editions, but felt the need to add chapters revealing the latest findings on avoiding the serious and feared health disorders that are so prevalent today. These include cancer, heart attack, stroke, high blood pressure, diabetes and Alzheimer's. I've also included a chapter on a new method of achieving permanent slimness that really works, and guidance as to whether you should take supplements. I have revised and updated these in this new 10th edition.

I welcome feedback, good or bad, on any aspect of this book.

"The first requirement of a good life is to be healthy."
                    Herbert Spencer 1820–1903, (English philosopher)

Flat 1. 980 High St, AVALON
Lower Hutt, WGTON. N.Z.
Tel. 5 6722 61.

(Steve, Ron's elder son brought
your letter up on Fri 1st. Dec.)
My Dear Stell. (from Petone)
            Very many thanks
for your letter.
    I am very concerned to
hear about your Pancreatic
Cancer, & am sending you this
book in the hope you will
find something helpful.
    My Dietician raved about it
& my Dr said it was an
excellent book, so you may
find something useful in it.
Vitamin D. on page 214 sounds
hopeful + Omega 3 also on 206.
        Will get this off to-morrow
Monday, if I can manage it.
        With much love to yourself
+ the family.
Have a very Happy Xmas.
(See pages 214, 206,   Peg XX
99, 102 + P.50, + 109.   P. T.O.

ALCALINE FOODS

Almonds, Apples, Apricots
Artichokes, Avocados-ie alligate
- Pears, Bananas, Beans,- dried
fresh string, green Lima, dried
Lima also known as Butter Beans in
the U.K. Kidney Beans & Soy Beans
Beets & Beet Tops, Bran Broccoli
Brussel Sprouts, Cabbage white, & red,
Cantaloup. Carrots & raw carrots,
also, Cauliflower, Celery & root,
Cherries, red & white, Cocoanut dried
natural, fresh & C. Milk, Corn, sweet &
dried, Cranberries, Cucumbers, Currants
dried (fresh are acid) Dates, Garlic,
Grapefruit, Guava, Herbs, Irish Moss,
Kelp Salt, Leeks, Lemons, Lentils
& Lettuce, Mango Milk- goats, Mushrooms,
onions, oranges, Parsley, Parsnips
Peaches dried (fresh are acid) Peas
fresh green & dried,

Acid Foods:

Asparagas, Barley, pearled, & whole grain also, Beef - lean dried, Beet Tops, Blueberries, Blackberries, Butter, Cashew Nuts, Cereals - whole grain, Cheese, chicken chocolate, cider, COCOA, Cod Liver oil, Cottage cheese, Currants - fresh (& dried, are alkaline) Egg whites & Yolks, Gooseberries, grapes, Halibut, Ham, Hazelnuts, Honey.

You need 20% acid in the diet & 80% alkaline food in your diet from Dr Bernard Jenson's book - Foods that Heal. Check this all out with a Diet-rician, or Nutritionish as things change; Don't forgot to listen to your body - in other words - Instinctive ~~Eating~~ Eating, your body's instinct will tell you what you need also,

Dr Linus Pauling 2 times
Nobel Prize winner.
" You can trace every
sickness, every ailment &
every disease to a mineral
deficiency. What minerals or
Vitamins are you lacking in?
Need a diet with 20% acid
& 80% Alkaline. (Need Dietician
or Nutritionist would help.
Starving Cancer with a
Ketogenic diet. page 206

Cod Liver Oil for Vit D. P.102
Flaxseed " Omega 3 help.
page 206.
And don't forget about CoQ.10.
on page 109.

Answers to your questions

You will find these and many more questions answered as you learn the latest findings of worldwide health research. Use the index at the back of the book to locate the information.

- How can I get rid of my arthritis pain?
- How can I lose fat quickly and stay slim permanently?
- How can I regain my lost energy?
- How can I improve my short term memory?
- How can I remain calm and relaxed without medication or alcohol?
- How can I avoid dementia and Alzheimer's in old age?
- What are the secrets of longevity?
- How can I restore my youthful libido?
- How can I avoid asthma attacks?
- How can I avoid or reverse type 2 diabetes?
- Should I take a cholesterol lowering statin drug?
- How can I prevent osteoporosis?
- How can I sleep peacefully all night, without medication?
- Should I drink eight glasses of water every day?
- I don't drink milk – how can I get enough calcium?
- How can I lower my high blood pressure without drugs?
- How can I cure my fibromyalgia?
- How do I protect myself against a heart attack or stroke?
- How can I stop needing to urinate frequently?
- My prostate is swollen and blocking my flow – what can I do?
- How can I regain my sexual potency?
- How can I avoid prostate cancer?
- How do I replace my gut probiotics destroyed by antibiotics?
- What do the food additive numbers on packaging really mean?
- Can good nutrition stop my hair turning grey?
- What is the cause of the explosion in autism nowadays?
- Is fluoride harmful to my body? What are the true facts?
- What nutrients will help me avoid feeling depressed?
- What minerals and vitamins prevent harm from taking the pill?
- What nutrients should I take to help me get pregnant?
- How can I get rid of my food allergies?

Doctors training

Doctors are often criticised for lacking in-depth knowledge of nutrition. However to be fair it should be remembered that doctors have obtained a degree in the field of medicine, not nutrition.

A medical degree covers the wide and complex field of pharmacology. Pharmaceutical drugs are designed to treat disease and relieve symptoms of discomfort, normally by artificially correcting abnormal body conditions. For years we have expected doctors to do the impossible and drug us back to health – but medications don't heal, nor are they designed to heal.

A doctor's extensive training also includes the physiology of the human body and diagnoses of numerous disorders. All of these fields are separate from nutrition and natural healing. It's unfair to expect doctors to be specialists in these fields also.

In the past, medical students were simply taught that a *'balanced diet provides all that is required for normal health'* but medical training in nutrition is now reported to be a little more comprehensive.

We should appreciate that medical doctors have high intellects, are normally dedicated for life to their profession and frequently work long hours, receiving little recognition for the stressful nature of their work.

Doctors also learn early in their careers that most patients have little interest in changing their eating habits, or doing any exercise. Can you blame a busy GP, with a full waiting room, who at the end of a consultation reaches for the prescription pad to prescribe a quick pharmaceutical drug fix for annoying symptoms? That is after all what a GP has largely been trained to do.

Human nutrition is a separate and highly complex field of study in itself, usually involving four or more years of study. If we want to try to avoid disease, or improve our health by good nutrition, we should consult a dietician or a nutritionist – or to treat a medically diagnosed disorder naturally, we should see a naturopath or a herbalist.

Unfortunately, in NZ the cost of visiting a natural practitioner is not subsidised by our taxes – neither are the supplements they may recommend. Perhaps they should be?

Nevertheless, many of the most useful sources consulted for this book came from former drug-prescribing medical doctors (such as the late Dr Robert Atkins). Every one of these doctors appeared greatly enthused by the results they were obtaining from nutrient therapy.

It is clear from my years of research, that there are three main causes for nearly all common health disorders:

- emotional stress
- poor diet
- lack of exercise

In other words, the so-called 'western lifestyle'.

Drugs won't heal these disorders, however, with the exception of advanced old age, our body is designed to be self-healing – all it requires is sound sleep, love, affectionate touching, self respect, freedom from anxiety and negativity, wholesome food and exercise.

However, along with a little self-discipline and perhaps the guidance of a sympathetic GP, dietician or natural health practitioner, the information in this book should help you maintain or greatly improve your health. Try to choose a health professional who enjoys his or her work, and if a medical doctor, one who is reluctant to prescribe drugs (except in emergencies). Moreover, choose one who has a warm reassuring smile and a cheerful, caring attitude. These personal qualities are healing in themselves.

"Man lives on one quarter of what he eats. On the other three quarters lives his doctor."
Old Arab proverb

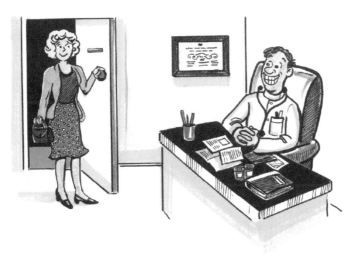

Try to choose a doctor who has a warm, reassuring smile.

Layout of this book

The first part of this book looks at the major food items – alcohol, food energy, carbs, sugars, fibre, fats, cholesterol, water and protein. Then we explore in detail, one by one, each of the vitamins and minerals necessary for good health. The format is simple and consistent so you can use the book as a handy reference.

Each vitamin and mineral section also has a food table that shows you how much of each vitamin or mineral is provided by typical servings of New Zealand (NZ) foods. Each section also provides you with interesting facts about each nutrient under the following headings:

Role in our body

This heading lists the roles played in our body by that particular nutrient as far as nutritional science understands it today.

Too little

Here you find listed the most commonly reported symptoms of a lack or deficiency of that particular vitamin or mineral. Not every symptom will show up in any one person. Some symptoms – low energy for example, are common to deficiencies of a range of nutrients.

The word 'factor' after a symptom means that a deficiency only contributes to the symptom and is not the primary cause.

Too much

This is a list of symptoms of too high an intake. Some nutrients can be toxic in high doses – vitamin A for example, and the minerals phosphorus, copper and iron.

Cooking losses

This lists cooking losses, if any. Cooking food, except for boiling veges and then tipping the water down the sink, normally does not significantly reduce the availability of nutrients (except for vitamin C). In some vegetables it enhances their availability.

Frying, baking, steaming and microwaving retain most of the nutrients in food – however, heat-sensitive enzymes can be destroyed by any cooking method.

The RDI (Recommended Daily Intake)

At the top of each food table you will see listed the **RDI** or **RDA** (Recommended Dietary Allowance) as it is known in some countries). This tells you how much of that vitamin or mineral needs to be in your diet each day to maintain good health.

In order to keep things simple, a food serving is only listed when it provides 10% or more of your recommended daily intake or RDI.

The RDI is the amount of that particular nutrient to maintain the health of 98% of the population, or as medical jargon puts it *'sustenance or avoidance of deficiency states.'* These are not necessarily optimum figures.

Many factors can hinder the absorption of nutrients, such as poor digestion due to emotional stress, lack of useful gut bacteria (probiotics), the birth control pill and pharmaceutical medications, especially stomach acid reducers such as Losec. Ironically, it can be during times of stress that we have our greatest need for nutrients.

For RDI purposes the average adult is defined as a male weighing 76kg (168 lb) and female 61kg (134 lb), although the NZ 2009 Nutrition Survey listed current male/female average weights at 89 kg (196 lb) and 75 kg (165 lb). However weight is not critical to nutrition requirements – fat is only stored energy. Height is a better indicator – the taller you are, the more nutrients you need to maintain your body. So the RDI is set for an average male height of 178 cm (5 ft 10) and female of 164 cm (5 ft 4).

The RDI (or RDA) is reviewed every few years as more nutritional knowledge becomes available. NZ and Australia share the same RDI. It was last revised in 2006. The RDI - RDA is similar for most nations.

Where a NZ RDI has not been officially set, an estimated figure has been used, averaged from reliable nutritional sources.

Some nutrients have special RDI's for children, but most are calculated on a weight pro-rata scale, ie, a 38 kg (84 lb) boy – half the average adult male weight of 76 kg (168 lb) would require 50% of the adult RDI.

Pregnant and breast feeding women have higher requirements than normal, generally around 20% more. This is mostly taken care of by increased appetite, although folate (folic acid) and vitamin C need to be almost doubled, and the intake of iron tripled.

Final chapters

The second part of the book contains some chapters on maintaining good health, based on the latest research. These include how to avoid heart attack and stroke, high blood pressure, cancer and Alzheimer's. Also information on the nutritional treating of health disorders and a look at whether we should take health supplements.

Then there is a chapter on becoming permanently slim for the rest of your life, revealing an effective (and even enjoyable) way to this elusive state. This could interest many of us – the 2009 Nutrition Survey found that 75% of NZ men and 63% of NZ women were overweight.

Also included in this second part of the book is a chapter on health and religious beliefs which takes an interesting look at the impressive health statistics from American studies of the Amish Mennonites, Seventh Day Adventists and Church of Jesus Christ of Latter Day Saints (Mormons), all of whom practice dietary laws that clearly promote superior health and longevity.

To summarise there is a **Conclusions** chapter, to try and arrive at some dietary and lifestyle recommendations from the information covered – also in the chapter headed 'My own health' I briefly outline my daily routine, something I'm often asked about.

A food additive chapter lists all the ingredient codes we see on processed food packaging and explains what they really are. The ones that are known to have caused health problems are marked with an *, and those that are particularly problematic **.

You might also decide to try the four healthy but tasty recipes I've developed in my passion for health.

Finally the book ends with a comprehensive index to help you find the information you want quickly.

"You are what you eat."   **Traditional proverb**

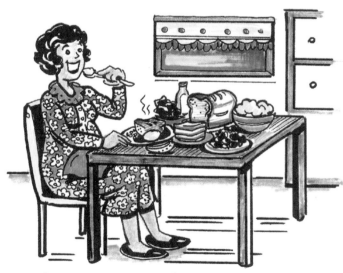

Higher RDI requirements for pregnant women are mostly taken care of by increased appetite.

Using the food tables

The food tables list the mineral and vitamin content of NZ foods and show you which foods will give you the recommended daily intake (RDI or RDA) of the minerals and vitamins you need.

For example, we New Zealanders have one of the lowest levels of selenium in the world – so you might decide to start by turning to the information in the **Selenium** section (page 168).

Firstly you'll read interesting facts about selenium, next the role of selenium in the body, and then a list of symptoms of too little or too much selenium in our diet – then comes the selenium food table.

Here you'll find listed all the foods containing useful amounts of selenium – those that give you at least 10% of your RDI in a typical serving. For example, this food table shows you that if you eat two eggs, you will get 15 mcg (micrograms) of selenium.

In the box at the top of the food table you will see the RDI of selenium, also in mcgs. This is the amount you should be getting from your diet every day. You'll see that it lists 70 mcg for men and 60 mcg for women.

Now run your eyes down the table and look for the foods that you normally eat in a typical day – then add up the mcgs of selenium in those foods and compare it to the RDI.

Let's assume you're a male and find you're only getting about 30 mcg a day of selenium from your food. This is less than half the RDI amount of 70 mcg you require for normal energy, health and some immunity from cancer – you're 40 mcg short each day.

So look again through the food table for good sources of selenium. You'll see that brazil nuts are a rich source – 210 mcg for 5 nuts, or 42 mcg per nut. So all you need do is eat one brazil nut a day and this will make up your daily selenium deficiency. Problem solved – it's that simple.

There are similar sections for each mineral and vitamin you need.

Measures and abbreviations

Listed below are measures and abbreviations you will find in the food tables (and elsewhere in the book).

g	gram – one thousandth of a kilogram
mg	milligram – one thousandth of a gram
mcg or **μg**	microgram – one thousandth of a milligram
tsp	one level teaspoon – 5 millilitres (ml) or about 5 grams
tbsp	one level tablespoon – 15 millilitres (ml) or about 15 grams

15

cup 250 mls – 1 metric cup, (8 oz)
pints US (not imperial)
cals kilocalories (4.2 kilojoules) – units of food energy
med medium size
svg typical serving (what will fit in the palm of your hand *)
std standard

RDI / RDA recommended dietary intake – average daily requirement

 * Serving sizes are defined as follows – 1 medium size fruit or potato or
 2 smaller fruit. ½ cup of diced fruit or vegetables. 1 cup of leafy vegetables. ¾ cup
 of fluid.

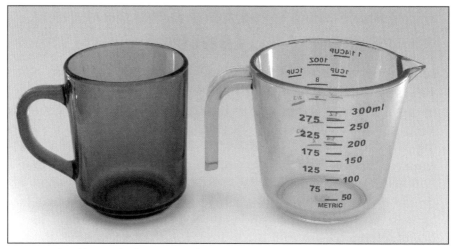

*A standard household mug (left) holds about 220 ml. A metric cup, used
as a food measure guide in the food tables of this book, holds 250 mls,
or 8 fluid ounces.*

Also bear in mind that –

- Meat can vary in nutritional value according to cut, so an average
  figure has been used.
- Fish also varies somewhat from species to species, but to keep things
  simple, an average figure has been calculated using the most
  common varieties, but not including shellfish.
- 100 g is about 3½ ounces, or a quarter of a pound. This is a common
  serving for many protein foods.
- Yoghurt nutrients are virtually identical to milk and have therefore
  not been listed separately.
- Nutrient figures given for canned baked beans, are for the navy
  variety, but can generally be applied to other varieties.

16

- Fruit juices listed are pure and not concentrated – the figures for canned fruit include the juice.
- Trim milk, reduced-fat milk and non-fat milk typically contain about 20% more milk solids than regular milk and are therefore correspondingly higher in some nutrients.
- Most supermarket bread sold as wholemeal (or wholegrain) contains only white flour and bran unless wheatgerm is mentioned on the label. This also applies to wholemeal flours purchased from supermarkets – they are normally just a re-mix of white flour and bran. The highly nutritious wheat germ has been removed, as it greatly reduces the shelf life of wheat flour products (the oil in wheatgerm begins to go rancid in two weeks when exposed to air).
- Therefore the figures quoted for wholemeal bread are normal commercial varieties that do not include wheat germ. Stone ground wheat flour from health shops does include the wheatgerm, but needs to be sealed and stored in the refrigerator or freezer immediately for maximum life.
- One bun on average is equivalent to two slices of bread.

Note for American readers

The New Zealand metric system use of 100 g (grams) for larger food portions in this book may be unfamiliar, but 4 oz is a near enough conversion, and elsewhere 1 oz = 25 g. Same with fluids – 1 litre (1l) = 2 pints.

Nutrition figures for foods are far from exact and vary wildly according to source and growing practices. The figures used in this book are New Zealand averages, tested from several sources.

To list all available foods, especially the vast variety available in America is impractical in a simple-to-use book of this nature, however there should be enough variety presented in the food tables to make intelligent guesses – one brand of hamburger or ice cream does not vary greatly from another in nutritional content.

Milo is a popular NZ chocolate-malt drink powder, Weetbix is a popular rectangular-shaped breakfast cereal whole-wheat biscuit and Marmite is a dark brown, salty, yeast extract savoury spread.

You may notice a few spelling differences in the text, such as colour for 'color' – New Zealand does have a strong English heritage.

"I pass with relief, from the tossing sea of cause and theory, to the firm ground of result and fact."   Sir Winston Churchill

Alcohol

Pure alcohol is a spirit similar to petrol – racing cars can run on it, yet our liver is still able to convert it into energy.

Two tablespoons of alcohol contain about 70 calories, so it can be fattening, as many 'beer-bellied' men amply demonstrate.

Alcohol is similar to sugar – a food high in calories and empty of nutrients. So calories from alcohol displace nutritious food that we might otherwise eat.

Excess alcohol stresses the liver and hinders the absorption of some important vitamins and minerals, particularly folate, pantothenic acid, magnesium and zinc. As a result malnutrition is more common among alcoholics than any other group of people.

Around 90% of alcoholics are deficient in folate – a vitamin that contributes to a calm mind and smooth muscle action. The resulting increased tension and anxiety make it all the more difficult to break the addiction.

Most alcoholics first began drinking to calm anxiety. Many researchers believe there is a cause and effect link between nutritional deficiencies and alcoholism – especially the B group vitamins that play a key role in our emotional calmness.

In one hospital study, 60% of alcoholics benefited from a niacin (vitamin B3) supplement and 20% maintained complete sobriety afterwards, compared to none with conventional treatment.

The muscle tremors or 'shakes' of the chronic alcoholic are usually caused by a deficiency of both niacin and magnesium.

Although alcohol can be very toxic to our body, there appears to be no adverse health effect as a result of light drinking. In fact some positive health benefits have been reported from a single beer or wine a day, probably due to the anxiety-dulling effects of alcohol. There could also be some antioxidant activity from fruit used in making alcoholic drinks.

Pure alcohol kills bacteria when applied directly to skin and can deactivate viruses. Methylated spirits (which is mostly alcohol) is widely used for this purpose. Alcohol can also kill our friendly gut bacteria.

"I have four good reasons for being an abstainer – my head is clearer, my health is better, my heart is lighter and my purse is heavier."
Thomas Guthrie, (Scottish philanthropist 1803–1873)

Food energy (Calories and Kilojoules)

Calories (or the metric equivalent kilojoules) are a measure of the amount of energy our bodies can extract from food. Generally about 70% of our calorie intake is used to maintain our body temperature, 20% our brain and heart function, and 10% for muscle energy and digesting our food.

Severe cold can triple requirements – 8000 calories a day is not unusual for Arctic trekkers. A doctor, Mike Stroud, pulling a heavy sled in Antarctica calculated his daily need at an impossible 11,650 calories a day – about 8000 was all he could manage to eat, from high fat foods.

Winter cold therefore increases our energy need, and inactivity and summer heat decrease our need. This is why we New Zealanders can easily pack on the weight due to warm weather and over eating during our Christmas and New Year.

For purists, the correct term for calories is kilocalories (1000 calories) but common usage has shortened it to calories, or the abbreviation 'cals'. A rough conversion to the metric kilojoules (kJ) is to multiply by 4, ie, 100 cals equals approx 400 kJ. The true conversion rate is 4.18.

Carbs and protein provide about 4 cals per gram, alcohol about 7, and fats and oils about 9 – 1 kg of body fat contains about 9000 calories.

Listed on the next page are typical energy or calorie needs of lightly active people according to age, sex and height. You'll see that merely standing on our feet uses nearly double the calories we use sitting or lying down – a brisk walk uses over four times as many.

Despite calorie tables, your unique environment and energy output best determine your calorie needs. Provided you are maintaining normal weight, not feeling the cold unduly and eating just enough to satisfy your appetite, your calorie intake should be correct, no matter how low it may seem.

Energy intake and health

Whenever our energy intake exceeds our needs, we open the door to numerous unpleasant health disorders. These include –

- allergies
- anxiety
- diabetes
- obesity
- insomnia
- colds and flu
- heart disease
- arthritis
- cancer

A medical phenomenon occurred in Europe during the close of World War II, as a result of widespread starvation – doctors noted a dramatic fall-off in the incidence of all the above listed disorders and conditions.

Also, despite sleeping in cold, wet outdoor conditions for weeks at a time, army troops reported a complete absence of colds among whole divisions while living on restricted rations.

Repeated experiments have shown that a 25% calorie restriction in mice can extend their lifespan by 50% – to 120 years in human terms.

Fattening and non-fattening calories

Calories from different food sources can have vastly different effects on our weight – protein calories are the most satiating, followed closely by fat calories. In other words, eating protein or fat keeps us feeling full longer, as they are much slower to digest than carbs.

On the other hand, carb calories, especially sugars and white flour are digested quickly and converted to glucose (blood sugar) our body's energy fuel. Surplus blood glucose is stored as fat. (More on this later.)

Average daily calorie needs

The figures below are for typical light activities, including a lot of sitting.
Increase by 10% during pregnancy.
Increase by 12% if you spend much of your day on your feet.
Increase by 20% if you do heavy work or have a highly active lifestyle.
Decrease by 10% during warm summer months.
Decrease by 25% if you are infirm, bedridden or walk infrequently.

	Age/Height	Male	Female	
Babies	1 year	80	80	(cals per kg)
Children	1 - 2 years	950	910	
	3 - 5 years	1400	1300	
	6 - 8 years	1700	1600	
	9 -11 years	2000	1800	
Adolescents	12 -14 years	2400	2100	
	15 -18 years	2900	2300	
	160cm / 5ft 3"	2450	2100	
Adults	170cm / 5ft 7"	2600	2300	
19-65 years	180cm / 5ft 11"	2800	2450	
	190cm / 6ft 3"	3000	2650	
	200cm / 6ft 7"	3200		
	160cm / 5ft 3"	2200	2000	
Adults	170cm / 5ft 7"	2300	2100	
over 65 years	180cm / 5ft 11"	2500	2200	
	190cm / 6ft 3"	2600	2300	
	200cm / 6ft 7"	2800		

Food energy – calories and kilojoules

20

Typical calorie usage (calories per hour)

Sleeping	65	Walking briskly 7 km/hr*	300
Sitting	70	Climbing stairs	350
Standing	125	Hiking with a small pack	420
Light work on feet	150	Jogging on flat	500
Walking a dog 3 km/hr*	175	Swimming normally	560
Garden weeding	210	Skipping slowly	840
Walking normally 5 km/hr*	230	Steady running on flat	875
Active work on feet	245	Cross trainer (vigorous)	900
Vacuuming	265	Cycling uphill	975
Mowing a lawn	280	Running uphill	1050
Cycling on a flat road	280	Sprinting	1260

* 3 km/hr = 2 mph   5 km/hr = 3 mph   7 km/hr = 4 mph

They all count

To burn off the 125 calories of just four pieces (individual squares) of a bar of chocolate you would need to –

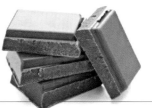

- sit for 108 minutes
- work lightly for 50 minutes
- walk briskly for 25 minutes
- run for 9 minutes

HEALTH HINT   The 4 laws of nutrition

'Never eat when not hungry'
'Sit down to at least one meal a day with an appetite'
'Skip a meal if not hungry'
'Avoid eating between meals'

"Dine with little, sup with less, do better still, sleep supperless."
Thomas A. Edison

Food energy – calories and kilojoules

Calories (to convert to kilojoules multiply by 4)   100 g = approx 4 oz

Food energy – calories and kilojoules

BEVERAGES		Cals
1 can	Beer (350 ml)	140
1 can	Beer (low alcohol)	100
1 glass	Wine	70
1 nip	Spirits	40
1 glass	Fruit juice (pure)	80
1 glass	Fruit cordial	90
1 can	Cola/fizzy drink	160
1 can	Cola/fizzy drink (diet)	5
1 cup	Milo (all milk)	215
1 cup	Milo (¼ milk)	100
1 cup	Tea/Coffee (black no sugar)	2
1 cup	Tea/Coffee (milk & sugar)	40

DAIRY / EGGS / FATS		
1 tbsp	Butter/margarine	110
1 slice	Cheese (4 mm)	60
2 tbsp	Cream	110
½ cup	Ice cream	120
1 lge	Ice cream cone	120
1 cup	Milk (standard)	160
1 cup	Milk (trim)	110
1 cup	Milk (non-fat)	90
1 cup	Milk (soy full fat)	158
1 cup	Milk (soy light)	112
1 cup	Custard	280
1 pot	Yoghurt (sweetened)	150
1 pot	Yoghurt (natural low-fat)	75
1 med	Egg (boiled)	75
1 med	Egg (fried)	120
1 tbsp	Beef dripping	110
1 tbsp	Vegetable oil	125
2 tbsp	Salad dressing	100

FRUIT		
1 med	Apple	80
1	Apricot	30
½	Avocado	190
1 med	Banana	100
½ cup	Berry fruit	40
5	Dates	100
1	Feijoa	15
½ cup	Fruit salad (canned)	125
10	Grapes	35
1	Grapefruit	70
1	Kiwifruit	50
1	Nectarine	60
1 med	Orange	70
1 cup	Pawpaw	125
1	Peach	50
½ cup	Peaches (canned)	100
1	Pear	100
1	Persimmon	65
½ cup	Pears (canned)	100
½ cup	Pineapple (canned)	100
2 med	Plums	50
5	Prunes	90
¼ cup	Raisins/Sultanas	130
½ cup	Rhubarb (stewed, sugar)	100
5	Strawberries	35
1	Tamarillo	20
1/8	Watermelon	50

GRAINS		
½ cup	Flour (wheat)	205
½ cup	Flour (soy)	190
1 slice	Bread (thin)	50
1 slice	Bread (med)	70
1 slice	Bread (med buttered)	170
1 slice	Bread (thick)	90
1	Bread roll	140
1	Sandwich (avg)	190
1	Bun (cream)	190
1	Bun (currant)	240
1	Scone (buttered)	230
1	Doughnut (plain)	170
1	Eclair	160
1	Crispbread (rye)	20
1	Biscuit (small plain)	40
1	Biscuit (choc coated)	60
1	Biscuit (icing filled)	60
1	Shortbread	65
1	Biscuit (home baked)	90
1 svg	Cake (plain)	160
1 svg	Cake (fruit)	165
1 svg	Cake (sponge with jam)	180
1 svg	Cake (iced)	300
1 svg	Cake (rich - iced)	440
1 svg	Steam pudding	235

1 svg	Christmas pudding	390		1	Milkshake	290
1	Pikelet (med)	60		1	Ice cream sundae	260
1	Pancake	110		150 g	Potato crisps	260
½ cup	Rice (cooked)	130		50 g	Potato crisps	85
½ cup	Rice pudding	170				
¾ cup	Spaghetti (canned)	130				

FISH

100 g	Fish (baked)	80
3	Fish cakes	240
100 g	Fish (canned in oil)	220
6	Oysters (battered)	310
6	Oysters (raw)	80
3 tbsp	Fish paste	30

NUTS

1/3 cup	Peanuts (salted, oiled)	300
1 tbsp	Peanut butter	105
1/3 cup	Other nuts (avg)	280
½ cup	Coconut flesh	165
1 tbsp	Coconut (shredded)	40

VEGETABLES (cooked)

¾ cup	Baked beans	130
5 slices	Beetroot (canned)	65
1 med	Carrot (raw or cooked)	15
5 slices	Cucumber	5
½ cup	Green Beans	10
1 med	Kumara (sweet potato)	120
½ cup	Lentils	95
3 leaves	Lettuce	5
6 med	Mushrooms (microwaved)	10
6 med	Mushrooms (fried)	160
1	Onion	40
½ cup	Peas	45
2 med	Potatoes (boiled)	170
1 cup	Potato (mashed/butter)	200
¾ cup	Pumpkin	35
½ cup	Silverbeet (chard)	10
1 cup	Soup (avg)	110
½ cup	Sprouts (raw)	30
¾ cup	Sweet corn (canned)	140
2 cobs	Sweet corn (15cm cob)	125
1 med	Tomato (raw)	20
¾ cup	Vegetables (mixed)	50
½ cup	Yams	85

MEAT (cooked)

100 g	Beef (grilled or stewed)	200
100 g	Beef (corned)	220
100 g	Beef (roasted)	222
100 g	Chicken (baked)	160
100 g	Chicken (baked w/skin)	220
100 g	Lamb (grilled)	220
100 g	Lamb (roasted)	265
2 slices	Bacon (fried)	140
100 g	Pork (grilled)	250
100 g	Pork (roasted)	280
1	Sausage (grilled)	225
3	Sausage rolls (med)	545
3	Meat pasties	420
100 g	Mince	210
100 g	Lasagne	150
2 slices	Luncheon	115
2 slices	Meatloaf	120
2 tbsp	Gravy	30

SWEETS

1 tsp	Sugar (white)	30
1 tsp	Sugar (raw)	25
1 tbsp	Honey	60
1 tbsp	Jam	50
1	Meringue (with cream)	170
1 svg	Cheese cake (190 g)	550
¾ cup	Jelly	135
1 cup	Trifle dessert	405
1 tbsp	Milo (dry)	30

FAST FOOD

100 g	Chicken (fried KFC)	310
1	Hamburger	250
1	Hamburger (Big Mac)	550
1	Eggburger	520
1	Cheeseburger	500
1	Hot dog	430
100 g	Fish (fried in batter)	300
1 cup	Potato chips (fried)	115
½	Pizza (23 cm diameter)	450
1 cup	Potato salad	240
½ cup	Coleslaw	85
1	Meat pie (small)	350
1	Fruit pie	240

2	Chocolates	40
50 g	Chocolate bar	260
120 g	Chocolate bar	630
1	Mars bar	265
1	Muesli bar	130
2	Peppermints	30
2	Toffee lollies	45
1 cup	Pop corn (candied)	40
1	Ice block	60

HEALTH FOOD

1 tbsp	Brewers yeast	10
100 g	Liver (stewed)	200
1 tsp	Marmite (yeast extract)	10
2 full tsp	Malt extract	90

1 tbsp	Molasses	50
1 mg	Stevia (plant sweetener)	1
½ cup	Tofu	110
2 tbsp	Wheat germ	60
2 tbsp	Wheat bran	10

BREAKFAST CEREALS
(With standard milk and sugar)

1 plate	Muesli	250
2	Weetbix	200
1 plate	Porridge	200
1 plate	Wheatflakes	200
1 plate	Rice bubbles	150

HEALTH HINT Tame that sweet tooth

A sweet tooth is mostly an acquired taste. You can usually restore your taste buds to normal by drastically restricting your sugar intake for one month. This also enhances your enjoyment of the more subtle flavours of vegetables.

You can also generally halve the sugar content of most traditional recipes for cakes, biscuits and desserts without significantly affecting the taste. In fact, taste is often heightened as the more delicate flavours are accentuated.

See also the Health Hint **Salt and sugar cravings** on page 175.

"Leave something on your plate ... 'better to go to waste than to waist."
Michael Pollan, (author "Food Rules: an eater's manual")

Carbs (carbohydrates)

Carbs are grains (flour, bread, rice, cereals, biscuits etc) and fruit, vegetables and nuts.

Sugars are also carbs, but are known as 'simple carbs' as opposed to the 'complex carbs' above. Sugars can have such a profound effect on our health that they are covered separately in the next chapter.

Carbs release energy (glucose) and other nutrients into our blood comparatively rapidly. However, if we don't use the energy right away, insulin stores the glucose as fat.

Sports research has shown that complex carbs (preferably unrefined) along with plenty of water, make an ideal food for quick sustained energy. It was previously assumed that protein such as meat and eggs were better, but proteins are slow to digest, and therefore like fats, slow to convert into energy. (However in recent years, some athletes are now preferring fats.)

Glycemic index and Glycemic load

Carb foods have been ranked from 0 to 100 by the speed at which they can be converted to glucose for our body to use as energy. This ranking is called the glycemic index or GI – pure glucose is rated top at 100.

The glycemic index is useful to know, as it shows the comparative risk of a food spiking our blood sugar and also how long it takes before we feel hungry again. The lower the number, the lower the spiking effect, and longer the time that food will keep our hunger at bay.

However, because the glycemic index is based on 100 g (4 oz) portions of food and does not take into account the non-carb portion of our food, it is of limited use. For example, 100 g of watermelon is ranked at a GI of 72 – the same as bread, but it's nearly all water (91%) and only 7% carb, so it contains little energy compared to bread which is 50% carb.

To overcome this problem, the index has now been replaced with a better system called the glycemic load or GL – this rates the energy content of each food, and uses a typical serving size instead of standard 100 g portions.

By using the new glycemic load system, watermelon drops from 72 to 4 which more accurately predicts the effect on our blood glucose.

Below is a typical glycemic load list for common foods – the lower the figure, the less the risk of the following problems – blood sugar spiking, fat gain, type 2 diabetes, insulin resistance, hypoglycemia, cardiovascular disease and many other sugar-related disorders.

Glycemic load chart   100 g = approx 4 oz

Carbs

SUGARS

100 g	Glucose	100
100 g	Sugar (white)	70
100 g	Sugar (brown)	60
100 g	Honey	50
100 g	Molasses	45
100 g	Fructose	20

BEVERAGES

1 can	Soft drink (soda)	32
1 can	Cola drink	20
1 can	Fruit juice	18
1 cup	Apple juice	10
1 mug	Milo (made with water)	9
1 can	Tomato juice	6

DAIRY / EGGS / FATS

150 g	Ice cream	18
1 cup	Milk (soy)	7
125 g	Yoghurt (sweetened)	5
1 cup	Milk (std & trim)	3
4 tbsp	Whey protein (25 g)	2

FRUIT

1 pkt	Raisins	20
1	Banana	15
5	Dates	15
5	Prunes	13
½ cup	Grapes	11
½ cup	Peaches (canned)	9
1 cup	Watermelon	8
1	Kiwifruit	5
2	Plums	5
1	Orange	5
½ cup	Rockmelon	4
1	Apple	4
½ cup	Strawberries	1

FISH

3	Fish fingers	11
100 g	Fish (all types)	0

VEGETABLES (cooked)

1 cup	Kumara (sweet potato)	26
2 med	Potatoes	23
2 cobs	Sweet corn	20
¾ cup	Baked beans	18
1 cup	Taro root	7
¾ cup	Pumpkin	6

1 cup	Tomato soup	6
½ cup	Hummus	6
¾ cup	Bean sprouts	5
½ cup	Peas (green)	4
¾ cup	Carrots	2

GRAINS

1 cup	Spaghetti canned	25
1 cup	Rice (white cooked)	24
4 slices	Bread (white)	24
1 plate	Rice bubbles	22
2	Pancakes	21
1 plate	Cornflakes	20
4 slices	Bread (wholemeal)	20
1 plate	Coco Pops	20
1 cup	Noodles (instant)	19
80 g	Banana cake	18
1	Muffin	17
2	Scones	14
1	Muesli bar	13
1 plate	Bran flakes	13
1 plate	Porridge	12
2	Weetbix	12
1 plate	Muesli	11
3	Cracker biscuits	10
¾ cup	Lentils	6
½ cup	Baby food	5
1 bag	Popcorn	8

NUTS

50 g	Coconut	4
50 g	Peanuts (salted)	3
2 tbsp	Peanut butter	2
50g	Most other nuts	0

MEAT (cooked)

1 med	Meat pie	21
2	Sausages	2
100 g	Meat (unprocessed)	0

FAST FOOD

150 g	French fries	22
200 g	Pizza	16
50g	Potato crisps	10

SWEETS

1	Lamington cake	25	1	Fruit bar		10
1	Mars bar	25	1 tbsp	Honey		9
50 g	Chocolate	13	1 tbsp	Jam		7

The higher the number, especially above 19, the more fattening the food (ie, extra insulin is released, increasing the risk of diabetes and other disorders).

Complex carbs far more nutritious than sugars

Complex carbs provide both energy and nutrients, whereas sugar provides mostly energy only – so when using that energy (which requires nutrients) the body becomes deficient in nutrients.

Even if we have eaten enough calories from sugary foods to supply our energy needs, the body will generate further hunger to obtain the nutrients it needs – especially potassium and magnesium.

See a comparison below of 200 calories of nutritious complex carbs in a potato and 200 calories of empty carbs of sugar in a soft drink (soda).

	Potato	**Soft drink (soda)**
Protein	5000 mg	0 mg
Potassium	850 mg	0 mg
Vitamin C	22 mg	0 mg
Calcium	10 mg	0 mg

The pattern is similar throughout the nutrient range.

Recommended daily percent of carbs, protein and fat

By examining diets that people will actually keep, nutritionists in developed countries (ie, 'low exercise countries') have now modified the recommended ratio of carbs, protein and fat for health and weight control. These are listed below (although the World Health Organisation now recommend only 10% of our calories be from sugars).

Complex carbs	25% of daily cals
Simple carbs (sugars)	15% of daily cals
Protein	30% of daily cals
Fat	30% of daily cals

Protein at 30% of our daily calories is higher than desirable, but keeps weight gain down as it is slow to digest and also uses calories in the process. For active people, reducing your protein intake to 15% and increasing your complex carbs to 40% is healthier.

The NZ 2009 Nutrition Survey revealed the following actual intakes:

Complex carbs	34% of daily cals
Simple carbs (sugars)	14% of daily cals
Protein	15% of daily cals
Fat	37% of daily cals

So New Zealand is reasonably close to the recommendations, we need just a little more protein and a little less fat.

Carbs generally make up the bulk of our food, (protein and high fat foods are higher in calories but much less bulky). Vegetables and whole grains are the most nutritious. Fruit is also nutritious (but normally contains a lot of sugar which can be surprisingly fattening). Purchasing carb foods in their natural perishable form is always best – if bugs thrive on it then so will we.

HEALTH HINT **Overcoming wheat allergy**

If you have a wheat gluten allergy, your digestive system may be able to handle the lesser amount of gluten found naturally in whole wheat or sprouted flour, which you can normally buy freshly ground, from a health shop. Whole wheat has not had extra gluten added by flour manufacturers (to increase rising qualities). You could try a whole wheat cereal such as the NZ staple Weetbix as a test.

Recent Spanish research has linked wheat/gluten allergies (including autoimmune celiac disease) to missing or imbalanced friendly gut bacteria (probiotics) of the bifidobacterium family, especially the bifidum strain. They suspect this may be due to the use of oral antibiotics. These friendly bacteria can be replenished using a high quality multi-probiotic.

(See also Health Hint on **How probiotics can help you,** page 113.)

Modern, high-yield wheat strains are faster digesting (ie, they spike your blood sugar more readily) and are higher in gluten than the pre-1970 varieties and have been linked to a higher incidence of diabetes and obesity.

You might wish to try older varieties of wheat – einkorn, spelt, emmer, monad or durum. Einkorn (*Triticum monococcum*, or *sifon* in Hebrew) is the original Biblical wheat – it is highly nutritious, tasty, light to bake with and particularly low in gluten. Unfortunately it can be expensive as it's not grown widely, as yields are low, and it's difficult to harvest.

"Do not let either the medical authorities or the politicians mislead you – find out what the facts are, and make your own decisions about how to live a happy life and how to work for a better world." Dr Linus Pauling

Sugar and sweeteners

Sugar is a fast-digesting carb and one of the most serious health threats we face. This is because sugar –

- Is highly addictive
- Suppresses our immune system by acidifying the body
- Can fatten us faster than any other food
- Can destabilise our mind through fluctuations in blood sugar
- Can cause cardiovascular disease
- Feeds yeast infections and cancer cells

According to the 2009 Nutrition Survey, most sugar in the NZ diet comes from sweetened beverages such as soft drinks (sodas) and fruit juices. Daily sugar intake by males has increased from less than a teaspoon a day (in 1900) to a whopping 28 teaspoons a day (120 g) in 2008. Female intake follows close behind at 23 teaspoons a day (96 g).

Sugar provides few, if any nutrients, only calories. Even honey which is widely regarded as a health food, contains only tiny amounts of nutrients. Molasses is an exception – this dark syrup residue of processed sugar is rich in minerals. Maple syrup also contains useful minerals.

Hidden sugar

The high levels of sugar in modern processed foods are often underestimated (one teaspoon is 4 g). A few examples:

1 can	soft drink (soda)	10 teaspoons of sugar
1 glass	fruit juice	8 teaspoons of sugar
1 bar	chocolate (small 50 g)	6 teaspoons of sugar
1 slice	iced fruit cake	6 teaspoons of sugar
1 slice	chocolate cake	3 teaspoons of sugar
1 svg	apple pie	4 teaspoons of sugar
1	Mallowpuff biscuit	3 teaspoons of sugar

How much sugar should you have each day?

There is no RDI for sugar. In fact the energy content of nearly all carb foods is eventually converted to sugar (glucose) by our bodies anyway.

Much of the harm from sugar comes from the white refined variety, which is devoid of nutrients, especially chromium which is essential for sugar to be safely managed in our bodies.

Harm is also caused from the spiking of our blood glucose by consuming large amounts of sugar at any one time, especially in liquid form on an empty stomach.

The World Health Organisation recommends that only 10% of our total calories come from added sugar, so this would provide the following daily maximums, based on our total daily calorie intake:

2000 calories = 50 g sugar - 12 tsp	2600 calories = 65 g sugar - 16 tsp
2200 calories = 55 g sugar - 14 tsp	2800 calories = 70 g sugar - 17 tsp
2400 calories = 60 g sugar - 15 tsp	3000 calories = 75 g sugar - 19 tsp

Glucose

Ordinary table sugar is approximately half glucose and half fructose, (more about fructose shortly). Glucose is the energy fuel that runs every cell in our bodies – rather like petrol runs a car. The glucose portion of sugar doesn't need to go through the digestive process and can be used 'as is' by the body. It's therefore rapidly absorbed and can spike our blood sugar level within minutes, producing a 'sugar energy rush'. We often see this in children at a birthday party after consuming drinks high in sugar.

Surplus glucose turned into body fat

A little understood fact is that our body fat is made from excess glucose – this occurs when too much glucose from food enters our bloodstream at any one time – ie, more energy than we can reasonably burn off. This is usually the result when we consume sweet drinks and fast digesting carbohydrate food – in other words, drinks and food with a high glycemic load rating, as listed in the chart on page 26.

If our blood glucose level is allowed to get too high, it can cause serious diabetic problems, so the surplus glucose needs to be rapidly withdrawn from our blood. This is done by insulin, which converts the surplus glucose to fat. This fat is stored around our waistline or other convenient places to be used for possible future energy needs. It is then able to be converted back to energy again by the liver.

Fructose can be even more fattening

Fructose (fruit sugar) is the other half of table sugar. Fructose needs to be converted to glucose by our liver before it can be used by the body.

However new research has discovered that when a large amount of fructose is consumed at once, one third of the converted glucose is not used for energy, but directly converted to fat. Dr R. Lustig, Endocrinology Division, University of California, states – *"120 calories of fructose results in 40 calories being stored as fat."*

Too much fructose can interfere with leptin – our appetite regulator, resulting in overeating. It can also lead to a serious and common condition called insulin resistance – a major cause of cardiovascular disease, type 2 diabetes and even brain disorders such as Alzheimer's. Insulin resistance also raises uric acid levels and can trigger gout.

Research Professor Gerald Reaven, a diabetes specialist of Stanford University states – *"If you want to cause insulin resistance in laboratory rats, feeding them diets that are mostly fructose is an easy way to do it. It's a very obvious, very dramatic effect."*

Fruit also contains fructose, but eating whole fruit in moderation is fine, as whole fruit needs to be digested first, and does not flood the liver with large amounts of fructose, like soft drink (soda) and pure fruit juice. However sweet fruit can still be fattening, as NZ wood pigeons attest. In fact eating too much fruit can be downright dangerous. Some years ago, a friend of mine in Whangarei, to save food costs lived for some days mostly on oranges growing on his property. He eventually collapsed into a coma and was taken to hospital and diagnosed with advanced type 2 diabetes – yet he had formally enjoyed normal health. It was an apparent case of fructose overload, causing insulin resistance.

In another instance, a Tauranga man wanting to use up his frozen grapefruit juice to make room for his currently ripe crop, began drinking the juice to the equivalent of over 30 grapefruit a day – he too collapsed and was taken to hospital.

Excess sugar creates bad fats

The very experienced Dr Robert Atkins has said, *"For 25 years I've been warning people that long-term consumption of sugar is the surest way to create disease. Avoid sugar, it will create bad fats when consumed beyond what the body needs. Sugar is broken down into small molecules and reassembled as fats. These fats are called triglycerides. These are the fats that impair blood flow inside blood vessels and raise the risk of coronary artery narrowing. Our cholesterol ratios also worsen, with HDL falling and LDL rising."*

Other sugar disorders

High sugar intake also provides an ideal environment for tongue and mouth ulcers – along with gum disease, candida, thrush, yeast and infections. Furthermore, it increases sensitivity to asthma, hay fever and allergies of all kinds. The following are other common sugar-related health disorders:

Hypoglycemia (low blood sugar) – This common disorder is initially caused by high sugar consumption. It happens when a large spike of glucose in the blood, from excess sugar consumption, triggers the release of a large amount of insulin to lower the glucose level and protect the body from high blood sugar. Insulin is our blood sugar regulator.

However before the abnormally large amount of insulin can all be withdrawn again from the blood, it can lower blood glucose too much, affecting brain function and energy levels.

Symptoms of hypoglycemia (low blood sugar) are a sudden drop in energy, shaky legs and hands, muscle weakness, craving sweet food, feeling depressed, blurred vision, poor memory, panic attacks, aggressiveness, irritability, heart palpitations and in severe cases, coma.

Normal fasting blood glucose levels are 4 to 6 mmol/L (70 to 110 mg/dl) Symptoms of hypoglycemia usually begin below 3.2 mmol/L (57 mg/dl).

If you ever feel shaky and depressed, which are common hypoglycemia symptoms, you can test your blood glucose level at home with a diabetic finger prick test kit. These only cost around $25 in NZ.

Surveys have found up to 95% incidence of hypoglycemia among alcoholics and 65% among schizophrenics. Occurrence is also high among drug addicts, violent criminals and 50% of all American psychiatric patients. A Norwegian study of teenagers found the worst mental health in the 10% of males who drank four or more soft drinks (sodas) a day.

Hypoglycemia is thought to be the root cause of most anti-social behaviour in the world today. This theory was tested in some prisons by restricting sugar consumption. However results were mostly indifferent, except when the sugar restriction was combined with nutritious meals. Then significantly better behaviour is noticed after three months – one prison reporting a 40% drop in breaches of discipline.

Tooth decay – This major and expensive problem is caused by eating sugary foods which are highly acidic. One of the worst foods for tooth decay is chocolate, as it can leave a brown acid residue in the hollows of our molars for over an hour after eating. I learned this myself the hard way many years ago – from age 18 to 25 I developed no new cavities in my teeth. Then I began finishing my lunch each day by eating two squares of a chocolate bar. Less than a year later, at my annual dental check up, the dentist found five new cavities. I will now eat a piece of dry bread immediately after any chocolate to remove the residue.

Tooth decay is not only caused by direct sugar contact – dentist Dr R. Steinman of Loma Linda University injected a glucose solution daily into the stomachs of mice. What he found was astonishing – over time, every one of the test animals developed severe tooth decay.

Cardiovascular disease – This deadly disorder can also be caused by excess sugar (some researchers say it's the main cause) especially by white sugar, which lacks chromium. Excess sugar always raises blood triglycerides (the medical term for blood fats) which are a high risk factor for heart disease.

During the Korean War, doctors performing autopsies on young American soldiers killed in battle, noticed that many had significant plaque deposits in their arteries, while the Koreans killed in battle did not. Also, 78% of American soldiers killed in Vietnam had signs of coronary artery blockage. (Stress can be a major factor in artery plaques.)

Diabetes – Researchers at Columbia University discovered that deaths from diabetes increased 400% in some American cities between 1900 and 1920 – coinciding with a 400% increase in sugar intake.

Natural and processed sugars

Glucose – The simplest sugar and the fuel all body cells prefer for energy. Solid carb food is converted into glucose by the body through bacterial action and digestive enzymes in the gut or liver.

Fructose – A naturally occurring plant sugar, 70% sweeter than glucose and usually found combined with similar amounts of glucose.

Dextrose – A term used for glucose derived from grain.

Sucrose (common table sugar) – Made by refining the juice of sugar cane or beets – contains approx equal portions of glucose and fructose.

White sugar – Dried and crystallised sugar cane or sugar beet syrup from which almost all nutrients and 'impurities' have been removed.

Castor sugar and icing sugar – Finely ground white sugar.

Raw sugar – White sugar with a thin coating of unrefined sugar syrup to give it a browner appearance (mostly for marketing purposes). It looks healthier but is virtually the same as white sugar.

Dark brown and demerara sugar – Generally just white sugar crystals coated or soaked in molasses.

Soft brown sugar – A blend of darker, less refined sugar crystals with finely powdered white castor sugar to lessen stickiness. It has more flavour and nutritional value than white sugar and twice the chromium content (lack of chromium in refined white sugar hinders the pancreas which helps control blood glucose levels).

Golden syrup and treacle – A thick liquid, extracted during the refining of cane sugar before drying, retaining some of the mineral content. Treacle does not go through a decolouring process and therefore has a stronger flavour than golden syrup.

Molasses – A thick dark syrup – the final by product of the sugar refining process. Unlike refined sugar, molasses is rich in plant minerals, especially potassium and also magnesium and calcium.

Lactose and galactose – Found mostly in milk products and made up of equal parts glucose and galactose. Galactose needs to be digested by probiotics (friendly bacteria) in the intestines – if we lack these friendly bacteria we can be intolerant to dairy.

Maltose – Found in malt barley and other cereals – it's all glucose but in a slightly different form from that found in table sugar, nevertheless it's readily absorbed into the bloodstream and can cause a rapid rise in blood sugar.

Corn syrup – Extracted from maize and usually left in liquid form. It is typically around 35% glucose and 65% fructose but can be blended to different percentages. Because corn syrup is extra sweet due to its high fructose content and so cheap to produce in the US, it has become the most popular sweetener for processed foods and drinks in that country.

Honey – Processed by bees from flower nectar and 35% sweeter than sugar. Honey is made up of 37% glucose, 46% fructose, 9% maltose and 8% other sugars and elements. Like most sugars it is an active bacteria killer and can help preserve foods.

Maple syrup – The sweet sap of maple trees grown in cold climates, mostly Canada. Like molasses, it contains useful amounts of minerals especially potassium and also calcium. It is expensive, so imitations are often made from flavoured sugar syrup.

Sorbitol (**420**) – A sugar alcohol obtained by the chemical modifying of glucose or fructose and also occurring naturally in many fruits. Sorbitol is about 50% as sweet as white sugar.

Mannitol (421) – A plant sugar found in abundance in nature, particularly in exudates from trees – it's named after the biblical manna. Nowadays it's mostly refined from various sugar syrups. Mannitol is widely used in the food industry as a dusting powder as it does not absorb moisture.

Xylitol (**967**) – A natural plant sugar, nearly as sweet as table sugar but with 40% less calories. It does not decay teeth or raise insulin levels in the blood and helps maintain a healthy probiotic balance in the gut.

Stevia (960) – A very sweet natural sugar, up to 250 times sweeter than table sugar. It is extracted from the leaves of the Stevia plant and normally refined to a white powder. Stevia is increasing in popularity worldwide due to its safety and naturalness. It is very popular in Japan and has become the main sweetener used in commercial foods. Stevia can have a lingering aftertaste in many foods, if not combined with sugar or other sweeteners.

Thaumatin (957) – A natural protein, 3000 times sweeter than sugar,

34

extracted from the Katemfe fruit of West Africa. It's not used much as it has a delayed onset, liquorice-like taste which lingers.

Erythritol (968) – A natural fruit sugar, 60% as sweet as table sugar but with 95% less calories. It's made commercially by fermenting yeast and glucose and normally used as a filler for an intense sweetener like stevia, to provide a texture and flavour similar to table sugar.

Chemical sweeteners

Acesulfame (950) – 200 times sweeter than table sugar and made from a potassium compound. Brand names are Sunett and Sweet One. It is not absorbed by the body, but can still cause a release of insulin into the blood.

Aspartame (951) – 200 times sweeter than sugar. Brand names include NutraSweet, Equal, Spoonful and Equal-Measure. Huge numbers of adverse reactions have been reported for aspartame due to the aspartate it contains. Aspartate is an excitotoxin that can damage human nerve neurons. A 10 year study by University of Texas Health Science Center found that those who drank two or more aspartame-containing diet drinks a day, increased their waist size six times greater than those who drank regular, sugar sweetened soft drink (soda). Aspartame is also reported to break down to the neurotoxin formaldehyde when heated – however there appears to be a lack of convincing evidence for this harmful effect.

Cyclamate (952) – 40 times sweeter than sugar and often combined with saccharin to improve taste. Brand names are Sucaryl, Assugrin and Sugar Twin.

Saccharin (954) – 350 times sweeter than sugar and the oldest of the chemical sweeteners (discovered as a coal tar extract in 1879). Brand names are Sweet'N Low, Sweet Twin, and Necta Sweet.

Sucralose (955) – 600 times sweeter than sugar. Brand names include Splenda, Sukrana, SucraPlus, Candys, Cukren and Nevella. It is manufactured chemically from sugar and is the most heat stable of the artificial sweeteners, but can alter the natural pH of the intestines and unbalance friendly bacteria. Has less aftertaste than other chemical sweeteners.

Neotame (961) – 8000 times sweeter than sugar. A newer and claimed 'safer' version of aspartame. Both neotame and aspartame are said to stimulate appetite by increasing the release of the hormones insulin and leptin. A report from India claims animals fed food containing neotame (Sweetos) consume more fodder.

"Sugar scares me."   Professor Cantley (Director: Harvard Cancer Center)

Fibre

Fibre is the insoluble, mostly indigestible part of food that our body cannot absorb as a liquid through the colon walls, so it passes through our intestinal tract largely unchanged, but retains water. This water helps keep fecal matter soft and adds bulk, allowing for an easier and faster bowel action. Even so called soluble fibre is not absorbed by the body. Fibre is essential for a healthy probiotic population in the gut.

Not all food fibre is dry and rough in texture like bran – foods like oranges, pears and carrots are also high in fibre. On the other hand, there is virtually no fibre in meat, dairy, eggs, sugar and most liquids.

Psyllium seed husk powder is very high in fibre and swells greatly in the presence of water. It's often used in detox supplements designed to flush out the bowel system.

Fibre is very filling and low in calories – for example try eating six high-fibre medium size carrots in one sitting. Yet six carrots (a total of 150 cals) contain less than half the calories of just one sausage (330 cals) which is low in fibre.

Fibre was long believed to protect against colon cancer, but two large studies involving over 100,000 men and women, found that while it reduced constipation, it made no difference to colon cancer rates. However, they did discover that adequate folate (vitamin B9) decreased the risk of colon cancer about 75%.

Too little fibre is a major cause of constipation which affects the majority of New Zealanders over 60 years of age. The 2009 Nutrition Survey found that we are about a third short (8 g) of the recommended amount of fibre to ensure good bowel regularity and health. Actual intake was 22 g for men and 18 g for women, mostly from bread and vegetables. (The RDI / RDA is 30 g for men and 25 g for women.)

Constipation leads to hemorrhoids, stomach pain and sometimes the complication of diverticulitis – a bulging of the colon walls.

Cereals are a good source of fibre – however research has shown that cereal bran eaten alone, can bind minerals such as calcium, zinc and magnesium and hinder them from being absorbed by the body. In one study, 50% less mineral absorption was found when a heaped table-spoon of bran was taken with every meal by elderly people – serious evidence that most foods are best eaten in their natural, whole state.

Large amounts of high fibre food in our diet do not appear to be harmful once our body adapts, however temporary gas and diarrhea can occur. So can constipation when reverting from a high-fibre diet back to a low-fibre diet. A large, early morning glass of warm water helps bowel elimination in both cases.

White flour has on average 75% less fibre than wholemeal flour, and also far fewer nutrients. Greater awareness of this fact has led to a increasing demand for wholegrain bread in recent years.

Role of fibre in our body
- Necessary for proper functioning of our digestive system.
- Promotes a healthy probiotic (gut bacteria) population.
- Produces a feeling of fullness that curbs overeating.

Too little fibre
- Constipation. Stomach pain. Hemorrhoids (piles). Diverticulitis.
- Unhealthy probiotics in the gut. Asthma attacks.
- Diabetes and cardiovascular disease.
- Obesity through overeating.

Too much fibre
- Extracted grain fibres (like bran flakes) can bind diet minerals.
- No long term harmful effects if consumed naturally in food.

Cooking losses
- Cooking does not significantly affect fibre.

HEALTH HINT   **Avoiding constipation**

Constipation and its two cousins – hemorrhoids and varicose veins are often caused by too much sitting, even when we're getting sufficient fibre in our diet.

As a general guide we should ideally spend about a third of our waking hours on our feet and moving. We should not sit longer than three hours at a time, without compensating for about half an hour with some activity using our legs and abdomen muscles. Brisk walking is excellent.

Correct breathing is also important – we should breathe using our lower abdomen rather than our upper chest (watch a sleeping child). This produces a continual massaging or palpitating effect on our intestines, similar to walking.

"There is so much we do not understand about the subtleties of nutrition that we are essentially shooting in the dark when we start to alter and process our foods."   Dr Gabriel Cousens, (Physician and Homeopath)

RDI · FIBRE

Child:	20 g	Woman:	25 g
Teenage boy: 28 g Teenage girl: 22 g		Pregnancy:	28 g
Man:	30 g	Breastfeeding:	30 g

FRUIT

		grams
½ cup	Fruit salad (avg)	5.0
½ cup	Raspberries	5.0
1	Pear	4.8
½ cup	Blackberries	4.5
1 med	Apple	4.0
1	Orange	4.0
5	Dates	3.6
1/3 cup	Sultanas/raisins	3.5
½ cup	Apricots (dried halves)	3.0
½ cup	Rhubarb (stewed)	3.0
4 slices	Beetroot (canned)	3.0
1	Passionfruit	2.9
1	Persimmon	2.9
1	Peach	2.6
5	Prunes	2.5
1	Nectarine	2.3
1	Guava	2.1
1	Tamarillo	2.0
1 med	Banana	1.9
2	Plums	1.6
1	Kiwifruit	1.6
½	Avocado	1.5
½ cup	Strawberries	1.5
1	Apricot	1.1
1	Feijoa	1.0

MEAT

2	Sausages	3.4

GRAIN / NUTS

½ cup	Flour (wholemeal)	8.0
4 slices	Bread (wholemeal)	6.4
1/3 cup	Peanuts	4.0
2	Weetbix	3.2
4 slices	Bread (white)	2.8
1/3 cup	Other nuts (avg)	2.5
½ cup	Flour (white)	2.1
1 plate	Porridge	2.0

VEGETABLES (cooked)

2 cobs	Sweet corn	12.0
¾ cup	Baked beans	7.0
½ cup	Peas	6.5
¾ cup	Broccoli	5.0
6 med	Mushrooms	4.2
¾ cup	Carrots	3.7
¾ cup	Pumpkin	3.6
2 med	Potatoes	3.6
¾ cup	Cabbage	3.0
1 med	Kumara (sweet potato)	2.9
1 cup	Cauliflower	2.6
½ cup	Coleslaw	2.2
3 slices	Beetroot	2.2
¾ cup	Parsnips	1.9
1 med	Tomato	1.6
1	Onion	1.6

HEALTH FOOD

1 plate	Bran cereal	6.3
1/3 cup	Oat bran	6.2
1/3 cup	Wheat germ	5.2
1 plate	Muesli	4.8
1	Muesli bar	1.6

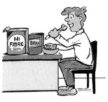

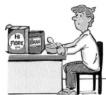

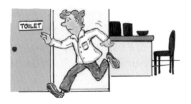

Fats (oils, fatty acids, lipids and triglycerides)

If you want to dramatically lower your risk of the modern plagues of cancer, heart disease, stroke, depression, allergies and inflammatory disorders like rheumatoid arthritis, this chapter may be the most important one of all for you.

There have been so many new findings on fats and oils in recent years that old beliefs are having to be discarded.

The four families of fats

There are four types or families of fats – saturated, polyunsaturated, monounsaturated and trans fat. Nearly all fat from food is a blend of the first three families, but in varying proportions.

Trans fat is not found in significant amounts in supermarket food nowadays, but is still in unlabelled commercial baking and frying fats.

How much fat do we need?

Fat is essential for health and is also desirable to enhance the taste and texture of our food. According to the 2009 Nutrition Survey, the fat content of the average NZ diet, measured in calories, is about 37%. This is just a little higher than the recommended maximum of 35%.

Most of it (18%) surprisingly comes from fried vegetable foods like chips, followed by butter and margarine (9%) and chicken 6%.

If our mix of fats is good (it seldom is), 37% of calories from fat should not harm us in any way, nor cause obesity. (More about the reasons for this later in the book.)

However, in the survey, the top scoring 10% of middle aged males consumed an almost unbelievable 80% of their diet calories in fat. This 80% figure is possible because fat has around three times the calories of grains and 30 times that of vegetables.

Saturated fat

The highest percentage of saturated fat is found in animal, nut and coconut products, but the saturated fat family is complex – there are 34 known types. The four most common saturated fats are: 1. Palmitic – found in butter, cream, eggs, salmon, beef, nuts and dark chocolate. 2. Lauric – found in coconut oil. 3. Stearic – also found in dark chocolate. 4. Myristic – found in coconut oil.

Saturated fats are named such, as they are saturated with hydrogen atoms – the more hydrogen atoms in a fat, the more solid it is at room temperature. For example solid butter is 53% saturated fat, but liquid olive oil is only 13%.

Saturated fat has an undeserved reputation for being harmful and until recently was believed to be a major cause of heart disease. However modern research has found that the diseases once thought to be due to saturated fat, are in fact due to a lack of omega 3 fat.

This makes sense – people have eaten saturated fats for centuries and suffered little or no cardiovascular disease.

However, modern farming and chemical fertilising methods have almost eliminated the omega 3 content in animal fats, but fish still remain a good source, as the sea still contains all the required nutrients.

Saturated fat in moderation is surprisingly good for the body – it's the most rapidly absorbed fat, and delivers sustained energy and less hunger for long periods of time. It's also required for the body to absorb the vitamins A, D, E and K, which are all fat-soluble.

Saturated fat also increases the absorption of calcium and magnesium, which is why natural milk contains cream.

Polyunsaturated fat – omega 3 and omega 6

The polyunsaturated fat family, or PUFA (polyunsaturated fatty acids) contains two sub-families – omega 3 and omega 6.

Omega 3 fats are found mostly in fish, nuts, seeds, algae and leafy greens. There are 11 known kinds of omega 3, but the three most important ones are – EPA (eicosapentaenoic acid), DHA (docosahexaenoic acid) and ALA (alpha-linolenic acid) – from these three fats (or essential fatty acids) a healthy digestive system can make the other 8.

Omega 6 fats are found mostly in bean, seed and grain oils. The three main kinds of omega 6 fat are – LA (linoleic acid), GLA (gamma-linolenic acid) and AA (arachidonic acid).

Monounsaturated fat – omega 9

The omega 9 (or monounsaturated) fat family is made up of six types – the two main ones are oleic and erucic acid. Omega 9 is found along with saturated fat in natural foods such as red meat, whole milk, nuts, and high-fat fruit such as olives, oil palms and avocados.

Omega 9 from food is not generally lacking in our NZ diet, nor does eating too much appear to cause any problems. A healthy digestive system can also make omega 9 from saturated fat.

Omega 9 helps maintain a healthy blood sugar level and prevent insulin resistance.

Olive oil is about 75% omega 9, avocado oil 74% and canola oil 61%. These are generally the best oils for cooking as they can stand higher temperatures before being damaged (ie, they have a higher smoke point). Canola oil (modified rapeseed oil) is heated during processing to deodorise the smell, but is generally regarded as acceptable for cooking.

Omega 9 was once believed to be a principal reason for the superior health and long life of Mediterranean people. They have a 50% lower early death rate, from all causes, than other developed nations. However this health advantage is now believed due to the higher level of omega 3, and lower level of potentially harmful omega 6 fat in their diet.

Omega 3 fat – powerful health protection

In 1989 the respected medical journal 'The Lancet' reported on a health study trialling an omega 3-rich fish oil diet, during which the death rate dropped an impressive 29%.

This result appeared to be due to the anti-blood clotting qualities of omega 3, and the lowering of blood fats (triglycerides), which are formed mostly from excess sugar and white flour.

The best sources of omega 3 are fish, flaxseed, walnuts and the extracted oils of these foods, (omega 3 is obviously an important fat, frequently lacking in our modern diet).

Three grams a day of omega 3 has successfully healed inflammatory disorders such as cardiovascular disease, arthritis, asthma, Crohn's disease, lupus and MS, as well as inflammatory skin diseases such as eczema and acne.

Depression and other psychiatric disorders also respond well to a diet rich in omega 3 – even cancers have responded when omega 3 has been combined with high levels of vitamin C given intravenously and optimum levels of vitamin D maintained.

Omega 3 is easily oxidised however – if you take an omega 3 supplement, check the label to make sure it contains an antioxidant such as vitamin E, or CoQ10. (Refrigeration will also extend its life.)

The ALA form of omega 3 from seed oils

Omega 3 from plant seed oils is a type called ALA and is found mostly in flaxseed and kiwifruit seeds. ALA needs to be converted by the body into the biologically usable forms of omega 3 – EPA and DHA (as found in fish oils which have already been converted by the host fish). This is similar to the vitamin A found in plants and called carotene – it needs to be converted to the retinol form before being used by the body.

Some people however, especially the sick and elderly can have difficulty in converting the ALA plant form of omega 3 to EPA and DHA – it may therefore be safer for them to rely on fish oil for their omega 3.

Freshly ground flaxseed contains about one third oil, which is rich (around 60%) in the ALA form of omega 3. Ground flaxseed can be mixed with flour for baking, or added to porridge. If you use it in baking, you can omit an equivalent amount of cooking oil or butter – ie, one third of the weight of the flaxseed. Ground flaxseed is cheap and readily available from health stores. (Store it in the freezer to prevent it going rancid.)

Omega 6 fat – too much causes health problems

Omega 6 fat is essential for energy, and for our body to make use of omega 3 fat. However it's now clear, that excess omega 6 from seed oils in our modern diet has become a massive health problem.

There are several kinds of omega 6, but the most common type is LA (linoleic acid) extracted from plant seeds such as soybean and safflower. This is normally referred to as 'vegetable fat' or 'vegetable oil' on processed food labels. Supermarket oils (with the exception of olive, avocado and canola oils) are high in this kind of omega 6.

It is over-consumption of this LA form of omega 6 that is strongly linked with the two major killers of today – cancer and cardiovascular disease.

The problem dates back to 1955 when health authorities mistakenly concluded that saturated animal fat caused cardiovascular disease. They therefore recommended a wholesale changeover to poly-unsaturated vegetable fats (which are mostly high in omega 6). Margarines are made from polyunsaturated vegetable oils and are about 24% omega 6, whereas butter, which is largely saturated fat, is only 3%.

With hindsight, it's now clear this recommendation was a major mistake. As a result, in America by 1980, three times more omega 6 fat was being eaten. Heart disease however continued to soar, and although the pro-portion of men who were smokers dropped from 75% down to 30%, the number of lung cancer deaths have soared 60 times higher – other cancers have also skyrocketed. (Smoking is not the only cause of lung cancer.)

This omega 6 problem only appears to apply to the LA form of omega 6, not to the GLA form found in evening primrose seeds and borage, nor the CLA form found in animal fat (more on this below).

Dangerous ratios of omega 6 to omega 3

The reason for serious health problems from excess omega 6 has now become clear – when the omega 6 to omega 3 fat ratio in our diet exceeds 9 to 1, the human immune system begins to shut down.

This allows cancer cells and inflammation causing infection disorders to gain the upper hand – these also include cardiovascular disease, asthma and rheumatoid arthritis.

LA omega 6 and increased incidence of cancer

The suppression of the human immune system from excess omega 6 was accidentally discovered in the 1980's when surgeons were hunting for a cure to the problem of tissue rejection of organ transplants. They found one effective way to suppress the human immune system was to inject large dosages of LA omega 6 intravenously into the blood of the patient (in excess of 25 parts to 1 part of the patient's omega 3 intake).

Surgeons soon however became astonished to see how quickly their patients developed cancers.

This same principle is now occurring in the modern diet – the ratio of omega 6 to omega 3 is estimated to be around 16 to 1 in NZ. The resulting suppression of the human immune system is believed to be one of the principal reasons for the numerous inflammatory diseases and the increased incidence of cancer we see all around us.

Excess omega 6 linked to many modern diseases

Dr Ray Peat Ph.D. a biological researcher has devoted his life to the study of physiology (living systems) and states – *"An excess of the polyunsaturated fats (PUFA's) is central to the development of degenerative diseases – cancer, heart disease, arthritis, immuno-deficiency, diabetes, hypertension, osteoporosis, connective tissue disease, and calcification."* Omega 6 is a PUFA or polyunsaturated fatty acid.

In the early 20th century, before the huge rise in the use of margarine and other processed vegetable fats from seed oils, death rates from cancer were only about 6%. Death rates have since increased five-fold to around 30% in NZ today.

Cardiovascular disease rates would be even higher were it not for the reduction in smoking, and anti-blood clotting medications like Clopidogrel. Warfarin (Coumadin) should be avoided as it works by blocking vitamin K.

Excess LA type omega 6 fat is also believed largely responsible for the alarming increase in melanoma skin cancers in NZ and Australia. Dr Ray Kearney, a professor in the Department of Infectious Diseases and Immunology, University of Sydney has written – *"Vegetable oils which are rich in linoleic acid (LA omega 6) are potent promoters of tumour growth."* Int Clin Nutr 1987; 7:157. The sun is popularly blamed for melanoma tumours, but unlike other skin cancers, melanoma occurs more frequently on areas not exposed to the sun.

Despite current medical treatment, cancer has now become the leading cause of death in NZ. Processed, additive filled meat also plays a major role in causing cancer. (See also the later chapter titled **Avoiding Cancer**.)

Fats

Avoiding excess omega 6

Common sources of LA omega 6 in our diet are from margarines, commercial baking fats (shortening) and frying fats. These high omega 6 fats are widely used in baked products (bread, cakes biscuits, etc), and fast foods.

Food labels, when available normally just list them as 'vegetable fat'. Where possible, calculate the omega 6 to omega 3 ratio.

Omega 6 levels are very high in supermarket oils, especially safflower, corn and soy oils. These should be avoided, or balanced with a higher omega 3 intake to keep your ratio to 9 to 1 or less. A healthy ratio is 4 parts omega 6 to 1 part omega 3 – this is the Japanese ratio. Healthier still is 1 part omega 6 to 1 part omega 3.

Studies have shown that a ratio of 4 to 1 omega 6 to omega 3 results in a 70% decrease in cardiovascular disease, and has a beneficial effect on asthma. (A ratio of 3 to 1 suppresses rheumatoid arthritis.)

CLA – cancer-protecting omega 6 (from animal foods)

There is however a form of omega 6 that is particularly healthy and is found in eggs and the fat of grass eating animals – it is called CLA (conjugated linoleic acid). It differs only slightly from the LA seed oil forms of omega 6, but this small difference gives it powerful anti-cancer properties.

Even at only 1% of calories in our diet, it is protective against breast cancer, colon cancer and melanoma. The best sources are dairy products (especially cream), eggs, and the fat on beef.

Theories in the past linking red meat to cancer came from the US, where they regularly trim off the fat which contains CLA – further evidence of natural fats being good for human health. It is the processed, mostly heat damaged fats that can be harmful.

Trans fats – not all bad

Trans fat, which is formed in partly-hydrogenated (processed) oils has been strongly linked to the following disorders:

- Cardiovascular disease
- Immune system suppression
- Breast cancer (75% higher risk)
- Infertility (73% higher risk)
- Depression (48% higher risk)

Due to public concern, trans fat in table margarines has been reduced or eliminated in recent years. However it is still found in commercial baking fats (shortening) and deep frying oils, as it extends shelf life by protecting against rancidity. (Trans fat is not normally tested for in NZ foods.)

It is possible that trans fat is taking much of the blame for the similar health problems resulting from excess, heat-damaged omega 6 fat.

However, the trans fat found in natural animal fat (dairy products normally contain about 2%) appears to be beneficial for health and helps prevent rancidity.

Supermarket cooking oils

Popular supermarket cooking oils, with the exception of virgin cold-pressed oils, while not as heat damaged as margarines and commercial baking fats, have generally been subjected to chemical extraction processes involving heat. These refined oils are nevertheless, generally better for frying than virgin cold-pressed oils, due to their higher smoke point. However, it still may be best to choose cooking oils low in omega 6, such as olive or avocado oil.

Cold-pressed oils

Better quality, virgin cold-pressed oils are supplied in dark containers to protect against oxidation and rancidity from light. These are best used and consumed at room temperature and added after cooking. There is little advantage in using these higher priced oils for cooking, as the heat destroys most of their health benefits. Cold-pressed oils mostly have a low smoke point.

Oils are damaged when heated to smoking point

Oils become toxic and unhealthy when heated to their blueish smoking point, and an even more toxic chemical called acrylamide is formed when fat is burnt past its smoking point. Burning oil can also create trans fat.

High smoking point cooking oils

Cooking oils and fats that generally have a high smoking point are light olive, clarified butter (ghee), coconut, lard, rice bran, refined soy, refined safflower, grape seed, palm, and the best but priciest, avocado oil.

Margarine vs butter

When liquid vegetable oils are processed (hydrogenated) into firm fats like margarine and shortening, much damage is done. The oil is heated to a very high temperature for several hours and then injected with hydrogen, along with certain chemicals.

Nearly all nutritive value is destroyed in this process. Trans fat is also created when the hydrogenation is only partial (to give a longer shelf-life). Margarine is usually also high in LA type omega 6.

Butter retains its nutrient value during processing as no heat or chemicals are involved.

> ## Cardiologist never saw a heart attack before 1928
> Dr Dudley White, a cardiologist writes, *"I began my practice as a cardiologist in 1921 and I never saw an MI (heart attack) patient until 1928. Back in the MI-free days before 1920, the fats were butter and lard, and I think that we would all benefit from the kind of diet that we had at a time when no one had ever heard the words 'corn oil'."*

My own daily fat choices

One of my proofreaders, somewhat perplexed by the complexity of the facts in this chapter, suggested I describe my own fat intake as a guideline for beginners on this subject.

My own diet fats are dairy (from butter and cream), nuts, flaxseed, salmon oil, and avocados in season. When I occasionally fry fish or roast pumpkin seeds, I use light olive oil. There is also in my diet, some unavoidable high omega 6 vegetable fat from processed supermarket foods, but I try and keep this to a minimum.

My percentage of fat calories would be around the NZ average of 30-35%. I don't normally worry about fat intake, so long as I can keep my omega 6 to omega 3 ratio within the recommended 4 to 1.

Role of fat in the body – all types
- Maintains healthy skin, hair and bones.
- Protects organs against shock damage.
- Suppresses hunger for long periods (when in food).
- Maintains body warmth by insulation (body fat).

Role of saturated fat in the body
- Acts as a long-lasting energy food.
- Helps the liver make cholesterol for cell building and repair.
- Helps strengthen the immune system.
- Required for manufacture of sex hormones and digestive enzymes.
- Helps incorporate calcium into the bones.
- Needed by the body to absorb vitamins A, E, D, K1 and K2.
- Assists the body to better utilise omega 3 fat.

Role of omega 3 fat in the body
- Essential for development and protection of brain and nerve cells.
- Helps maintain mental clarity and emotional well being.
- Important for healthy eyes.
- Helps regulate blood pressure.
- Important for regulation of blood clotting.
- Helps prevent fibrillation (erratic heartbeat).

- Required for an effective immune system.
- Helps maintain healthy body weight and normal appetite.
- Required for joint health.
- Helps maintain healthy menstruation.
- Helps maintain optimum HDL/LDL cholesterol levels.
- Promotes balanced triglyceride (blood fat) levels.
- Needed to maintain healthy bone density in the elderly.
- Helps keep skin moist and supple.

Role of omega 6 fat in the body (at 4 to1 ratio to omega 3)
- Assists with omega 3 functions.
- Helps regulate normal brain function.
- Regulates normal growth and development.
- Helps transport nutrients to the cells.
- Helps regulate blood pressure (GLA form from evening primrose).
- Strengthens the immune system (CLA form from animal fat).
- Helps regulate the immune system.
- Assists in the manufacture of hormones.

Too little fat (20% or less of calories) all fats except noted
- Frequent desire for fatty foods, especially those with carbs and sugar.
- Unhealthily low body weight.
- Increased risk of obesity/diabetes (due to overeating of carbs).
- Blood clots. Heart attack. Stroke. (omega 3 only)
- Reduced long term endurance energy.
- Unhealthy dry skin. Rosacea. Dull hair (GLA form of omega 6).
- Poor absorption of fat-soluble vitamins – A, D, E and K.
- Depression and other psychiatric disorders (omega 3 only).
- Increased risk of cancer (lack of omega 3 only).
- Lower levels of protective HDL cholesterol (especially omega 3).
- Sub-optimal health of cells and hormone regulation.
- Hardening of arteries (omega 3 only).

Too much fat (35% or more of calories) all fats except noted
- Excess weight gain.
- Increased risk of blood clots (LA type omega 6).
- Double the risk of macular degeneration in eyes (LA type omega 6).
- Suppressed immune system (LA type omega 6).
- Eczema.

Cooking losses
- Fats will generally go rancid if left exposed to light and air, but there are no significant cooking losses unless heated to the smoking stage, when toxins are created.

RDI | FATS

Omega 3			
Child:	900 mg	Woman:	800 mg
Teenage boy: 1200 mg	Teenage girl: 800 mg	Pregnancy:	1000 mg
Man:	1300 mg	Breastfeeding:	1200 mg
Omega 6	Four times the amount of omega 3 (optimum three times)		
Omega 9	Not critical - can be made by the body from omega 3 and 6		
Saturated fat	Not critical provided RDI of omega 3 met and total fat does not exceed 35% of calorie intake		
TOTAL FAT	Maximum 35% of calorie intake (Minimum 20%)		
	2000 cals/day = max 220 g fat		
	2500 cals/day = max 280 g fat		
	3000 cals/day = max 330 g fat		
	(See page 20 for recommended calorie intakes)		

Foods with 10 g (1/3 oz) or more fat per serving
(1 gram of fat = 9 calories) (100 g = approx 4 oz)

Serving size	Food	TOTAL FAT grams	Satur fat grams	Omega 3 grams	Omega 6 grams	Omega 9 grams
1/4 svg	Quiche (22cm)	65	36	0	5	24
1 slice	Cheese cake	60	37	0	2	21
2 pces	Fish (fried in batter)	59	29	1	6	23
150 g	Omelette cheese (2 eggs)	36	22	0	2	12
4	Savouries	33	19	0	2	12
1 svg	Chips (deep fried)	32	17	0	3	12
1	Pie (meat)	32	16	0	2	14
100 g	Chocolate	30	19	0	1	10
1 slice	Cake (thickly iced)	29	18	0	2	9
1	Cheese sandwich	29	15	0	5	9
1	Hot dog (battered)	29	15	0	1	13
100 g	Bacon fried	27	10	0	3	14
1 svg	Christmas pudding	27	14	0	2	11
1/3 cup	Nuts mixed	27	5	0	8	14
1	Lamington	26	21	0	1	4
1/3 cup	Nuts, macadamia	26	6	0	1	19
1/3 cup	Peanuts (salted)	26	4	0	10	12
2	Sausages (boiled)	26	13	0	2	11
1 svg	Bread and butter pudding	25	13	0	4	8
4	Sausage rolls	25	13	0	2	10
3	Fish cakes (crumbed)	24	3	1	10	10

Serving size	Food	TOTAL FAT grams	Satur fat grams	Omega 3 grams	Omega 6 grams	Omega 9 grams
100 g	Lamb	**24**	13	0	1	10
2	Meringues with cream	**24**	17	0	1	6
2	Sausages (grilled)	**23**	11	0	2	10
50 g	Nuts (avg)	**23**	3	0	5	5
1 svg	Cream sponge	**22**	13	0	2	7
2 pces	Chicken (KFC)	**22**	7	0	3	12
151 g	Omelette plain (2 eggs)	**22**	12	0	2	8
1 cup	Potato salad	**22**	3	0	14	5
½	Avocado	**21**	3	0	3	15
5	Chicken nuggets	**21**	6	0	4	11
1	Fishburger	**21**	9	1	5	6
2 tbsp	Margarine	**21**	5	1	7	8
1	Spring roll (deep fried)	**20**	10	0	2	12
1	Eggburger	**19**	9	0	2	8
2 lge	Eggs (fried)	**19**	5	0	5	9
1 slice	Cake (thinly iced)	**18**	6	0	5	7
50 g	Cheese	**18**	13	0	1	4
3 tbsp	Cream	**18**	12	0	0	6
1	Hamburger	**18**	7	0	2	9
1 svg	Lasagne	**18**	9	0	1	8
5	Oysters (battered)	**18**	4	1	5	8
1 bag	Potato crisps (50 g)	**18**	9	0	2	7
2	Cakes, cream (small)	**17**	11	0	1	5
1	Cheeseburger	**17**	6	0	2	9
200 g	Chicken (home cooked)	**17**	7	0	2	8
1 cup	Ice cream	**15**	11	0	0	4
1 svg	Apple crumble	**14**	3	0	3	8
1 cup	Trifle dessert	**14**	8	0	1	5
1 cup	Coleslaw	**13**	2	1	7	3
2 tbsp	Peanut butter	**12**	2	0	4	6
1	Apple pie	**12**	6	0	1	5
1 slice	Cake (not iced)	**11**	3	0	3	5
2 lge	Eggs (boiled)	**11**	3	0	1	7
1 slice	Meat loaf	**11**	5	0	1	5
1	Muffin	**11**	3	0	5	3
1 svg	Pizza	**11**	6	0	1	4
100 g	Beef	**10**	5	0	0	5
3 med	Biscuits, chocolate or iced	**10**	2	0	4	4
1 cup	Milk (whole)	**10**	7	0	0	3

Fat types – in common oils and fats (%)

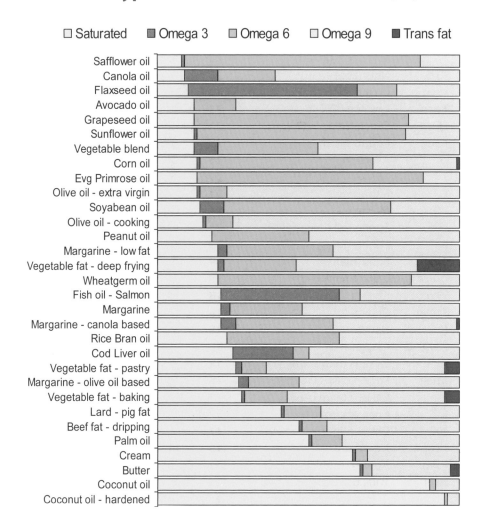

Legend: ☐ Saturated ■ Omega 3 ▨ Omega 6 ☐ Omega 9 ■ Trans fat

Fats (vertical axis label)

Safflower oil
Canola oil
Flaxseed oil
Avocado oil
Grapeseed oil
Sunflower oil
Vegetable blend
Corn oil
Evg Primrose oil
Olive oil - extra virgin
Soyabean oil
Olive oil - cooking
Peanut oil
Margarine - low fat
Vegetable fat - deep frying
Wheatgerm oil
Fish oil - Salmon
Margarine
Margarine - canola based
Rice Bran oil
Cod Liver oil
Vegetable fat - pastry
Margarine - olive oil based
Vegetable fat - baking
Lard - pig fat
Beef fat - dripping
Palm oil
Cream
Butter
Coconut oil
Coconut oil - hardened

"Margarine eaters have twice the rate of heart disease as butter eaters."
Nutrition Week (22 Mar 1991 21:12)

Cholesterol

Cholesterol is a soft, waxy substance, needed for countless functions in every cell of our body and brain – we would die without it.

About 80% of cholesterol is made by our liver (about 1 gram daily), the other 20% is normally supplied by protein food such as eggs.

Misconceptions about cholesterol

Cholesterol is essential for life, but in the minds of most people it has the image of a stealthy killer – why is this?

Cholesterol's negative image began back in 1948, when 5,209 residents of the town of Framingham, Massachusetts (aged 30 to 62 years) were selected by the US Health Service for a 20 year study into the causes and treatment of cardiovascular disease – it was called the Framingham Heart Study.

Many facts were gained from this study, but one of the most 'media-worthy' findings was that many who had cardiovascular disease also had high blood cholesterol. It was therefore assumed at the time, that cholesterol must be the principal cause of cardiovascular disease.

This appeared plausible – the plaque build up in artery walls contains cholesterol (although it also contains fat, calcium and many other substances). This news made major headlines and so, in the minds of the general public, the image of cholesterol as a killer was born.

Since then however, numerous clinical trials have found no evidence of high blood cholesterol causing heart disease. In fact, half of all heart attacks take place in individuals with normal cholesterol levels.

In 1992, a review of 26 major cholesterol studies concluded that – *"Lowering serum cholesterol concentrations does not reduce mortality and is unlikely to prevent coronary heart disease. Claims of the opposite are based on preferential citation of supportive trials."* (In other words, only results that supported a particular point of view had been selected.)

Researchers at the University of San Diego School of Medicine went even further and pointed out that, rather than being harmful, high overall cholesterol in those aged over 75 is protective of health and linked with a clearer mind and lower risk of Alzheimer's.

However it depends on what form of cholesterol we are talking about.

High density and low density cholesterol

Essentially there is only one kind of cholesterol in our body, but it takes on different characteristics as it combines with proteins for its various roles. The two main types are HDL (which stands for high density lipoprotein) and LDL (low density lipoprotein).

HDL cholesterol   Healthy HDL cholesterol (think of H for healthy) is essential for every cell in our body. HDL is called 'good' or 'healthy' as one of its roles is to carry used repair debris away from body cells for recycling. This includes removing excess LDL cholesterol and clotted blood from artery repairs. Artery repairs are usually required because of inflammation damage.

This removal of debris formed during artery repair, greatly reduces our risk of blood clots from accumulations of this material breaking away. Generally, the higher our level of HDL cholesterol, the safer we are from cardiovascular clots.

LDL cholesterol   This type of cholesterol is also essential for every cell in our body, especially as mentioned above, to repair artery inflammation and other damage.

LDL cholesterol carries fats *to* the body cells for repairs (rather than *from* the cells, as does HDL). It is often called 'bad' or 'lousy' cholesterol (mostly incorrectly) as it is only old, oxidised LDL, lodged in the walls of narrowed arteries that is harmful – a problem that only arises when our levels of healthy HDL are insufficient to carry away the used LDL from the repaired areas. Or as one of my readers aptly put it, *"LDL is the repair man, who after plastering the cell's walls, leaves a mess – HDL is the rubbish man who picks up after him."*

A high blood level of LDL cholesterol – above 3 mmol/L (120 mg/dl) is generally a sign there is not enough HDL cholesterol circulating in our blood to remove the excess LDL.

Researchers have found that when LDL is not cleared fast enough from the inner linings of our artery walls, it begins to break down and oxidise. These oxidised cholesterol particles are called oxysterol and cause further inflammation, attracting even more LDL cholesterol to repair the damage. This destructive cycle is a major root cause of cardiovascular disease. Cholesterol generally only blocks arteries when it has been oxidised and hardened.

It is important to realise that LDL cholesterol, in its unoxidised normal state, is not a cause of artery damage, just one of the repair materials, (mostly from healing inflammation).

Cholesterol blood tests – what are good levels?

These days, cholesterol blood tests look more at the ratio of HDL to LDL cholesterol, known as the TC/HDL ratio (total cholesterol divided by HDL cholesterol). The lower your TC/HDL ratio the better; 2.5 or less is good – this indicates a good level of HDL.

A high TC/HDL – above 2.5 is an indicator of inflamed arteries being repaired by LDL (inflammation is the main cause of artery disease, leading to heart attacks and stroke). There's more about this in the later chapter **Avoiding a heart attack or stroke**.

A cholesterol blood test will normally also measure your level of blood fats known collectively as triglycerides. These fats transport surplus glucose, which insulin has converted into fat, to the fat storage cells of the body. Generally the lower our triglyceride reading the better.

The optimum levels to look for in a cholesterol blood test are –

HDL cholesterol 2.0 mmol/l or higher (80 mg/dl USA)
LDL cholesterol 2.0 mmol/L or lower* (80 mg/dl USA)
Total cholesterol to HDL (TC /HDL ratio) 2.5 or lower
Triglycerides 1.7 mmol/L or lower (150 mg/dl USA) **

* LDL is nearly always higher than 2.0 mmol/L. This can still be acceptable however, as long as your HDL cholesterol is 40% or more of your total cholesterol. For example, if your LDL is high at 3.0, but your total cholesterol is 5.0, your HDL will be 2.0 (5.0 – 3.0 = 2.0). This still gives an acceptable TC/HDL ratio of 2.5 (5.0 ÷ 2.0 = 2.5).

**Conversion from mmol/L to mg/dl is scaled differently for cholesterol and triglycerides due to density – mmol/L is volume-based and mg/dl is weight-based.

Too low HDL cholesterol can be dangerous

HDL cholesterol levels below the minimum of 2.0 mmol/l (80 mg/dl) have been linked to depression, anti-social behaviour and drug addiction.

A very low HDL cholesterol level, below 1.0 mmol/l (40 mg/dl), or less than 20% or 1/5th of your total cholesterol, is a serious risk factor. Not only for cardiovascular problems, but for heart fibrillation (an abnormal beating rhythm). An abnormal heartbeat is the main cause of death following a non-fatal heart attack.

What causes low HDL cholesterol?

The following factors all tend to lower healthy HDL cholesterol levels:

- constant anxiety
- anger
- excess sugar and white flour
- excess iron
- smoking
- lack of exercise
- excess LA type omega 6
- lack of omega 3

Also lack of some essential nutrients, in particular –

- fibre
- vitamin K2
- iodine
- potassium
- niacin
- CoQ10
- chromium
- selenium
- inositol
- calcium
- zinc
- vitamin C
- magnesium
- manganese

Healthy levels of HDL cholesterol are often found in areas where the drinking water is hard – most often from the minerals magnesium and calcium. These two minerals work together and have a relaxing effect on our body and mind.

Anger and anxiety lowers HDL

A 10-year study of 374 young adults, found that the 17% who scored above average on a psychological test for anger, accumulated over 100% more cholesterol repair deposits in their arteries than the below average scorers. Anger lowers HDL cholesterol by releasing adrenalin and other companion stress-related hormones, such as cortisol, into the blood stream.

A significant American study also found higher LDL cholesterol in shift workers who had different co-workers during each shift, compared with those who worked with familiar faces each shift – another obvious stress and anxiety factor.

What causes high LDL cholesterol?

High levels of LDL are usually the result of low levels of HDL. This is because there is less than the required amount of HDL cholesterol circulating in the blood to carry away used LDL cholesterol, along with the repair debris from arteries. This is a dangerous condition, as repair deposits in arteries can easily become large and break away, causing a blockage in blood flow.

Should I take a cholesterol lowering drug?

Numerous independent studies have found that taking a drug to artificially lower the liver's production of cholesterol, has only a minor effect on cardiovascular deaths. This is a logical outcome when cholesterol's 'repair role' in artery inflammation is understood.

Cholesterol lowering drugs (such as Lipex, Lipitor, etc) are known as statins and are currently the world's most heavily prescribed medication.

In a small percentage of people, statins have reduced the number of heart attacks or strokes, however this is now believed to be due to a side effect of statins in raising nitrous oxide levels in the blood. Nitrous oxide relaxes arteries, allowing them to widen and carry more blood. (Nitroglycerin-based angina inhalers and warm sunshine on our skin, produce the same effect.)

Even allowing for this effect, 100 people would have to take a statin drug for more than three years to avoid just one heart attack. There are far more cost-effective (or free) means to reduce the occurrence of heart attacks.

Statins also cause numerous health problems – sore weak muscles (the heart is also a muscle), a dementia-like 'fogged up' mind (ie, no longer able to reconcile the bank statement) and long term liver damage.

These side effects are believed to be mostly due to the typical 40% reduced output by the liver of a health-promoting hormone/enzyme known as CoQ10. (There's further information on CoQ10 in a later chapter.)

Because of these side effects, about 70% of people give up statins within a few months.

Information on the proven heart medications of nitroglycerin and blood anti-coagulant medication can be found in the chapter on **Avoiding a heart attack or stroke.**

Conclusions

Taking into account what is currently known about cholesterol, leads to five logical conclusions:

1. Our total cholesterol level is almost worthless in determining our risk of heart attack or stroke – what is important is that we have a naturally low level of LDL cholesterol (indicating an absence of artery inflammation) that is 2.0 mmol/L (80 mg/dl) or lower. Whatever the LDL figure, our HDL cholesterol should be 40% or more of our total cholesterol reading.

2. A high triglyceride reading – above 1.7 mmol/L (150 mg/dl) can be a greater risk factor than high LDL cholesterol. Realise that these extra blood triglycerides are pure fat, converted from excess glucose, on their way to be stored somewhere in the body, usually around our middle. Excess glucose is due to eating more calories from carbs (especially sugar and white flour) than we expend in energy.

3. We require a dietary intake of the full RDI of all vitamins and minerals.

4. Anxiety can have a profound effect on our LDL cholesterol level.

5. Artificially lowering cholesterol manufacture by our liver, using a statin drug, is not effective in preventing the causes of cardiovascular disease. It just means inflammation is repaired more slowly.

For a fuller treatment on avoiding cardiovascular diseases, see the chapter **Avoiding a heart attack or stroke**.

"Cholesterol is a vital component of every cell membrane on earth. In other words, there is no life on earth that can live without cholesterol."
Dr Ron Rosedale MD, (anti-ageing researcher)

"The odds are very high, greater than 100 to 1, that you don't need drugs to lower your cholesterol." Dr Joseph Mercola

Water

Water makes up about 65% of our body – about 40 litres (85 pints). As little as 2% loss of our water (dehydration) or just under a litre (2 pints) can begin to cause health problems. These include constipation, dry mouth, headaches, and the risk of kidney stones. Physical and mental performance also begins to drop, and dehydration can raise our blood pressure, due to thickened blood – an 11% loss of water is normally fatal.

Our daily requirement for water, not including perspiration, is about 2.5 litres (10 cups) a day. Half of this is lost in evaporation from our lungs (as we breathe) and from our skin. The other half is lost in urine and stools.

Perspiration during summer, or during physical exertion can increase our water need from half a litre an hour to over 2 litres (8 cups) an hour, and even more in extreme conditions.

Fruit, vegetables and other food typically supply about 25% of our daily water intake. The rest comes from drinks, except surprisingly, our body creates about a cup of water each day as a by-product of oxidation when burning calories for energy.

Should you drink eight glasses of water a day?

Millions of people around the world, particularly women, claim that drinking eight glasses of water a day (about 2 litres) has improved their health. They strongly maintain that they feel much better, have increased energy, more regular bowel movements, less weight problems and better looking skin.

Others (mostly men) feel it's unnatural to force water down when they don't feel thirsty, especially during winter.

Research has come up with scant evidence that drinking more water than normal thirst dictates, can improve health. Researchers suggest that the reported health benefits are due more to what is not being drunk, rather than the additional water itself (ie, fewer drinks containing sugar and caffeine).

A 2004 study of identical twins found no difference in skin hydration when one twin drank 2 litres (8 cups) of water a day for a month, while the other twin drank just half a litre a day (2 cups).

The often reported weight loss benefit of drinking more water appears to be due to eating less calories – a glass of water can instantly eliminate a hunger pang. For the purposes of weight control, the extra water is best drunk first thing in the morning.

Dehydration

As far as dehydration is concerned, a healthy body will normally trigger massive thirst cravings long before dehydration becomes serious – however, it's not uncommon for the elderly to lose their natural perception of thirst. Diuretic drugs and laxative use are often part of the problem, but generally it's regarded as a side effect of dementia.

We can safely assume we're well hydrated, when our urine stream is colourless, or light yellow and we have normal levels of saliva. Dark yellow urine is a sign of dehydration.

However, due to the wealth of empirical evidence, it would appear better to err on the side of too much, rather than too little water. (Most nutritionists recommend four glasses of water a day during winter, in addition to normal food fluid.)

Role of water in the body

- Dissolves nutrients and oxygen and carries them to the cells.
- Regulates body temperature.
- Moistens skin, eyes, mouth, nose, etc.
- Lubricates joints.
- Flushes out waste products.
- Keeps blood viscosity normal.
- Helps prevent constipation.

Too little water

- Reduces physical and mental performance.
- Headaches.
- Overheating and delirium. Fainting.
- Dry mouth from decreased saliva. Dry skin.
- Morning sickness and nausea in pregnant women.
- Constipation.
- Asthma.
- Raised blood pressure due to thickened blood.
- Lower back pain.
- Increased risk of kidney stones.
- Increased risk of bladder and colon cancer.

Too much water

- Can flush out electrolyte minerals, such as potassium and sodium.

"Beware of mindlessly drinking several glasses of water per day without considering your diet, exercise habits, climate, and sense of thirst – and when you do find yourself in need of water, remember that you can get it from liquids and/or whole foods that are rich in water." Dr Ben Kim

RDI WATER

Recommended daily total fluid intake in litres, including
food sources, but not additional perspiration requirements

Child : To 8 yrs	1.2 L/day (5 cups)	Woman:	2.1 L/day (8 cups)
9-12 yrs	1.6 L/day (6 cups)	Pregnancy:	2.3 L/day (9 cups)
Teenager:	2.2 L/day (9 cups)	Breastfeeding:	3.5 L/day (11 cups)
Man:	2.6 L/day (10 cups)		

HEALTH HINT   Muscle power from water

As the muscle protein in our body requires water to work efficiently, we should drink plenty of water before any strenuous work or athletic performance.

Even mild dehydration can reduce muscle efficiency by 25%.

HEALTH HINT   Back pain and stress

A major reason for the sudden onset of lower back pain, especially when no heavy lifting has been done, is emotional stress.

When we bend our backs, many small muscles need to work in sequential order, one after the other.

When we are under stress and flustered, the signals from an overloaded brain to these muscles, can get out of sequence, resulting in two or more muscles working against one another and tearing slightly. This can result in considerable pain until they heal.

One way to reduce this stress is to consciously slow down our breathing.

I highly recommend this daily morning back exercise, developed by world-renowned NZ therapist Robin McKenzie OBE, CNZM:

First, stand and arch your back backwards, stretching hard as you can. Then, while keeping your legs stiff, bend over and do your best to touch the floor with your finger tips, 20 times. Keep pushing downward until you can touch the floor before your 20 bend over exercises are complete.

This is an excellent exercise, which if persistently done should keep your spine and back muscles fully stretched, flexible and pain free.

"The best doctor gives the least medicines."   Benjamin Franklin

58

Protein

Protein is made up of 20 different building blocks known as amino acids. Our body uses these building blocks for a huge range of functions, just as we use the letters of the alphabet to make words and sentences. Protein is used to form all body cells and enzymes.

Eggs and dairy whey protein contain all 20 building blocks, but most other protein foods have a few of the blocks missing. Our liver however acts as a storehouse to recombine the various blocks in the correct proportions as required. Our liver can also manufacture 12 of the 20 building blocks – the other eight have to come from our diet.

We normally think of protein food as coming from animal sources – meat, eggs, milk, cheese, etc, but plants are also a major source of protein. Meat and dairy foods are, after all, created from grass growing in a farmer's paddock.

Our muscles are largely protein, but increasing the amount of protein in our diet won't build bigger muscles – only heavy exercise can do that.

Surprisingly the NZ 2009 Nutrition Survey found that most protein in our diet comes from white bread, followed closely by chicken and milk. The average intake by men was 102 g, much higher than the RDI of 64 g. Average intake by women was 71 g (RDI 46 g).

Our human need for protein is not very high – human breast milk contains only 1% protein, the lowest of any mammal, whereas cow's milk is three times higher at 3%. (Rat's milk is highest at 12% protein, but rats grow 50 times faster than a human.) Elderly humans need a little more protein to help minimise muscle wasting.

Protein is not an efficient energy food as it is slow to digest. Most athletes perform better, at least in the short term, on carbs which are quickly converted to glucose, the energy fuel of our body.

Because protein is slow to digest and uses twice as many calories as carbohydrates in the process, it can help us avoid obesity. Also, like fat, it provides satiety, or a feeling of fullness – in other words it can keep our hunger satisfied for long periods.

High protein, low-carb weight loss diets do work, but they can cause depression and irritability if they don't contain sufficient carbs to provide enough glucose (blood sugar) for our brains to function properly.

Too much animal protein has been blamed for almost every disease known to man, and the high cure rate of fasting has been used to support these claims. However excess carbs are more likely to be the cause of the diseases blamed on too much protein, for there is little convincing evidence that excess protein alone is harmful. Nevertheless, the high phosphorus content of most protein food, especially meat, can upset the acid-alkaline balance of our body. Meat lacks calcium to buffer the acidity of phosphorus. However unless we are a bodybuilder, or over 70, we should not exceed 1 g of protein per 1 kg of lean bodyweight (our weight less our fat percentage, which is normally too high, typically around 22% for men and 35% for women).

Lack of protein is still a problem in the poorer countries of the world. Rice is a poor provider – one cup of cooked rice yields only 5 g of protein (just 8% of the RDI for an adult male).

Role of protein in our body
- Provides the building material for our body cells.
- Required for muscle building and wound healing.
- Helps regulate brain function.
- Helps regulate our reproductive system.
- Helps regulate our immune system.

Too little protein (below 10% of daily calories)
- Lack of growth and development in children.
- Muscle wasting in adults, especially the elderly.
- Dull hair that can pull out easily.

Too much protein (above 30% of daily calories)
- Depression and irritability, if not balanced with carbs.
- Excess cell acidity if the high acidic phosphorus content of most protein foods is not buffered with calcium.

Cooking losses
- No significant losses.

DANIEL IN BABYLON

The King assigned them a daily portion of the rich food which he ate and of the wine which he drank – but Daniel resolved not to defile himself with the King's rich food or the wine which he drank.

So Daniel said to the King's steward, "Test us for ten days – let us be given pulse (peas, beans, lentils, etc) to eat, and water to drink, then compare our appearance with that of the young men who eat the king's food."

At the end of ten days it was seen that Daniel and his three companions looked healthier and better nourished than any of the young men who ate the King's rich food.

Bible Book of Daniel 1:4-16

RDI PROTEIN

Child:	1-3 yrs	14 g	Man over 70:	81 g
	4-7 yrs	20 g	Woman:	46 g
	8-12 yrs	30 g	Woman over 70:	57 g
Teenage boy:		65 g	Pregnancy:	60 g
Teenage girl:		45 g	Breastfeeding:	67 g
Man:		64 g		

Protein

DAIRY / EGGS		gm	VEGETABLES (cooked)		
25 g	Whey protein powder	24	¾ cup	Baked beans	10
2 cups	Milk (std or trim)	17	2 cobs	Sweet corn	10
2 med	Eggs	13	**MEAT / FISH**		
25 g	Cheese	7	100 g	Meat (white)	28
GRAIN / NUTS			100 g	Meat (red)	24
1/3 cup	Nuts	10	100 g	Fish	16
4 slices	Bread (wholemeal)	10	100 g	Meat (processed0	14
4 slices	Bread (white)	8			
½ cup	Flour (wholemeal)	8			
1 svg	Pizza	8			
½ cup	Flour (white)	6			

HEALTH HINT Grains, beans and nuts

Grains require milling, rolling, cooking or sprouting before they can be properly digested and their nutrients absorbed. Also, the high phosphorus content of raw grains (known as phytate) can prevent around 40% of their zinc, magnesium, manganese and iron being absorbed. This is mostly overcome by the traditional bread-making methods of fermenting with yeast, or sour dough, or sprouting the grain before drying and milling to flour. Sprouting greatly enhances the nutritional value of a grain.

Food like muesli often contain raw grains that cannot be fully utilised by our digestive system. Beans also contain high levels of phosphorus and are best sprouted or soaked overnight before cooking.

Nuts need thorough chewing before swallowing – if nuts are not thoroughly chewed they will pass through our digestive system largely undigested.

"Medicines are only palliative (symptom-relieving), for back of disease lies the cause, and this cause no drug can reach."

Dr Weir Mitchell MD (1829 –1914)

61

Vitamin A – Carotene and Retinol

Vitamin A is an antioxidant that plays a major role in the health of our eyes, skin, teeth and bones. It also helps protect us from infections and cancer – numerous studies show that a deficiency in vitamin A is linked with cancer of body organs and basal and squamous cell skin cancers.

Our body makes vitamin A from carotene, an orange-yellow plant pigment found in orange coloured foods such as carrots, pumpkin and apricots, and also in dark green foods like silverbeet (chard). There is no danger from too much carotene, except temporary yellow skin colouration in extreme cases.

After carotene is converted by our body to vitamin A, it is known as retinol and is stored in our liver. Our body needs dietary fat to make this conversion. Some children in Denmark went blind during World War II when that country's butter and cream was all exported, as dairy had been their main source of fat to make vitamin A from carotene.

As you will see from the food chart, it's not difficult to obtain all the carotene we need to make vitamin A from vegetables and fruit – one carrot a day will suffice. However despite this, the NZ 2009 Nutrition Survey found deficiencies in all age groups, some serious. About a third of all teenage boys had a deficient intake of carotene, also half of all Maori and Pacific Island teenage girls, and Pacific Island women over 50. The overall average deficiency was 17% for all age groups.

In poorer countries of the world, where fresh vegetables and fruit are unaffordable, millions of children die of infections from vitamin A deficiency, as children's bodies can hold only small reserves of vitamin A. Low income NZ families have higher rates of infectious diseases.

The already converted retinol form of vitamin A can be obtained from dairy products, eggs and liver, also cod liver oil is a rich source. However, too much vitamin A in this form can be harmful, if our vitamin A body stores are already full. In the 16th century, a group of Dutch seamen ate polar bear liver, which is extremely high in retinol, they were shocked a few days later to see their skin dry up and begin to flake off.

As with most nutrients that are toxic in excess, body size makes a difference – a rowing crew once took huge doses of retinol vitamin A, but the only one who developed overdose symptoms was the lightly built coxswain, who sits in the back of the boat calling the strokes.

In New Zealand, about 40% of our vitamin A is obtained from retinol in dairy foods, eggs, margarine or health supplements – the remaining

60% must be made by the body using carotene from plant foods.

Prolonged stress, especially from bodily injury, has been found to deplete the body's vitamin A levels dramatically, particularly after surgery.

Our skin is very dependent on vitamin A. Dr Robert Atkins wrote, *"For almost 100% of the skin conditions I treat, I prescribe vitamin A."* He found nearly all acne sufferers to be low in vitamin A, and typically prescribed a therapeutic size catch-up dose of 100,000 mcg a day of retinol for three to four months. Psoriasis also improves at the same dose, when taken with additional vitamin D.

Role of vitamin A in our body

- Helps maintain clarity and lubrication of our eyes.
- Assists our eyes in adapting to darkness.
- Helps maintain the lubrication of internal linings and outer skin.
- Needed for healing wounded body tissue.
- An antioxidant to help maintain youthfulness of body cells.
- Assists our immune system to kill infections.
- Protects against organ and skin cancer.
- Necessary for normal development and strength of bones.
- Helps regulate spacing and straightness of teeth in children.
- Helps regulate blood sugar.

Too little vitamin A

- Irritable, inflamed, dry, dull, or rough-feeling eyes – blindness in severe cases. Cataracts. Reduced night vision. Free radical damage.
- Weak, easily broken bones and easily decayed teeth.
- Stunted growth and crooked or malformed teeth in children.
- Low immunity to infections, especially children. Tuberculosis.
- Body organ cancer. Basal and squamous cell skin cancers.
- Oily or coarse skin on the face and back, sometimes with acne.
- Dull hair. Excessive dandruff.
- Duodenal ulcers.
- Psoriasis.

Too much vitamin A (over 55,000 iu daily – retinol only)

- Itchy, dry, sometimes flaking skin, with raised hair follicles.
- Osteoporosis due to interference with vitamin D.
- Birth defects if over 6000 iu of retinol taken during pregnancy.
- Yellow tinge to skin, especially on palms (carotene form only).

Cooking losses

- No significant losses.

RDI · VITAMIN A (Retinol converted form)

1 mcg vitamin A = 3.6 iu of Carotene or 0.3 iu of Retinol
RDI figures below have been converted to Retinol

Child:	600 mcg (2200 iu)	Woman:	700 mcg	(2500 iu)
Teenage boy:	900 mcg (3200 iu)	Pregnancy:	800 mcg	(2900 iu)
Teenage girl:	700 mcg (2500 iu)	Breastfeeding:	1100 mcg	(4000 iu)
Man:	900 mcg (3200 iu)			

DAIRY / EGGS		mcg
3 tbsp	Butter	450
3 tbsp	Cream	200
2 cups	Milk (std)	170
2 med	Eggs	140
3 tbsp	Margarine	100
½ cup	Ice cream	75

FRUIT		
2	Apricots (small)	465
5	Apricots (dried halves)	325
1 cup	Cantaloupe	270
1	Persimmon	180
1 cup	Pawpaw	170
2	Plums	140
¾ cup	Peaches (canned)	120
1	Tamarillo	115
1	Peach	110

½	Avocado	105
1	Nectarine	85

VEGETABLES (cooked)		
½ cup	Silverbeet (chard)	2500
¾ cup	Pumpkin	2000
1	Carrot (med)	1850
2 cobs	Sweet corn	405
½ cup	Spinach	170
1 cup	Broccoli	165
1 med	Tomato (raw)	120

FISH		
100 g	Eel	1900
100 g	Orange Roughy	100

HEALTH FOOD		
100 g	Liver	13,000
1 tbsp	Cod liver oil	3600
100 g	Kidney	320

HEALTH HINT   Antioxidant supplements

The sale of antioxidant supplements is big business. Antioxidants can be important for our long term health, but there is no need to pay excessive prices for them. Nor does research indicate that taking antioxidants in supplement form is particularly effective, if at all, with the exception of natural vitamin A and vitamin C, two of the most active antioxidants of all.

There appears to be little understood substances within natural foods in which antioxidants are found, that are necessary for them to work effectively. We should be able to obtain all the antioxidants our body can use from a range of brightly coloured natural foods – each predominant colour, blue, purple, red, green, brown, etc, contains different antioxidants. (The main ones are listed on page 65.)

Surprisingly, uric acid, which is naturally produced by our body, is the most powerful antioxidant of all.

Antioxidant rich food

The ORAC test measures a food's antioxidant activity. Dieticians recommend 4000 ORAC units per day for optimum long term health (the average person gets only about 1400). You need to vary food colours to obtain all varieties of antioxidants.

Below is a list of ORAC values from antioxidant rich foods.

Antioxidant rich food	Serving	ORAC value
Chocolate (baking dark)	50 g	31,000
Turmeric powder	2 tsp	16,000
Cinnamon powder	1 tsp	13,000
Gogi berries	½ cup	12,500
Chocolate bar (dark)	50 g	11,000
Plums dark red skin & flesh (med)	2	9700
Cocoa powder	2 tsp	8200
Plums green flesh (med)	2	8200
Prunes	½ cup	7300
Beans red (cooked)	¾ cup	6900
Raspberries	1 cup	6100
Apple (red skin)	1	5900
Apple (green skin)	1	5400
Curry powder	2 tsp	4800
Blueberries	½ cup	4500
Cranberries	½ cup	4500
Gala apple	1	3900
Blackberries	½ cup	3800
Strawberries	½ cup	3000
Ginger powder	1 tsp	1400
Cherries	¼ cup	1200
Garlic cloves	3	500

HEALTH HINT   Change your diet gradually

To avoid temporary nutritional deficiencies occurring, major changes to your diet should be phased in gradually to allow your digestive system time to develop the necessary enzymes and probiotics to properly digest the new food.

For similar reasons, we should where possible, eat the same types of food at the same time each day – our bodies thrive on regularity.

"An ounce of prevention is worth a pound of cure." Traditional proverb

Vitamin B1 – Thiamine

Thiamine B1 is the first of the B family of vitamins – the B family work in unison and are often found together in food.

As you will see in the sections ahead, B group vitamins have a marked effect on our emotional and mental states. Lack of thiamine for example can open the mind's door to depression, apathy and confusion, along with feelings of impending doom. If that were not enough, severe deficiency can result in panic attacks, rapid heartbeat and eventual death.

Low levels are often found after surgery, especially in the elderly which can result in temporary mental confusion.

Thiamine is one of the most commonly deficient vitamins in the world, particularly among people whose diet is predominantly refined white rice. Refined rice is quicker to cook than the more nutritious unrefined brown rice, but in removing the outer bran during refining, 70% of the thiamine in rice is lost. Wheat also loses 60% of thiamine when refined into white flour.

Surveys have found widespread thiamine deficiencies among females, especially pregnant women (over 50% in an Australian survey) and among alcoholics and people with psychiatric disorders.

The 2009 Nutrition Survey estimated that 28% of NZ women are deficient and 13% of men. They only measured dietary intake, but excess sugar and alcohol are known to deplete body reserves. Dr Robert Atkins found the real life situation to be far worse than supposed and wrote, *"The person who doesn't require additional thiamine is a rare find."*

The elderly do not absorb thiamine well and diuretic drugs like frusemide can soon deplete the body of thiamine.

Like most of the B group vitamins, thiamine is harmless in excess – being water soluble it is flushed out of the body in the urine.

Lack of thiamine (or lack of absorption) has been linked to cot death – there was an Australian incident reported many years ago where an Aboriginal community, severely deficient in thiamine were experiencing a cot death rate of 40% among breast-fed babies. This was able to be immediately reversed by supplementing both mothers and infants with the vitamin.

Travellers in lands infested with biting bugs sometimes take large doses of thiamine (5000 mcg daily) to discourage bites.

Role of thiamine in our body

- Promotes the clarity and calmness of our brain and nerves.
- Assists in the body's manufacture of fats and acids.
- Helps transport glucose and oxygen to needed areas.
- Helps maintain heart health.
- Helps regulate the growth of children.
- Helps control our immune system and removal of lead from our body.

Too little thiamine

- Depression. Nervousness. Panic attacks. Insomnia. Mental disorders.
- Numbness and tingling in hands and feet – eventual loss of feeling.
- Prickly, painful muscles in lower legs.
- Irregular or rapid heartbeat (fibrillation), breathlessness.
- Apathy. Confusion. Poor memory. Dementia symptoms.
- Anti-social behaviour. Alcoholism. Anorexia nervosa. Lead poisoning.
- Low energy. Loss of appetite. Weight loss. Constipation.
- Attention disorders and/or slow growth and learning in children.
- Increased risk of cot death among infants.
- A weakened immune system.

Too much thiamine

- No known toxic effects.

Cooking losses

- Heat destroys thiamine and about 70% is lost from peanuts when they are roasted. Boiling food in water can destroy and leach out about 35% the thiamine, but some of this can be recovered if the water is consumed.

HEALTH HINT   **Negative thinking and health**

A major cause of psychiatric and physical ill health is the habit of negative thinking. Insufficient B group vitamins such as thiamine can contribute to habitual negativity, which often leads to depression and other mental and physical disorders.

Psychologists say that a simple way to break this destructive habit is to remember every morning on awakening, a pleasant event that has occurred in your past, and doing your best to recall this happy memory from time to time throughout the day (writing it down helps). By doing this you can eventually break the negative thinking habit.

"A person's mental health can be measured by the amount of good he or she sees in the people around them."   Traditional maxim

RDI VITAMIN B1 THIAMINE

Child:	700 mcg	Woman:	1100 mcg
Teenage boy:	1200 mcg	Pregnancy:	1400 mcg
Teenage girl:	1100 mcg	Breastfeeding:	1400 mcg
Man:	1200 mcg		

DAIRY / EGGS		mcg
2 cups	Milo (using all std milk)	860
2 cups	Milk (std)	360
2 cups	Milk (trim)	160

FRUIT		
1 cup	Orange juice (pure)	180

GRAIN / NUTS		
1/3 cup	Peanuts (raw)	450
1 plate	Cornflakes (with milk)	390
½ cup	Flour (wholemeal)	260
4 slices	Bread (wholemeal)	240
½ cup	Flour (white)	150
1/3 cup	Other nuts (avg)	125
1/3 cup	Peanuts (roasted)	125
1 plate	Porridge (with milk)	120

MEAT / FISH (cooked)		
100 g	Pork	750
100 g	Trout (brown)	320
100 g	Lamb	130
100 g	Beef	120

VEGETABLES (cooked)		
2 cobs	Sweet corn	520
¾ cup	Peas	305
2 med	Potatoes	150
¾ cup	Baked beans	140
1 med	Kumara (sweet potato)	140
1 cup	Broccoli	100
1 cup	Brussels sprouts	100
1 cup	Cauliflower	100

HEALTH FOOD		
1 tbsp	Brewers yeast	1250
1 tsp	Marmite (yeast extract)	550
100 g	Kidney (lamb)	480
1 tbsp	Malt extract	480
1/3 cup	Oat bran	450
1 plate	Muesli (with milk)	380
3 tbsp	Sesame seeds	300
100 g	Liver (lamb)	260
100 g	Kidney (beef)	250
2 tbsp	Wheat germ	200
100 g	Liver (beef)	180

HEALTH HINT Work off stress or mild depression

The best antidote to stress or mild depression is vigorous exercise in the fresh air – it's been repeatedly proven to be more effective than a session with a psychiatrist.

"Homo Sapiens is the only animal that hasn't enough sense to stop eating when he is sick." Dr Ulric Williams (NZ surgeon turned Naturopath)

Vitamin B2 – Riboflavin

Riboflavin is a fluorescent yellow vitamin and is sometimes used as a food colouring (code 101) – this quality can also cause your urine to turn bright yellow after taking a vitamin capsule containing riboflavin.

Riboflavin, like vitamin A, is important for healthy eyesight. Research has linked long term riboflavin deficiency with cataracts. Elderly people who suddenly give up drinking milk, which is a good source of riboflavin, run this risk. Supplementing with riboflavin has been reported to reverse cataracts if caught early.

Riboflavin intake was calculated to be deficient in 17% of the over 70's in the NZ 2009 Nutrition Survey, but only 5% of the younger age groups – 23% of riboflavin intake came from milk.

Lack of riboflavin hinders our body's absorption of iron and can also weaken our thyroid gland.

Sunlight destroys riboflavin – 70% is lost from milk after 3½ hours in direct sunlight. Smoking, alcohol and the birth control pill can hinder absorption.

An active lifestyle increases our requirement for this vitamin.

Role of riboflavin in our body
- Helps us absorb nutrients from our food.
- Activates vitamin B6 and glutathione (a natural antioxidant).
- Helps regulate the growth of children.
- Helps maintain the health of our eyes, skin and nerves.
- Assists blood cells transport glucose to our muscles for energy.
- Helps our cells take up oxygen from the blood.

Too little riboflavin
- Irritable, bloodshot eyes. Over-sensitivity to bright light.
- Dark skin under the eyes. Red eyelids. Cataracts.
- Cracks on lips or at the corners of the mouth.
- Insufficient milk in breastfeeding mothers.
- Slow growth in children.
- Red greasy skin on the face.
- Red burning tongue or lips.
- Poor absorption of iron by the body.
- Weakened thyroid function.
- Eczema or scaly skin on the face and/or genitals. Itching skin.
- Excessive hair loss.

Too much riboflavin (supplement only)

- Bright yellow urine – no known toxic effects.

Cooking losses

- No significant losses, however baking soda, which is an ingredient of baking powder can destroy riboflavin on contact.

RDI	VITAMIN B2 RIBOFLAVIN			
Child:	600 mcg	Woman:	1100 mcg
Teenage boy:	1300 mcg	Woman over 70:	1300 mcg
Teenage girl:	1100 mcg	Pregnancy:	1400 mcg
Man:	1300 mcg	Breastfeeding:	1600 mcg
Man over 70:	1600 mcg		

DAIRY / EGGS		mcg
2 cups	Milo (all milk)	1240
2 cups	Milk (non-fat powder)	1100
2 cups	Milk (std or non-fat)	1000
4 tbsp	Whey protein powder	800
2 med	Eggs	300
½ cup	Ice cream	240

NUTS		
1/3 cup	Almonds	470

MEAT / FISH (cooked)		
100 g	Lamb	500
100 g	Venison	410
100 g	Eel	400
100 g	Mackerel	380
6	Oysters	360
100 g	Sardines (canned)	360
100 g	Trout (brown)	320

100 g	Pork	250
100 g	Salmon (canned)	180
100 g	Chicken	150
100 g	Beef	150
100 g	Fish (avg)	120

VEGETABLES (cooked)		
1 cup	Broccoli	330
2 cobs	Sweet corn	200
¾ cup	Peas	140

HEALTH FOOD		
100 g	Liver	3600
100 g	Kidney	2100
1 plate	Muesli (with milk)	700
1 cup	Soy milk (full fat)	480
1 tbsp	Malt extract	450
1 tsp	Marmite (yeast extract)	430
1 tbsp	Brewers yeast	340

HEALTH HINT   Milk a good source of riboflavin

Milk is a rich natural source of riboflavin. When food budgets are limited, non-fat milk powder can be purchased in bulk for about half the cost of the equivalent liquid milk. By mixing it a little richer than recommended, a pleasant tasting milk can be obtained that is higher in riboflavin than regular milk.

"I am come down to deliver them out of the hand of the Egyptians, unto a good land, a land flowing with milk and honey."

God speaking to Moses, (Exodus 3:8)

Are there dangerous pesticides and harmful minerals in New Zealand food?

As part of the NZ 2009 Nutrition Survey, 4000 food samples were tested for contamination by 241 agricultural pesticides and the harmful elements of arsenic, cadmium and mercury.

Only 0.4% of food tested had detectable residues, which was lower than previous surveys – ie, 1.4% in 1997 and 0.5% in 2003.

Of that tiny 0.4% proportion, 96% had less than one 1000th of the levels set by the World Health Organisation as the minimum standard for food safety. The remaining 4% had less than 100 times the minimum standard.

So despite widespread fears, there appears to be no reason for alarm regarding contamination during the growing stages of NZ foods.

A far more serious problem in our food, is the depletion of essential minerals in our soil, along with the inclusion of unhealthy additives during the manufacturing processes.

HEALTH HINT   **The power of affirmations**

It may feel foolish at times, but mental affirmations, repeated with enthusiasm several times daily, have proven to be a powerful and effective means of rapidly swinging our minds from unhealthy negativity, to health promoting positivity.

Affirmations are generally repeated mentally, spoken aloud, or written down and read.

One historic favourite is – *"Every day in every way, I am getting better and better and better."*

Another one to speed recovery to good health is – *"I feel well and healthy – full of energy."*

"Always rise from the table with an appetite and you will never sit down without one."   William Penn 1644–1718 (English Quaker statesman)

Vitamin B3 – Niacin

Niacin has a marked calming effect on our brain and emotions and helps avoid states of needless anxiety. Lack of niacin often leads to addiction to tobacco, alcohol, or anti-anxiety drugs.

The mellowing effect of niacin can increase our tolerance to stress so there is less adrenalin and cortisol coursing through our arteries during difficult times. This generally means most migraines can be avoided and healthy HDL cholesterol blood levels maintained. Also LDL cholesterol and blood fat (triglycerides) usually do not rise as much as they normally would, due to less inflammation from stress and food bingeing.

Symptoms of niacin deficiency appear to be widespread in NZ, yet the 2009 Nutrition Survey reported our intake of niacin (mostly from meat) appeared to be adequate, apart from a small deficiency among Maori and Pacific Island females.

Supplements of over 100 mg of niacin daily have been found to increase good HDL cholesterol 22%, reduce LDL cholesterol 20% and lower blood fat (triglycerides) by an astonishing 525%. This is far superior to any statin drug. Researchers have stated, *"To our knowledge, no other single agent has such potential for lowering both cholesterol and triglycerides."* Grundy, Mok, Zechs and Berman, 1981.

In a NZ study involving 34,000 children aged 5 to 8, niacin supplementation cut the incidence of type 1 diabetes by more than 50% (Dr Atkins' Vita-Nutrient Solution, 1998, pg 61). Also 100 mg of niacin daily for two weeks can be an effective treatment for youth acne.

A high dose of 500 mg of niacin, three times daily can decrease osteo-arthritic pain and improve joint mobility over a three year period, with benefits appearing after 3 months.

Very high supplements of niacin (up to 3000 mg daily) pioneered by Dr Abram Hoffer have been found to normalise most schizophrenics who often have higher than normal needs. In October 2012, Dr Joseph Mercola wrote of this, *"In studies using 3,000 milligrams of niacin a day, an astounding 80 percent of schizophrenia cases were resolved."* Similar results are obtained with other psychiatric disorders, especially ADHD. Niacin can also take the place of sleeping pills and tranquilisers.

A high 60% of alcoholics being treated in an American hospital study benefited from a rectification of their niacin deficiency which is almost universal among alcoholics – they reported a reduced craving for alcohol and 20% of them maintained complete sobriety after discharge, compared to none under previous treatments.

High doses of niacin however, produce a side effect of temporary but intense, hot itchy skin flush, especially to the face and neck. This does however, lessen day by day as the body gets used to it. The effect can be avoided by using a form of niacin known as niacinamide, but this form is only effective for treating osteoarthritis, not for reducing the need for LDL cholesterol and improving blood circulation. A better niacin alternative to avoid flushing is inositol hexanicotinate.

Role of niacin in our body
- Helps the body absorb nutrients from food to provide energy.
- Helps convert omega 3 from plants to usable DHA and EPA forms.
- Calms, protects and regulates the brain.
- Helps lower stress and maintain healthy cholesterol levels.
- Helps regulate blood sugar and blood fat (triglycerides).
- Helps maintain the health of our nerves, skin, joints, digestive and reproductive system.

Too little niacin
- Anxiety. Panic attacks. Insomnia. Schizophrenia. ADHD.
- Frequent urination. High blood sugar. Type 1 diabetes.
- High triglycerides in the blood.
- Low energy.
- Tobacco, alcohol and drug addiction.
- Migraine headaches.
- Anorexia nervosa. Bulimia nervosa.
- Poor general memory. Alzheimer's (factor).
- Low HDL and high LDL cholesterol. High blood pressure.
- Over sensitivity to cold temperatures.
- Red burning tongue. Gum disease.
- Darkened or red skin on the face and hands. Red eyelids.
- Osteoarthritis (factor).

Too much niacin (supplement only)
- Over 25 mg of niacin daily can produce a 15 minute, hot flush to the face and neck and itchy skin on the lower body. This effect reduces over time as the body gets used to it. The effect can be avoided if niacinamide or inositol hexanicotinate is used.
- Regularly taking over 2000 mg a day of sustained release niacin can cause liver damage or a stroke.

Cooking losses
- No significant losses.

"There has not been a death from a vitamin in America for 28 years."
     Dr Andrew W. Saul, (author of the book "Doctor Yourself" 2003)

RDI VITAMIN B3 NIACIN

Child:	10 mg	Woman:	14 mg
Teenage boy:	16 mg	Pregnancy:	18 mg
Teenage girl:	14 mg	Breastfeeding:	17 mg
Man:	16 mg		

BEVERAGES		mg
2 cups	Milo (all milk)	5.0
1 can	Beer	1.5

DAIRY / EGGS
2 cups | Milk | 4.2
2 med | Eggs | 3.8

FRUIT
1 cup | Honeydew | 2.1
1 cup | Pawpaw | 1.7
½ | Avocado | 1.5
1 cup | Cantaloupe | 1.4

GRAIN / NUTS
1/3 cup | Peanuts (roasted) | 9.3
1 plate | Cornflakes (with milk) | 4.5
4 slices | Bread (wholemeal) | 4.0
4 slices | Bread (white) | 3.2
1 plate | Wheatflake cereal | 3.2
½ cup | Flour (wholemeal) | 2.6
1/3 cup | Other nuts (avg) | 2.5
1 tbsp | Peanut butter | 2.4
½ cup | Flour (white) | 2.1
½ cup | Rice (brown) | 2.0

MEAT / FISH (cooked)
100 g | Chicken | 7.0
100 g | Lamb | 4.5
100 g | Beef | 4.0
100 g | Pork | 3.0
100 g | Fish | 3.0

VEGETABLES (cooked)
2 cobs | Sweet corn | 5.4
¾ cup | Peas | 2.8
¾ cup | Baked beans | 2.6
1 bag | Potato crisps (50 g) | 2.5
2 med | Potatoes | 2.0
1 cup | Broccoli | 2.0
1 med | Kumara (sweet potato) | 1.9

HEALTH FOOD
100 g | Liver (lamb) | 33.0
100 g | Liver (beef) | 20.0
1 cup | Tomato juice | 6.4
1 plate | Muesli (with milk) | 6.0
2 tbsp | Pumpkin seeds | 3.4
1 cup | Soy milk | 3.3
1 tbsp | Brewers yeast | 3.0
1 tsp | Marmite (yeast extract) | 2.5
1 tbsp | Malt extract | 2.0

HEALTH HINT   Cheerful people live 14% longer

If we cannot smile readily, we are probably under emotional stress.

A 30-year study of 30,000 adults by the University of Carolina found that people with a cheerful, sunny, optimistic personality lived on average 14% longer than frowning, negative-thinking pessimists.

This is in line with other findings by medical researchers who have clearly demonstrated that an optimistic outlook, even a simple smile, measurably strengthens our immune system.

Vitamin B5 – Pantothenic acid

Pantothenic acid, or vitamin B5 as it's now commonly known, is found in human breast milk and nearly all foods, but mostly in only tiny amounts. Fortunately, B5 can be made in our intestines, by enzymes and friendly probiotics when our digestive system is working properly.

Pantothenic acid is required by our immune system to prevent inflammation in the body. Inflammation is the cause of many, if not most of our serious health disorders including cardiovascular disease and arthritis. Pantothenic acid helps our body use omega 3 and protects friendly probiotic bacteria in the intestines from damage by antibiotics. It also protects against acne, gout and burning feet.

When taken as a 900 mg daily dose, studies have shown that B5 typically lowers high LDL cholesterol by 21% and high blood trigly-cerides (fats) by 32%. Like niacin, this is superior to any statin drug and without the side effects.

Dr Robert Atkins pioneered the use of large dosages of vitamin B5 as a natural healer. He claimed that pantothenic acid is *"the single best substance on the planet for restablishing optimal levels of cholesterol and triglycerides in the blood."*

Dr Atkins reported similar results with over 90% of his heart patients (more than 20,000 case histories). He would also tell his patients they could eat whatever they liked (except too many carbs) provided they took their pantothenic acid.

He also found that pantothenic acid had a spectacular healing rate with other inflammatory disorders, such as, arthritis, lupus, colitis, gout and Crohn's disease. He used B5 to replace the drug prednisone and found that the vitamin had none of the serious prednisone side effects. Excellent results were also obtained by treating yeast infections such as candida with pantothenic acid. His remedy for gout or 'burning feet' is 200 mg, four times a day.

Dr Atkins writes, *"Pantethine's results aren't just good. They're spectacular. I use Pantethine and Pantothenic Acid together, making them the number one nutrient used in my practice."* Pantothenic acid converts to pantethine in the body, but evidently taking pantethine together with pantothenic acid can double its effectiveness.

Vitamin B5 is also important for a healthy digestive system – 900 mg daily are sometimes prescribed by surgeons to get the stomach working again after an operation.

A lack of B5 in animals is known to cause grey hair, and correcting the deficiency restores the original hue – but experiments with large doses have failed to restore human hair to its former colour. Better results might be achieved with longevity – pantothenic acid at three times the normal intake, increased the average life span of mice by 20%, the human equivalent of 90 years.

Role of pantothenic acid in our body

- Helps maintain health of the brain, nervous system and skin.
- Regulates optimal levels of cholesterol and blood fats.
- Helps preserve friendly probiotic bacteria in the intestines.
- Needed by adrenal glands to produce anti-inflammatory hormones.
- Helps our body cells utilise omega 3.
- Helps protect living cells from the effects of radiation.

Too little pantothenic acid
(Smoking hinders manufacture by probiotics in the intestines)

- Inflammatory disorders – arthritis, lupus, colitis, arteries and allergies.
- Irritable bowel (IBS). Crohn's disease.
- Lowered immunity. Colds, flu and yeast infections. Candida.
- Loss of appetite. Indigestion. Low energy.
- Insomnia. Depression.
- Acne. Low resistance to radiation damage.
- High blood triglycerides and LDL cholesterol. Heart attack/stroke.
- Impaired absorption of omega 3.
- Gout. Burning sensation in the feet.

Too much pantothenic acid

- No known toxic effects.

Cooking losses

- About one third is destroyed if food cooked at a high temperature.
- Baking soda can also neutralise pantothenic acid in food.

HEALTH HINT   **Preventing acid stomach**

The discomfort of an acid stomach (which strangely is often linked with low stomach acid) is mostly the result of eating too much food too quickly, and in a state of anxiety.

Under stressful conditions, the upper valve or lid of the stomach does not appear to seal well. This allows stomach acid to leak past the valve (reflux) and burn the lower esophagus tube, which is not designed to resist acid. A tight belt can contribute to this leakage in men.

When eating during a stressful time, small, easily digested vegetable meals are best. Fasting is better still and has a calming effect.

RDI VITAMIN B5 PANTOTHENIC ACID

The figures below are for diet only – Vitamin B5 is also made naturally by intestinal probiotics and enzymes, according to the body's needs, when our digestive system is working properly

Child:	5 mg	Woman:	5 mg
Teenage boy:	7 mg	Pregnancy:	6 mg
Teenage girl:	6 mg	Breastfeeding:	7 mg
Man:	7 mg		

DAIRY / EGGS — mg
		mg
2 cups	Milk (trim)	1.9
4 tbsp	Whey protein powder	1.6
2 cups	Milk (std)	1.5
2 med	Eggs	1.2

FRUIT
½	Avocado	.9

GRAIN / NUTS
1/3 cup	Peanuts (roasted)	.9
4 slices	Bread (wholemeal)	.8

MEAT (cooked)
100 g	Chicken	1.4

VEGETABLES (cooked)
6 med	Mushrooms	1.4
1 cup	Pumpkin	1.2
¾ cup	Split peas	1.0
2 cobs	Sweet corn	1.0
1 cup	Broccoli	.8
1 cup	Cauliflower	.8
1 med	Kumara (sweet potato)	.8
1 cup	Honeydew	.8
2	Potatoes	.8

HEALTH FOOD
100 g	Liver (lamb)	7.6
100 g	Liver (beef)	5.7
100 g	Kidney (beef)	3.0
100 g	Kidney (lamb)	2.0

HEALTH HINT The power of words on our health

The B vitamins are not the only things that can markedly affect our sense of wellbeing – whether we feel positive, relaxed and healthy, or negative and tense is largely determined by the words we choose to speak.

How much better we would feel, and those around us if all the words we spoke first passed the test of being – **kind, true** and **necessary.**

"When we try to pick anything out by itself, we find it hitched to everything else in the universe." John Muir 1838 –1914 (Scientist)

Vitamin B6 Pyridoxine

Vitamin B6 (pyridoxine) is one of the most needed and yet most commonly deficient of the B vitamins – due mostly to the milling and refining of wheat which removes nearly all the B6 from white flour.

The 2009 Nutrition Survey found that 53% of NZ women aged over 70, 57% of Maori women over 50 and 20% of teenage girls had a deficient intake of vitamin B6.

Also 42% of Maori men over 50 were deficient and 28% of European men. Teenage boys were the only ones with an adequate intake, due mostly to a high potato-based food consumption – potato crisps perhaps? NZ crisps test surprisingly high in B6, possibly due to a food additive.

There are many sources of B6 as you'll see from the food chart, so there should be no need for such a widespread lack – it appears to be due to a diet heavily reliant on nutrient barren, white flour.

Vitamin B6 is important in regulating woman's hormones, so the above deficiencies might explain why so many NZ women have trouble in this area of health. Vitamin B6 helps relieve yeast infections, pre-menstrual tension, fluid retention, and nausea and pre-eclampsia (toxemia) during pregnancy. Convulsions in babies and cleft palates have also been linked to lack of B6 during pregnancy.

Vitamin B6 has numerous other roles in the body, especially blood sugar control. It's important in protecting against diabetes and linked to cardiovascular disorders – in particular, keeping our blood free of deadly clots. It also assists our digestive system to convert omega 3 from a plant sources to the EPA and DHA forms the body can use.

In an American study of 50,000 doctors, those with the lowest B6 blood levels had 50% more heart attacks than their peers.

Like other B vitamins, B6 has a profound effect on our mind – it helps produce a sense of wellbeing and guards against a range of psychiatric disorders including ADHD, autism and depression – in one study, 80% of depressed people lacked B6.

Some autistic children have become normal when a magnesium and B6 deficiency has been rectified. Dr Bernard Rimland, director of the Autism Research Institute states, *"No biological treatment for autism is more strongly supported in the scientific literature than the use of high dosage vitamin B6 (in conjunction with magnesium)."*

Magnesium and B6 can also improve memory function in old age.

Excess B6 can affect sleep quality

Not being able to remember dreams was once thought to be a sign of lack of B6. However dreams are only remembered when we wake up immediately after them. Lack of dream recall is now recognised as a sign of a good night's sleep – not a lack of vitamin B6.

In fact too much B6 from a vitamin pill – as little as 5 mg (5000 mcg) when we are not deficient, often acts as a mental stimulant, causing restless sleep and repeated awakenings during the night. Many dreams will be recalled, but sleep will be far from restful. On several occasions when I was younger, I recall lying awake for hours with a 'wired' mind after taking a vitamin pill high in vitamin B6 before bed. It was a relief to finally determine the cause.

Just 2 mg a day (2000 mcg) from a supplement is sufficient for a healthy person. Some supplement manufacturers put high levels of B6 into their products because of the caffeine-like mental stimulus B6 can give to the brain – but often a heavy price is paid, in insomnia.

Vitamin B6 is necessary for good digestion and in particular to allow our body to absorb vitamin B12 and the minerals iron and zinc. Often a low blood count (anemia) is caused by lack of B6 rather than lack of iron.

Excess coffee, smoking, the birth control pill and continued stress can deplete vitamin B6.

Role of vitamin B6 in our body

- Regulates female hormones and healthy pregnancies.
- Helps control blood sugar (glucose).
- Helps regulate optimum calcium and magnesium ratios.
- Helps convert omega 3 from plants to usable DHA and EPA forms.
- Calms and regulates the brain.
- Provides a sense of mental wellbeing.
- Helps the body absorb protein, iron, zinc and vitamin B12.
- A natural diuretic.

Too little vitamin B6

- Diabetes and other blood sugar disorders.
- Blood clots. High blood pressure. Heart attack. Stroke.
- Weak red blood cells (anemia). Pale skin.
- Cracks or sores at the corners of the mouth. Sore red tongue.
- Acne around nose or on the forehead. Red eyelids.
- Low appetite. Poor digestion. Nausea. Anorexia nervosa.
- Iron or zinc deficiency. Low energy.
- Calcium or magnesium imbalance.
- Fluid retention. Swollen legs.

- Yeast infections. PMT.
- Nausea and pre-eclampsia (toxemia) during pregnancy.
- Birth malformities. Convulsions in babies.
- ADHD and Autism.
- Anxiety, depression and irritability. Frequent urination.
- Twitchy eyelids.
- Poor short term memory in old age.
- Carpal tunnel. Stiff or swollen arthritic finger joints. Tendonitis.
- Numb or tingling hands, arms and legs.

Too much vitamin B6 (over 20,000 mcg/20 mg daily)

- Insomnia. Restless sleep. Tension. Over-vivid dreams.
- Nerve damage. Asthma. (over 50,000 mcg/50 mg daily)
- Magnesium – calcium imbalance.
- Supplements over 20,000 mcg/20 mg daily can also cause a dependency on the supplement, ie, the body may fail to extract vitamin B6 from food when the supplement is stopped.

Cooking losses

- Heat can destroy, and B6 can leach out into cooking water.

"When 25% of the diet calories are sugar, one is at risk of diabetes, glucose intolerance, heart attack, social problems, excess calcium in the urine, gallstones and mineral deficiencies."   **American FDA 1986**

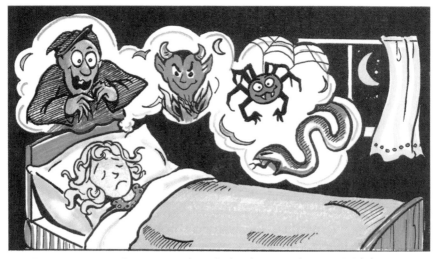

Excess vitamin B6 can produce light sleep and over-vivid dreams.

RDI VITAMIN B6 (PYRIDOXINE)

Child:	600 mcg	Woman:	1300 mcg
Teenage boy:	1300 mcg	Woman over 50:	1700 mcg
Teenage girl:	1200 mcg	Pregnancy:	1900 mcg
Man:	1300 mcg	Breastfeeding:	2000 mcg
Man over 50:	1700 mcg		

DAIRY / EGGS — mcg

2 cups	Milk (trim)	260
2 cups	Milk (std)	200
2 med	Eggs	200

GRAIN / NUTS

1 plate	Cornflakes (with milk)	550
½ cup	Flour (wholemeal)	250
½ cup	Rice brown (cooked)	190

MEAT / FISH (cooked)

100 g	Chicken	560
100 g	Liver	500
100 g	Salmon/sardines	460
100 g	Pork	420
100 g	Beef	240
100 g	Fish	200

FRUIT

1	Banana	650
1 cup	Honeydew	240
½	Avocado	210
1	Kiwifruit	160
1/3 cup	Raisins/sultanas	150

VEGETABLES (cooked)

2 cobs	Sweet corn	420
1 bag	Potato crisps (50 g)	400
1 cup	Brussels sprouts	280
¾ cup	Baked beans	240
1 cup	Broccoli	210
½ cup	Spinach	200
1 cup	Cauliflower	180
1 med	Kumara (sweet potato)	170
2 med	Potatoes	160

HEALTH FOOD

1 plate	Muesli (with milk)	950
1 tbsp	Malt extract	750
1 cup	Tomato juice	300
1 tbsp	Brewers yeast	200
2 tbsp	Wheat germ	200
1 cup	Soy milk	150

HEALTH HINT Are you lacking vitamin B6?

A quick test for a deficiency of vitamin B6 is to stretch your hand wide open, with your fingers close together. Now keeping your hand rigid, try and bend just the top half of your fingers down, to touch the bottoms of your fingers (where they join the palm). If you can do this, you are unlikely to be deficient in vitamin B6.

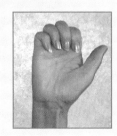

Vitamin B6

HEALTH HINT Three rules to minimise stress

Lack of vitamin B6 can result in us being less effective in handling stress. Long term stress greatly lowers our immunity to sickness and is a major factor in serious disease.

Most sources of stress involve three areas in our life –

- Family
- Finances
- Fellow workers

There are three simple, proven rules to minimise stress in these areas. They are as follows:

Family – forgive those who have offended you, either face-to-face or through a letter. In other words, to follow the Christian principle of handing the offence over to God to deal with justly, in his own time.

Finances – spend less than you earn and invest 10% of your income.

Fellow workers – if you can't wake up most mornings and look forward to your day's activities, you are in the wrong occupation. Why not work towards changing it for something you enjoy more and have an aptitude for, even if your income is lower at first?

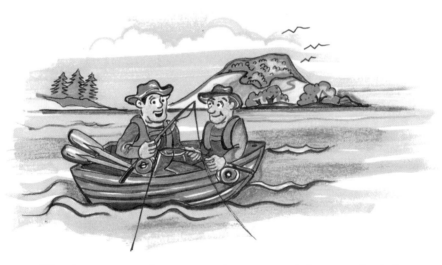

"The doctor warned me to avoid stress, so I didn't open his bill."

Vitamin B9 Folate (Folic acid)

Our vitamin status is only as strong as its weakest link. This important yellow vitamin has been one of those weak links, and was once among the most commonly deficient vitamins in NZ – especially among women and newborn babies.

Folate (also known as folic acid) is required by our DNA to control cell division and is especially important for the health of pregnant women and their babies. During pregnancy the need for folate doubles and deficiencies can result in problems such as pre-eclampsia, miscarriage, mental impairment, spina bifida and other malformities of children, especially cleft palate. NZ doctors recommend that women who plan to become pregnant take 800 mcg of folate daily for at least a month before trying to conceive, and for at least 12 weeks after conceiving.

So strong is the evidence for birth defects in newborn babies, along with numerous other adult disorders linked with lack of folate, that American health authorities require white flour to be fortified with folate. This has proven successful and was to be trialled in NZ bread beginning in 2009. However the decision was strongly opposed by many bakers (on cost) and the Green Party (on mass medication principle) and was placed on hold. Late in 2012 it was decided not to enforce the decision.

It may now not be as necessary – NZ folate intake reported in the 2009 Nutrition Survey had dramatically and mysteriously improved. Now only 2% of New Zealand adults overall, and 8% of teenage girls have low intakes. In the previous 1997 survey, 29% of teenage girls and 26% of women had low folate intake.

However some researchers believe the RDI is set too low for reliance on obtaining sufficient folate from our food, as cooking losses are high at 50%, even up to 90% in some instances. Excess alcohol, smoking, aspirin and the birth control pill are known to drain the body of folate.

Dr Robert Atkins, who used high doses of folate to treat many diseases successfully, recommended that folate be taken in supplement form as it is more reliably absorbed than from cooked food.

The large 1998 Nurses' Health Study found that adequate folate reduced the incidence of colon cancer by a massive 75% and a 9 year study by Baltimore Longitudinal Study of Aging found that taking 400 mcg of folate daily, lowered the risk of Alzheimer's by 55%.

A blood test is the best way to measure folate status – low folate is defined in the red cell test as below 317 nmol/L (140 ng/mL). The average reading in NZ is 900 nmol/L (400 ng/mL). The healthy range is 906 to 1400 nmol/L (400 – 620 ng/mL).

Lack of folate is a cause of elevated blood homocysteine levels, which in turn is a high risk indicator for cardiovascular disease. This is easily corrected with a folate supplement. Other diseases linked to high blood homocysteine are macular degeneration, Alzheimer's, multiple sclerosis (MS) and rheumatoid arthritis.

Lack of folate during times of severe anxiety has been linked with premature greying of hair. Interestingly, a large amount of folate can restore abnormally grey hair in an animal, to its natural hue, but like pantothenic acid, it doesn't seem to work with humans.

In treating menopausal women, Dr Robert Atkins found high temporary therapeutic dosages of about 50,000 mcg (50 mg) a day of folate, with adequate boron, substituted for hormone therapy and relieved menopausal discomfort without the side effects of prescription estrogen.

He also reported that this same high dosage, along with vitamin B5 (pantothenic acid), sufficient omega 3 fat, and a low-sugar diet, was 85% effective in treating Crohn's disease – and when combined with vitamin B12, the hard to cure skin complaints of psoriasis and vitiligo have also responded.

Muscle injections of folate can heal numb, tingling nerve pains in the arms and legs.

Folate is similar in action to B12 and appears to be equally important for psychiatric health. Low levels are commonly found in alcoholics, mentally slow children, depressed people, psychiatric patients and those suffering from dementia or Alzheimer's disease.

Many schizophrenics respond to a combined treatment of folate, niacin and zinc. Epileptics have been found to improve on folate and B12 supplements.

Gut probiotics – lactobacillus and bifidobacterium can manufacture small amounts of folate but most must be supplied from food.

Role of folate in our body
- Assists in the forming of body and blood cells from DNA.
- Vital for healthy development of the unborn child during pregnancy.
- Assists in protecting and maintaining normal brain function.
- Assists in maintaining clear arteries.
- Helps maintain the health of our eyes, ears, hair and skin.
- Helps maintain the health of our digestive system and bowels.
- Helps our body form and utilise protein.
- Helps control uric acid levels.

Too little folate

- Pre-eclampsia, premature birth, or miscarriage in pregnant women.
- Colon cancer. Cervical cancer.
- Irritable bowel syndrome (IBS). Crohn's disease.
- Malformed and/or mentally slow infants if mother is deficient.
- Post-natal depression, irritability and psychiatric disorders.
- Hot flushes during menopause.
- Alcohol, drug and tobacco addiction.
- Age-related hearing loss. Dementia symptoms. Alzheimer's.
- ADHD attention disorder in children.
- Macular degeneration in the eyes of elderly people.
- Weak red blood cells, pale skin, low energy (anemia).
- Chronic fatigue. Cold hands and feet.
- Narrowed arteries. Heart attack. Stroke.
- Numb or tingling nerve pains in arms and legs. Restless legs.
- Sore, smooth red tongue.
- Premature grey hair.
- Arthritis. Gout.

Too much folate (over 4000 mcg daily)

- Sleep and mental disturbances. Mild depression.
- Can mask a vitamin B12 deficiency.

Cooking losses

- High – usually around 50% when cooked at high temperatures.

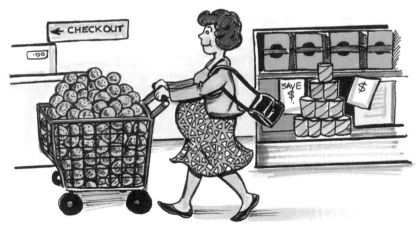

*The need for folate doubles during pregnancy –
oranges are a good source.*

RDI VITAMIN B9 FOLATE

Child:	250 mcg	Woman:	400 mcg
Teenager:	400 mcg	Pregnancy:	600 mcg
Man:	400 mcg	Breastfeeding:	500 mcg

Vitamin B9 Folate (Folic Acid)

DAIRY / EGGS		mcg
2 med	Eggs	40
2 cups	Milk (std or low-fat)	25

FRUIT		
1 cup	Honeydew	100
½	Avocado	55
1	Orange	50
1 cup	Rock melon	40
1 cup	Orange juice (pure)	20

GRAIN / NUTS		
1 plate	Cornflakes (with milk)	85
1/3 cup	Peanuts (roasted)	65
4 slices	Bread (wholemeal)	40
1/3 cup	Almonds/cashew nuts	40
½ cup	Flour (wholemeal)	35
4 slices	Bread (white)	30
2	Weetbix (with milk)	20

MEAT / FISH (cooked)		
100 g	Pipis (clams)	50

VEGETABLES (cooked)		
1 cup	Broccoli	180
1 cup	Brussels sprouts	145
½ cup	Spinach	120
2 cobs	Sweet corn	85
¾ cup	Green peas	75
1 cup	Cauliflower	70
4 slices	Beetroot	60
¾ cup	Baked beans	50
1 med	Kumara (sweet potato)	35
1 med	Tomato (raw)	30
½ cup	Green beans	25
2 med	Potatoes	25
1	Onion	25
½ cup	Coleslaw	20
1 cup	Lettuce (raw)	20

HEALTH FOOD		
100 g	Liver	260
1 tbsp	Brewers yeast	190
1 tsp	Marmite (yeast extract)	100
1 plate	Muesli (with milk)	95
1	Muesli bar	45
2 tbsp	Wheat germ	40
1 cup	Soy milk	25

HEALTH HINT   A healthy pregnancy

The need for folate doubles during pregnancy. This is more reliably achieved with a supplement in addition to natural foods. Therefore to help ensure a healthy baby, before and during pregnancy, mothers-to-be should eat plenty of green vegetables, yellow melons and oranges and take a folate supplement. (This also applies throughout breastfeeding.)

A long walk (most days) minimises the common risks of varicose veins and constipation during pregnancy.

"The best time to start feeding a baby is several years before it is born."
Brenda Sampson, (NZ allergy consultant and author)

Vitamin B12

Vitamin B12 (cobalamin) is a dark red vitamin – a deficiency is a major problem for those over the age of 60, and even those in their 40's. Dementia symptoms can be caused by lack of this important vitamin. Two monthly injections of B12 are often given to overcome this problem.

Absorption of B12 by our body typically drops off as we get older and needs to be supplemented or injected. President John F. Kennedy is widely quoted as saying he would *"never have become president without injections of B12"* – he was only aged 43 when elected.

Although it affects mostly the elderly, lower than optimal levels of B12 can be found in all age groups – when blood levels are measured overseas, up to 80% of city dwellers are typically deficient. The NZ Nutrition Survey found over 20% of NZ women had inadequate intake of B12 foods (levels of NZ men were fine), but absorption wasn't measured and this is where the major problem lies.

However, smoking, high sugar consumption and the birth control pill can lower body levels of B12 at any age. Metformin and stomach antacid drugs like Losec are also known to hinder absorption.

Dementia symptoms

Like the other B vitamins, B12 is an important brain nutrient and necessary for our sense of well being, alertness, concentration, memory and relaxation. Often symptoms of dementia such as slow thinking, poor memory, mental fog or confusion, shaky hands and legs and impaired balance are partly or entirely due to B12 deficiency.

Rectifying this deficiency by a B12 supplement or injection can bring about dramatic improvement.

The Japanese regularly monitor the B12 levels of their elderly and treat dementia symptoms with this vitamin. As a result, the Alzheimer's death rate in Japan is only 2.5%, ten times lower than the 25% death rate in the US. The NZ death rate is 15%, however, the dementia symptom rate for those aged 85 and over is 47% and increasing steadily.

In one American study, 61% of early dementia patients made a complete recovery with B12 supplementation, but there was little improvement in long term, full-blown Alzheimer patients.

Other disorders linked with lack of vitamin B12

Other disorders associated with lack of B12 are – poor sleep, nerve problems, tinnitus, hearing loss, multiple sclerosis, numb and tingling (pins and needles) disorders, burning feet, osteoporosis, arthritis, listlessness, food or chemical allergies and patchy loss of pigmentation in brown skinned people.

High oral doses of 30,000 mcg (30 mg) of B12 for two weeks have relieved asthma problems (10 out of 12 asthmatics in one study).

B12 also works with folate and B6 to prevent heart attacks and strokes, protect our nervous system, and help prevent bursitis, asthma, low blood pressure and auto-immune diseases.

Sources of vitamin B12

Unlike the other B vitamins, B12 is not found in fruit, grains or vegetables, but in animal products such as milk, eggs and meat. Liver, pipis (a common NZ clam shellfish) and sardines are rich sources.

As would be expected, deficiencies are common among vegetarians, but not so much in poorer countries. It's believed that B12, which is only required in tiny amounts, is obtained from insect life, especially eggs and insect feces consumed with plants and untreated drinking and cooking water, (not all people are as fanatical about food hygiene as westerners).

The mineral cobalt is part of B12, which is where the name cobalamin comes from. Some NZ soils are seriously low in this mineral and farm stock have suffered badly from lack of B12 in the past. Cobalt is now added to fertiliser where necessary.

Even when animal products are part of the diet, deficiencies of B12 are widespread among the elderly (especially the blue-eyed) due to the increased difficulty in absorbing B12 from food as we age.

Blood testing and supplementing

Blood tests are not a reliable way of determining B12 status – blood levels can be high, but absorption by body and brain cells poor.

A more reliable method is the MMA (methylmalonic acid) test. However to save the cost of testing, a simpler method is to just inject the vitamin and see if there is any improvement. The recommended medical protocol for this is to inject 1000 mcg of B12 cobalamin daily (usually into a muscle) for three days, then weekly for a month. If improvement is noted, then a one or two monthly injection of 1000 mcg is continued indefinitely.

However some studies have shown that high daily oral dosages (by pill) of 1000 mcg of cobalamin can be just as effective as injections. B12 is non-toxic to the body, however NZ law currently permits only 50 mcg per supplement, so 1000 mcg daily would be by prescription only.

Although the normal cobalamin form of B12 can be difficult for the elderly to absorb without being injected, there is another supplement form called methylcobalamin, which although expensive is much better absorbed by the digestive system.

Another recent development is to deliver B12 methylcobalamin under the tongue (sublingually) daily, using a lozenge or a spray bottle.

Role of vitamin B12 in our body
- Helps maintain brain health and a feeling of well being.
- Helps maintain the health of nerve fibres.
- Helps maintain blood health and prevent heart attack and stroke.
- Helps regulate the immune system to prevent auto-immune disorders.
- Processing of carbs and absorbing nutrients from food.
- Assists in regulating fat storage.

Too little vitamin B12
- Dementia/Alzheimer's symptoms. Psychiatric disorders.
- Slow thinking. Halting speech. Poor memory and concentration.
- Frequent confusion. Easily depressed. Listless.
- Difficulty in walking smoothly. Reduced sensory perception.
- Poor balance. Shaky hands or legs. Weak muscles.
- Weak, sore, poorly controlled muscles.
- Numb or tingly legs, feet or fingers. Burning feet.
- Difficulty in relaxing. Insomnia.
- Too low or too high blood pressure. High homocysteine.
- Shortness of breath. Low energy.
- Tinnitus. Hearing loss. Eventual deafness.
- Chronic fatigue. Weak red blood cells (anemia). Pale skin.
- Painful joints, sometimes with brown discolouration.
- Calcium growths. Osteoporosis and arthritis (factor).
- Damaged nerves. Multiple sclerosis (factor).
- Easy bruising.
- Dark red, sore tongue.
- Patchy loss of skin pigmentation in brown skin (vitiligo). Psoriasis.
- Food and chemical allergies.

Too much vitamin B12
- No known toxic effects.

Cooking losses
- No significant losses.

HEALTH HINT **Milk can supply your B12 needs**

If strict vegetarianism appeals, the minor compromise of two glasses of milk daily (whole or low-fat) can take care of your vitamin B12 needs.

RDI VITAMIN B12

Child:	1.2 mcg	Woman:	2.4 mcg
Teenager:	2.4 mcg	Pregnancy:	2.6 mcg
Man:	2.4 mcg	Breastfeeding:	2.8 mcg

DAIRY / EGGS		mcg
2 med	Eggs	2.0
2 cups	Milk (std/low-fat)	1.8
25 g	Cheese	.3
½ cup	Ice cream	.2

MEAT / FISH (cooked)		
100 g	Pipis (clams)	62.0
100 g	Sardines (canned)	28.0
6	Oysters	18.0
100 g	Salmon (canned)	4.0
100 g	Lamb	2.2

100 g	Beef	1.6
100 g	Chicken	.8
100 g	Pork	.7
100 g	Fish	.6

HEALTH FOOD		
100 g	Liver (beef)	110.0
100 g	Liver (lamb)	81.0
100 g	Kidney (lamb)	79.0
100 g	Kidney (beef)	31.0
1 tsp	Marmite (yeast extract)	.5

HEALTH HINT Nine ways to a good night's sleep

There's no better aid to both physical and psychiatric health than the rejuvenating effects of a good night's sleep – preferably seven unbroken hours. Generally speaking, no matter what else we do, we will never fully recover from a physical or mental disorder until we obtain regular restful sleep, for this is when our body and mind heal themselves.

Ideally, the only thing we should recall in the morning is laying our head on the pillow the night before, and perhaps just one dream from within the few minutes before we awoke.

Nine proven requirements for deep, refreshing sleep:

- No food or beverages three hours before bedtime.
- Some evening exercise, such as brisk walking.
- Winding down with non-stimulating reading, or writing a journal.
- A very dark room, without light from street lights or a clock.
- A mattress and pillow that aligns our body comparable to standing.
- Cotton or natural bedding material – no synthetics.
- Warm feet when getting into bed (or wear socks).
- No late night conversation and no computer work after 7pm.
- An unlit alarm clock (or two) on which you can rely.

"A merry heart doeth good like a medicine." King Solomon

Lecithin

Lecithin is a waxy, fatty type substance, usually yellow in colour and found in all our cells. It helps maintain a healthy brain and nervous system.

Food sources are mostly egg yolks and animal fats, but lecithin is also found in seed oils and plant proteins.

Human breast milk contains lecithin – a sure sign that it is essential for health.

One study found that taking a supplement containing 10 g of lecithin a day considerably improved the short-term memory of healthy adults.

Lecithin also appears to protect against inflammation of the arteries and therefore cardiovascular disease – LDL cholesterol normally drops and good levels of HDL blood cholesterol are maintained.

Lecithin can be made by our liver from good dietary fats when our body is healthy and well nourished, but adequate folate and vitamin B12 are necessary for this to occur. A low-fat diet increases the risk of lecithin deficiency, otherwise lack of lecithin should not be a concern.

Lecithin is widely used as an additive in processed foods (number 322) usually as an emulsifier, especially in margarine and ice cream to provide a smooth consistency.

Role of lecithin in our body
- Helps build and maintain the health of our body cells and brain.
- Helps build and maintain a healthy nervous system.
- Helps prevent artery inflammation.

Too little lecithin
- Impaired nerve and brain development in infants.
- Poor short-term memory.
- Nervous twitching.
- Increased risk of heart disease.

Too much lecithin (Supplements over 10,000 mg/10 g daily)
- Fishy body odour.

RDI	LECITHIN
RDI not set and NO FOOD TABLE as some lecithin is found in almost all plant and animal food and can be made by a healthy liver.	

Inositol

This lesser known B vitamin has been described as nature's tranquilliser, or sleeping pill. It's often found with lecithin but is a sugar-like carb rather than a fat. Not a lot is known about its role.

High levels of inositol are found in breast milk, so mothers should ensure that any infant formula they use contains this vitamin.

After testing inositol's calming influence on over 10,000 patients, Dr Robert Atkins wrote *"It eliminates the need for a whole category of potentially harmful drugs, tranquillisers and sleeping pills."* He found that supplements of about 6000 mg (6 g) daily for two weeks relieved even severe cases of anxiety and panic attacks without side effects. He recommended 1000 mg (1 g) at bedtime to overcome insomnia, and the same amount in the morning to relieve anxiety during the day.

This same dosage can reduce high blood pressure and high LDL cholesterol – two disorders strongly linked with anxiety. High doses of inositol can also help a reluctant body burn off excess fat.

Extra vitamin C helps the body retain inositol, whereas excess caffeine (more than 3 cups of coffee a day) is reported to deplete body reserves.

Good food sources are oranges, rock melon, beans, peas, broccoli, whole wheat products, beef and liver.

PABA is another B vitamin similar to inositol. As with inositol, not much is known about PABA except that it can help overcome infertility in women. Both inositol and PABA can be made by a well nourished body.

Role of inositol in our body
- Promotes calmness of the brain and a sense of wellbeing.
- Promotes deep, healthful sleep.
- Helps relax the bowel to avoid constipation.
- Assists the body to digest fats.
- Helps maintain health of the nervous system.
- Helps control blood pressure and cholesterol balance.

Too little inositol
- Anxiety. Panic attacks. Insomnia. Psychiatric disorders.
- High blood pressure and high LDL cholesterol.
- Constipation.

Too much inositol
- No known toxic effects.

Cooking losses
- No significant losses.

RDI INOSITOL (Limited data available)

Can also be made by healthy kidneys			
Child:	250 mg	Woman:	500 mg
Teenager:	500 mg	Pregnancy:	600 mg
Man:	500 mg	Breastfeeding:	700 mg

DAIRY / EGGS   **mg**

2 cups	Milk (std or low-fat)	100

FRUIT

1 cup	Orange juice (pure)	340
1	Orange	250
1 cup	Rock melon	250

GRAIN / NUTS

1/3 cup	Peanuts (roasted)	90
4 slices	Bread (wholemeal)	90
½ cup	Rice (brown cooked)	80
4 slices	Bread (white)	60
½ cup	Flour (wholemeal)	60
1 plate	Porridge	60

MEAT / FISH (cooked)

100 g	Beef	150
100 g	Chicken	50
100 g	Pork	50
100 g	Lamb	50

VEGETABLES (cooked)

¾ cup	Baked beans	320
¾ cup	Peas	190
1 cup	Broccoli	125
1 cup	Brussels sprouts	120
2 cobs	Sweet corn	120
1 med	Kumara (sweet potato)	100
½ cup	Spinach	90
½ cup	Silverbeet (chard)	85
1 med	Tomato (raw)	75
1 cup	Cabbage	75
1 cup	Lettuce (raw)	60
2 med	Potatoes	60

HEALTH FOOD

100 g	Liver (cooked)	340
2 tbsp	Wheat germ	120

"As our body ages we require more nutrients and fewer calories."
Jane Kinderlehrer, (American lecturer on nutrition)

"The doctor of the future will give no medicine, but will interest his patients in the care of the human frame, in diet, and in the cause and prevention of disease."
Thomas A. Edison 1847 –1931

Inositol

Vitamin C (Ascorbic acid)

Vitamin C is one of the few substances known to man that can destroy both bacteria and viruses. Mercury, silver, bleach and alcohol can do the same, but are not always safe. Vitamin C is also an anti-toxin vitamin – assisting our body in ridding itself of toxic metals such as cadmium, lead, mercury and organic poisons. It's also by far the major antioxidant in our body, along with uric acid. Its antioxidant effect can be demonstrated by applying vitamin C to the flesh of a freshly cut apple – it prevents oxidation browning.

Fruit and vegetables are essential in providing us with vitamin C. Lack of vitamin C has caused more suffering and death in the history of mankind than any other nutritional deficiency – especially from the horrible disease of scurvy.

Less than 250 years ago it was not unknown for two thirds of a ship's crew to die of scurvy during a long sea voyage. In 1577 a Spanish galleon was found drifting with all crew on board dead from this disease.

In 1740, Commodore Anson left England with six ships and over 1800 seamen. Four years later he returned with just one ship and only 188 seamen – this was due almost entirely to deaths from scurvy and other vitamin C deficiency disorders. The English navy later solved the problem with sauerkraut (fermented cabbage) and a daily one ounce dose of lemon or lime juice per man. In fact it became their secret weapon in mastering the seas and was largely responsible for the rise of the British empire.

However it was not only seamen who were affected, but entire nations, especially during winter and wartime. Scurvy was the underlying cause of the great plagues of Europe in the Middle Ages such as the Black Death, when a quarter of the population of Europe died.

The flu epidemic that swept the world after World War I and killed 50 million people (more than died from the war itself) was believed to be the result of lack of vitamin C from fresh fruit and vegetables, due to the war's disruptive effect on transport and crop growing.

When resistance to infection is lowered by a deficiency of vitamin C, diseases that are normally mild can rip through populations with incredible ferocity.

Vitamin C not a vitamin

Vitamin C is not actually a vitamin, which by definition means *'only required in tiny amounts'*. The label of 'vitamin' was acquired as a result of earlier misinformation that vitamin C was only required in tiny amounts – in fact it is more of a bulk blood salt, not unlike blood glucose in some ways.

Humans, apes, bats and guinea pigs are the only mammals that cannot make their own vitamin C (from enzyme action in the liver). We need to get it from our food. Interestingly, an adult gorilla in the wild obtains about 4500 mg of vitamin C each day in his or her food. Our human RDI is just 1% of this – 45 mg.

An estimate of the daily amount of vitamin C created in the body of a 70 kg animal is about 12,000 mg a day. Even a tiny mouse can make up to 19,000 mg a day in an emergency – that's about four teaspoons.

In one study of 44 sets of twins, 1000 mg of vitamin C daily resulted in 19% fewer natural colds, 38% less duration and 22% less severity.

The average intake reported in the NZ 2009 Nutrition Survey was double the RDI – a surprisingly high 99 mg, mostly from vegetables (41%) and fruit (22%). However about 10% of Maori and Pacific Islanders reported a daily intake of less than the RDI of 45 mg.

Vitamin C is found in human milk in useful amounts, and also in fresh cow's milk, but this is mostly destroyed by pasteurising. Bottle-fed infants therefore need to have their milk supplemented with vitamin C – this is normally provided in formula, or done by adding fruit juice.

Vitamin C can slow ageing

Another important role of vitamin C in our body is the maintenance of collagen – well-nourished collagen slows down the appearance of ageing by helping keep skin firm and wrinkle-resistant. Collagen is the protein that holds our body together – it supports our muscles, strengthens our bones, keeps our gums healthy and our teeth firmly in place, and helps wounds heal.

Collagen also strengthens our arteries and veins to prevent aneurysms and hemorrhages which cause strokes and other internal bleeding problems. Collagen cannot be formed without vitamin C, which is why the collagen dependent, joints, skin and heart eventually fail in scurvy.

Other health benefits

High amounts of vitamin C – over 500 mg a day have been found to lower LDL cholesterol levels approx 10%. Also to drop blood fats (triglycerides) around 40%, which in turn normally lowers high blood pressure.

Many experienced doctors nowadays recommend 600 mg of vitamin C a day, taken in three 200 mg doses by mouth – increased mental alertness is often reported with these high intakes. While massive dosages of vitamin C can be absorbed when given intravenously, recent studies have shown that 200 mg is the most our body can absorb at any one time when taken by mouth, unless the blood is seriously deficient.

Overseas surveys have found widespread vitamin C deficiencies among asthmatics, elderly men, 75% of cancer patients and up to 100% of psychiatric patients. Psychiatric health can often be restored with vitamin C – one study showed an average of six days for psychiatric patients to reach tissue saturation of vitamin C, compared to only one and a half days for a control group of normal people. It was also observed that the patients receiving the high doses of vitamin C smiled more, were more sociable and less tense. High dosages have also been successful in assisting drug addicts overcome their addiction.

Smoking destroys on average 27% of the vitamin C in the blood each day – this contributes to the haggard appearance of many smokers.

High intravenous doses

Numerous serious health disorders have been healed by extremely high doses of vitamin C. One American doctor, Fred Klenner discovered that an effective dosage for viral infections in a 70 kg adult was 10,000 mg of ascorbic acid, given intravenously (in a drip) every two to four hours around the clock – that's 100,000 mg (100 g or 25 tsp) per day. This amount went far beyond anything tried previously, yet he recorded one successful healing after another.

A NZ King Country farmer also made world headlines in 2010 when the same high intravenous dose of 100,000 mg daily of vitamin C brought him back from serious coma and certain death from swine flu.

Role of vitamin C in our body

- The body's major antioxidant (along with uric acid).
- Assists our immune system to kill infections and viruses.
- Assists our immune system to eliminate harmful metals and poisons.
- Helps convert omega 3 from plants to usable DHA and EPA forms.
- Helps the body absorb nutrients from food, especially iron.
- Assists the body in forming and maintaining collagen.
- Helps maintain the health of bones and teeth.
- Helps heal broken bones, bruises and wounds.
- Helps regulate cholesterol levels.

Too little vitamin C

- Rapid skin ageing, wrinkles, poor skin colour. Free radical damage.
- Low iron anemia (weak red blood cells). Low energy. Pale skin.
- Easy bruising. Purplish skin. Bed sores.
- Bleeding or abnormally red gums. Loose, easily decayed teeth.
- Cataracts. Glaucoma.
- Poor digestion of food. Weight loss. Bad breath.

- Food and chemical allergies.
- Increased levels of toxins in the body.
- Low immunity to colds, infections and poisons.
- Slow recovery from illness, fractures and wound injury.
- Scurvy. Painful joints and lower back. Bowed legs.
- Internal bleeding. Heart failure.
- Arthritis and muscle pain.
- High LDL cholesterol and triglycerides. High blood pressure.
- Oxidised LDL cholesterol. Hardened arteries. Artery inflammation.
- Pre-eclampsia (toxemia) during pregnancy. Kidney disorders.
- Insufficient milk when breastfeeding.
- Low fertility in males.
- Depression. Anxiety. Insomnia. Addiction. Psychiatric disorders.
- Cancer (factor). Asthma (factor).

Too much vitamin C

- Over 2000 mg daily by mouth can cause temporary wind, diarrhea, skin rashes or irritation of the urinary passage. This can be minimised if the dosage is spread throughout the day.
- Excess of the ascorbic acid form of vitamin C can lower body pH – this can be avoided by using the more alkaline sodium ascorbate.

Cooking losses

- Boiling food in water washes out much of the vitamin C but it can be recovered if the water is consumed.
- Vitamin C in freshly killed meat is destroyed during cooking.
- Long exposure of food to air and light destroys vitamin C.

HEALTH HINT   **High dose vitamin C healing**

If you suffer from any of the disorders listed below, you might like to try taking 200 mg of vitamin C three times a day (preferably the sodium ascorbate form to avoid excess acidity) and see if any improvement occurs – all are on record as having responded to high doses of vitamin C. (For higher dosages, intravenous drips are normally necessary.)

Infections	High blood pressure	High LDL cholesterol
Gum disease	Low energy	Rheumatoid arthritis
Anxiety	Insomnia	Psychiatric disorders

"Everyone has a doctor in him or her – we just have to help it in its work. The natural healing force within each one of us is the greatest force in getting well. Our food should be our medicine. Our medicine should be our food."
Hippocrates, (Greek physician 460 - 377 BC)

RDI VITAMIN C

Child:	35 mg		Woman:	45 mg
Teenager:	40 mg		Pregnancy:	60 mg
Man:	45 mg		Breastfeeding:	85 mg

BEVERAGES		mg
1 can	Beer	7

DAIRY / EGGS		
2 cups	Milk (std or low-fat)	7

FRUIT		
1	Kiwifruit	95
1 cup	Orange juice	90
1 cup	Honeydew	85
1 cup	Grapefruit juice	70
1	Orange	65
1 cup	Rockmelon/cantaloupe	45
1 cup	Apple juice	30
1 cup	Pawpaw	21
1	Tamarillo	20
1 med	Banana	13
1/8	Watermelon	11
1 med	Apple	10
1	Persimmon	10
½ cup	Pineapple (canned)	9
2	Passionfruit	8
2	Apricots	8
1	Peach	8
1	Nectarine	6
½	Avocado	6
½ cup	Peaches (canned)	5
2 med	Plums	3
½ cup	Grapes	3

VEGETABLES (cooked)		
½ cup	Green peppers	85
1 cup	Brussels sprouts	65
1 cup	Cauliflower	60
1 cup	Broccoli	55
1 med	Kumara (sweet potato)	35
½ cup	Coleslaw	30
1 med	Tomato (raw)	30
½ cup	Cabbage	30
1 bag	Potato crisps (50 g)	25
2 cobs	Sweet corn	24
2 med	Potatoes	20
¾ cup	Peas	20
½ cup	Spinach	15
¾ cup	Pumpkin	15
¾ cup	Parsnips	12
½ cup	Alfalfa sprouts (raw)	8
½ cup	Mung bean sprouts (raw)	7
1 cup	Lettuce (raw	7
1	Onion	7
½ cup	Green beans	5
½ cup	Silverbeet (chard)	5
3 slices	Beetroot	5
½ cup	Carrots	3

HEALTH FOOD		
1 tsp	Ascorbic acid powder	4000
1 cup	Lemon juice	100
1 tbsp	Rosehip syrup	60

HEALTH HINT   "An apple a day ..."

Researchers have discovered that eating just one unpeeled apple a day can provide as much antioxidant activity as 1500 mg of vitamin C taken as a supplement.

Evidently the phenolic acids, bioflavinoids and phytonutrients found in apple skin greatly enhance natural body antioxidant activity.

"Perfect health is above gold, and a sound body before riches."
King Solomon

Vitamin D (Cholecalciferol)

Vitamin D is formed by the action of ultra violet B (UVB) sunlight on our skin. Vitamin D is not actually a vitamin but a fat-soluble hormone that plays a huge role in the body. Vitamin D is known as D3 when in its active form in the body.

Sunblock preparations stop vitamin D from forming on the skin, and statin drugs and sleeping pills can also hinder it. For these and other reasons, vitamin D has become the most deficient vitamin in the developed world – this has contributed to widespread health disorders, especially bone fractures, heart attacks and organ cancers.

Blood testing of over 3000 adults for vitamin D was done during the NZ 2009 Nutrition Survey – overall, 27% of New Zealanders were found deficient, however this included an alarming 84% of the elderly and 80% of Maori and Pacific Islanders. Testing was done over the course of a year to even out seasonal differences. As might be expected, the lowest readings were found in the South Island during the winter months of August, September and October.

Food is not a viable source of vitamin D, except for a little from butter, eggs, pork and oily fish. The richest food source is cod liver oil.

Obviously nature intended this vitamin to come from the sun. The feel of warm sunlight on our skin can be one of life's free luxuries, and for most people it feels instinctively healthy and reduces anxiety and stress.

UVA rays age skin – UVB rays brown and burn

The fairer our skin, the more efficiently vitamin D is formed in the skin from sunlight – but it won't take place behind glass – the necessary UVB sunlight rays that tan do not pass through window glass. (You can remember the action of UVB by thinking B for *'browns and burns'*).

UVA sunlight rays however, do pass through window glass but do not form vitamin D in our skin. UVA ages our skin more severely than UVB as the rays penetrate deeply into our skin. (You can remember UVA as A for *'ageing'*). UVA rays can also cause skin cancer.

Nearly all of the sun's UV radiation is UVA (95%) and is relatively constant during all hours of daylight. So we can minimise damage to bare skin from ageing UVA rays, by doing any health related sunbathing rapidly during the middle hours of the day (11am to 3pm summer daylight saving time) when the vitamin D forming UVB rays are strongest. During these hours we only need a short exposure time to produce vitamin D. This minimises UVA ageing damage to our skin.

Vitamin D deficiency a serious problem

Because New Zealand is a sunny country, vitamin D deficiencies were long assumed to be rare, until a two year study found low levels of vitamin D among heart attack victims. It was also noted that these deaths were nearly 50% higher during the winter months – a follow up Australian study made similar findings.

As our vitamin D levels fall during winter, so does our bone density and our immune system vitality. Recent research has also found that men's testosterone and libido levels drop along with vitamin D blood levels.

Our bone health is heavily dependent on vitamin D, but also needs adequate calcium to do its job. An Austrian study concluded that 89% of people in Western Europe do not get enough vitamin D and calcium for optimum bone health (however the minerals boron, magnesium and iron are also important).

A nursing home experiment involving 3270 women with an average age of 84, reduced the number of hip fractures by 43% with daily supplements of 20 mcg (800 iu) of vitamin D and 1200 mg of calcium.

For best absorption into bones, calcium supplements over 500 mg should be taken in a 2 to 1 ratio with magnesium.

When optimum body levels of vitamin D, calcium and magnesium are found together, the incidence of cancer drops hugely – 60% in some studies. The Osteoporosis Research Center in Omaha reports – *"Improving calcium and vitamin D status substantially reduces all cancer risk in postmenopausal women."*

Pre-eclampsia during pregnancy can drop 40% with sufficient vitamin D. Another study showed the risk of type 1 diabetes developing in children dropped 80% when 50 mcg (2000 iu) of vitamin D a day was given to pregnant mothers and then to their children.

How to obtain sufficient vitamin D

We can provide sufficient vitamin D by exposing the bare skin of our face and arms (without sunblock) to outdoors sunlight during the times when the sun is high enough to cast a shadow shorter than our body.

To obtain maximum vitamin D formation in the skin takes about 20 minutes of midsummer sun for most European skin types, and up to an hour for darker Polynesian skin, or two hours for black African skin.

We should not wash with soap immediately after sunbathing as the vitamin D is still being absorbed from our skin oils and is easily washed off. Research has found that it actually takes two days to absorb vitamin D fully. Daily soapy washing is the reason that many deeply tanned people who spend hours outdoors, still test low in vitamin D. However, gentle washing with warm water only, can preserve the oils. Extensive swimming will also wash off the skin oil that makes vitamin D.

Unfortunately, after about age 65 the skin on our arms and face becomes less efficient at converting sunlight to vitamin D – by age 70, vitamin D levels have typically dropped 75%. For this reason, the RDI has recently been increased by 50% for those over 70.

So if you don't feel comfortable sunbathing, it would be wise to take a vitamin D supplement. These normally contain 25 mcg (1000 iu) of vitamin D. However, some experienced researchers recommend 75 – 150 mcg (3000 – 6000 iu) a day for optimum health. The toxicity level of vitamin D supplements is now accepted as being over 250 mcg (10,000 iu) a day for adults, and 100 mcg (4000 iu) a day for children. You cannot overdose on vitamin D from sunbathing.

A winter vitamin D blood test is advisable for the elderly and also for Maori and Pacific Islanders. A test in NZ costs about $45 if you pay for it privately, or free if your doctor requests it. Ideally your blood level should be around 120 nmol/L (48 ng/mL) – most New Zealanders and other developed nations have blood levels far below this.

Vitamin D is normally stored by our liver for about 6 months to get us through the winter.

Role of vitamin D in our body
- Helps absorb nutrients from food, especially the bone minerals calcium, phosphorus, magnesium, boron and iron.
- Forms and maintains the health of nerves, bones and teeth.
- Enhances the immune system and reduces the risk of cancer.
- Helps maintain testosterone hormone levels.

Too little vitamin D
- Lower bone mass. Eventual osteoporosis. Calcium growths.
- Brittle, easily broken bones in adults.
- Pre-eclampsia (toxemia) during pregnancy. High blood pressure.
- Weak bones in children, bowed legs and spinal defects (rickets).
- Cataracts in infants if mother is lacking during pregnancy.
- Poor muscle development in adolescents. Low sex drive.
- Tooth decay and gum disease.
- Types 1 and 2 diabetes .
- Calcium build up in arteries (hardening/atherosclerosis).
- Irregular heartbeat (arrhythmia). Heart attack. Stroke.
- Increased risk of cancer including melanoma.
- Nerve damage. Multiple sclerosis.
- Leg pain. Weak muscles.
- Yellow toenails.

- Dry flaky skin. Psoriasis. Vitiligo (factor).
- Crohn's disease (factor).

Too much Vitamin D (supplement only – over 10,000 iu daily)

- Loss of appetite. Nausea. Drowsiness. Frequent urination.

Cooking losses

- No significant losses.

RDI	VITAMIN D (1 mcg = 40 iu)		
Made by sunlight on skin. See chart over page for NZ sun exposure times			
Child:	5 mcg (200 iu)	Woman:	5 mcg (200 iu)
Teenager:	5 mcg (200 iu)	Woman over 50:	10 mcg (400 iu)
Man:	5 mcg (200 iu)	Woman over 70:	15 mcg (600 iu)
Man over 50:	10 mcg (400 iu)	Pregnancy:	5 mcg (200 iu)
Man over 70:	15 mcg (600 iu)	Breastfeeding:	5 mcg (200 iu)

FOOD SOURCES		mcg			
1 tbsp	Cod liver oil	360	3 tbsp	Butter/margarine	5
100 g	Fish (canned types)	12	100g	Pork (lean)	2
2 med	Eggs	2			

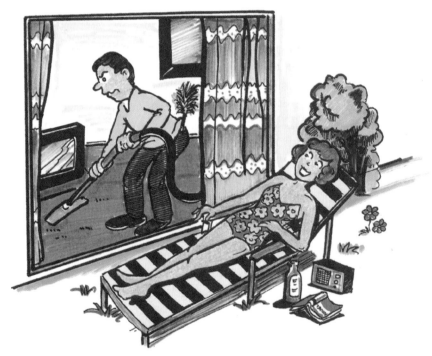

"But I must get my vitamin D, dear."

HEALTH HINT   Sunbathe to avoid cancer

We are constantly warned by the media to stay out of the sun to avoid melanoma skin cancer – the opposite is now known to be true.

Building up high levels of vitamin D by sunbathing (but not artificial sunbeds, which appear to promote all skin cancers) offers huge protection against nearly all cancer, including melanoma. The ideal blood level of vitamin D is around 120 nmol/L (48 ng/mL).

Australian beach lifeguards have a far lower incidence of melanoma than Australian office workers.

We should of course sensibly avoid sunburn, but if your skin tans, you can generally, with common sense, spend an hour or more in the summer sun without sunblock, when lightly tanned.

When you expose untanned skin and start to get slightly pink, you've reached the maximum limit of vitamin D formation and it's time to cover up.

Vitamin D from the sun in NZ when clothed

The chart below shows in minutes, the approximate time you need to be in direct sunshine (or partly cloudy conditions) between 11 am and 3 pm to get adequate vitamin D for two days.

The time is based on being fully clothed, but with bare arms, hands and face. For covered arms, multiply the time by 5. For overcast conditions multiply by 7.

The chart takes into account your skin type (fair, medium or dark) and the time of year. NZ has been divided into three geographical regions from North to South. North is from Taupo upward. Central is between Taupo and Christchurch. South is south of Christchurch to Invercargill.

(There are now free apps available for Android and Apple devices that will calculate this information for Australia – Google *sunsmart apps*.)

Skin	Summer Dec-Feb			Autumn Mar-Apr			Winter Jun-Aug			Spring Sep - Nov		
	Fair	Med	Dark	Fair	Med	Dark	Fair	Med	Dark	Fair	Med	Dark
North	1 min	2 min	4 min	3 min	5 min	7 min	6 min	9 min	19 min	1 min	2 min	4 min
Central	1 min	2 min	4 min	4 min	6 min	13 min	10 min	14 min	29 min	1 min	2 min	5 min
South	1 min	2 min	4 min	5 min	8 min	17 min	17 min	22 min	46 min	2 min	3 min	5 min

"Almost no one is being made sick by vitamin D toxicity, but literally millions are dying from vitamin D deficiency."

Dr Frank Garland, (vitamin D researcher)

HEALTH HINT   Blood testing for vitamin D

You can obtain a vitamin D blood test from most doctors or medical centres. Healthy levels range between 40 nmol/L (16 ng/mL) up to the ideal of 120 nmol/L (48 ng/mL).

Many New Zealanders drop to 16 nmol/L (6 ng/mL) during the winter months.

Some labs may tell you your vitamin D level is normal if you are 20 to 25 nmol/L (8 to 10 ng/mL). It may be normal as far as the deficient average person is concerned, but for optimum health your level should be between 80 nmol/L and 120nmol/L (32 to 48 ng/mL).

Readings in excess of 125 nmol/L (50 ng/mL) when taking a vitamin D supplement may be a sign of toxicity.

HEALTH HINT   High vitamin D levels in Italy

An Italian study showed that healthy blood donors from Rome had excellent average vitamin D levels of 120 nmol/L (48 ng/mL) during their summer. The NZ summer average is around 60 nmol/L (24 ng/mL).

Most Italians love the sun. An old Italian proverb states – *"Where the sun does not go, the doctor does."*

HEALTH HINT   Testosterone levels and vitamin D

Researchers at the Medical University of Graz in Austria found that men with the highest levels of vitamin D in their blood had much more testosterone circulating than those with less.

They also found the average amount of testosterone over the course of a year was subject to the same fluctuations as the vitamin D level – both drop during the winter months.

These findings back up previous research that found an hour of sunshine can boost a man's testosterone by 69%.

"Without health, riches, possession and fame are all mud."
Ed Wynn, 1886 –1966 (American radio comedian)

Vitamin E

Vitamin E is a blood conditioner that helps prevent clots. It's also an antioxidant that partners with selenium and vitamin C to protect our cells from the damaging and ageing effects of oxidation.

An example of oxidation damage can be seen in the browning effect when a sliced apple is left exposed to the air. Food manufacturers use vitamin E as a preservative to slow down the oxidation of food oils.

Vitamin E – found in 8 different forms

Vitamin E is an oil based vitamin and found naturally in eight forms – four tocopherols and four tocotrienols. These are named after the first four letters of Greek alphabet – alpha, beta, gamma and delta.

All eight have different roles, but the alpha-tocopherol form has long been regarded as the most active form for humans. It's also the cheapest to extract from oils and is used almost universally in vitamin supplements.

However, modern research is now discovering that the other seven forms of vitamin E also have significant effects, especially as anti-oxidants and in clearing clogged arteries and preventing cardiovascular disease and cancers.

For example alpha-tocotrienol is 45 times stronger as an antioxidant than the common alpha-tocopherol.

Studies over the years, using just the single alpha-tocopherol form of vitamin E (in supplement form) have invariably produced disappointing results. It is now becoming clear that the full spectrum of vitamin E is required for true health benefits, not just the one alpha-tocopherol segment of this eight-part vitamin.

Wheat germ oil has by far the richest concentration of full spectrum vitamin E from food.

Protects against heart attack and breast cancer

Full spectrum vitamin E from food (ie, all eight forms) is a powerful health protector as it helps keep our red cell platelets separated. A low level of this vitamin is consistently found in heart attack victims.

A 1996 study of 35,000 women aged over 50 found that those whose diets provided the most vitamin E (from food only) had 62% less likelihood of dying from cardiovascular disease than those whose diets provided the least. Women in the same study who took vitamin E in supplement form (alpha-tocopherol) continued to suffer heart attacks at the average rate.

Another study of 5000 women also demonstrated that full spectrum vitamin E from food is critically important as an immune support vitamin. Researchers found the risk of breast cancer was five times higher when vitamin E intake from food was low.

Increased intake of vitamin E from food was also found to improve hormonal balance in women and relieve the cramps, sore breasts and leg swelling suffered by many women prior to menstruation. Also to reduce excessive bleeding during menstruation.

Another study, reported in the *British Medical Journal* found an almost 400% greater risk of type 2 diabetes when vitamin E intake was low.

The NZ 2009 Nutrition Survey showed that vitamin E intake appeared to be generally adequate, mostly from butter and margarine. Average intake was 11 mg for men (RDI 10 mg) and 9 mg for women (RDI 7 mg). However, as around a third of vitamin E is destroyed when fats are heated, there is a serious question mark over the quality of vitamin E from margarine – the original seed oils are heated to damaging high temperatures during hydrogenation.

Smoking, excess alcohol and strenuous exercise deplete body reserves of vitamin E.

Whole wheat a good source

Wheat germ oil is the richest natural source of quality vitamin E, and it's regrettable that the highly nutritious wheat germ is removed during the milling of wheat into white flour, to extend shelf life. Even the wholemeal flour commonly sold in supermarkets has had the wheat germ removed for the same reason – it's only a re-mixing of white flour and bran.

Freshly ground wheat flour from health shops retains the wheat germ, or you can grind your own wheat at home, as I do myself. One 25 kg bag can last me a whole year as I am the only one in my family that uses it. A fast, electric wheat grinder is expensive at about $700 but should last a lifetime (WonderMill is a good brand). In New Zealand you can currently order bags of organically grown wheat from Ceres Whole-foods Stores, Auckland or Chantal Organic Wholesalers, Napier.

Gluten sensitivity problems can be greatly reduced by using freshly ground whole wheat flour, or even eliminated by lightly sprouting and drying the grains before grinding. (Extra gluten is commonly added to white flour by millers and bakers to improve rising characteristics.)

Role of vitamin E in our body
- Necessary for healthy blood and to prevent internal clots.
- Antioxidant to protect body cells and fats from oxygen damage.

- Assists in wound healing, and growth and development of children.
- Balances hormones in women.
- Assists the immune system to protect against cancer.
- Assists immune system to kill infections and eliminate poisons.

Too little vitamin E
- Increased risk of blood clots resulting in heart attack and stroke.
- Hardened arteries. Poor blood circulation, especially to legs.
- Difficulty in breathing. Asthma.
- Type 2 diabetes.
- Birth defects. Growing pains during adolescence.
- Cataracts.
- Low energy and concentration. Weak red blood cells (anemia).
- Prostate cancer in men. Breast cancer in women.
- Pre-menstrual tension in women (PMT). Excessive bleeding.
- Low immunity to infections. Bed sores.

Too much vitamin E (over 200 mg daily, supplement only)
- May increase blood clotting time if on anti-coagulation medication.
- Increased risk of prostate cancer by inhibiting selenium.
- Can deplete vitamin A stores in the body.
- Nausea. Diarrhea.

Cooking losses
- Can be high, about a third, when nuts are roasted or foods are fried.
- Exposure to air diminishes the vitamin E content of plant oils.

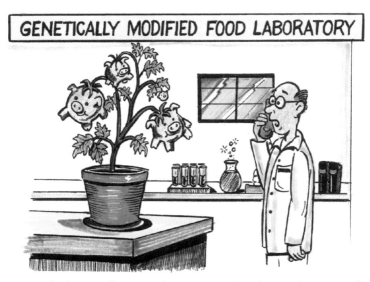

"Yes sir, the bacon flavoured tomato project is coming on well. One minor problem ...."

RDI VITAMIN E (1 mg = 1.5 iu)

Child male:	7 mg	Man:	10 mg
Child female:	6 mg	Woman:	7 mg
Teenage boy:	10 mg	Pregnancy:	7 mg
Teenage girl:	8 mg	Breastfeeding:	11 mg

DAIRY / EGGS

		mg
3 tbsp	Butter	3.5
3 tbsp	Margarine	3.5
1 cup	Soy milk	2.0

FRUIT

½ cup	Blackberries	2.5
½	Avocado	2.0
1	Kiwifruit	1.5
1	Peach	1.5

GRAIN / NUTS

1/3 cup	Almonds (raw)	12.5
1/3 cup	Peanuts (raw)	5.0
1/3 cup	Pecan nuts (raw)	2.5
2 tbsp	Peanut butter	1.5

MEAT / FISH (cooked)`

100 g	Eel	5.0

VEGETABLES (cooked)

1 med	Kumara (sweet potato)	5.0
6 med	Mushrooms	4.0
½ cup	Yams	3.5

1 cup	Taro root	3.0
1 bag	Potato crisps (50 g)	2.5
1 tbsp	Cooking oil (soy)	2.5
1 cup	Squash	2.5
½ cup	Asparagus	2.0
2 med	Potatoes	2.0
½ cup	Silverbeet (chard)	2.0
½ cup	Spinach	1.5
¾ cup	Baked beans	1.5

HEALTH FOOD

1 tbsp	Wheat germ oil	20.0
1 tbsp	Sunflower seed oil	7.0
2 tbsp	Sunflower seeds	6.5
1 tbsp	Olive oil	6.3
1 tbsp	Cod liver oil	3.0
1 plate	Muesli cereal	3.0
2 tbsp	Wheat germ	2.5
2 tbsp	Corn/maize oil	2.5
1 cup	Tomato juice	2.5

"If I could live my life over again I would devote it to proving that germs seek their natural habitat, diseased tissues – rather than being the cause of disease. In other words, mosquitoes seek the stagnant water, but do not cause the pool to become stagnant."

Dr Rudolf Virchow, 1821–1902 (German pathologist)

CoQ10 (Coenzyme Q10/Ubiquinone)

This bright orange-yellow enzyme is needed by every cell in our body to fire up energy. It acts rather like the spark plug in a petrol engine – helping generate over 90% of the body's energy. Our hard working heart muscles use twice as much CoQ10 as other muscles.

CoQ10 (Coenzyme Q10) boosts our immune system, acts as an anti-oxidant and slows down the ageing of our skin and brain. CoQ10 is so universally required by our body it is named ubiquinone, which means *'required by every living cell'*.

CoQ enzymes have other numbers besides 10 – there's also CoQ7, CoQ8 and CoQ9, which are found in fatty foods. A healthy body will use these three other CoQ enzymes to make CoQ10 – provided our blood selenium levels are adequate.

Nevertheless, once we pass age 30, we gradually lose the ability to make CoQ10 and our body levels begin to drop, (this is one of the ways our body ages). When CoQ10 drops to 75% of normal levels, health problems begin to appear – these include gum disease, muscle wasting, diabetes, cancers, cardiovascular disease, low energy and skin wrinkles. The high incidence of gum disease in NZ (about 90%) is overwhelming evidence of a general deficiency of CoQ10.

When our CoQ10 drops to 25% of normal levels, serious disease and mental deterioration is inevitable. Diabetics on average have less than half the CoQ10 levels of a healthy person. Cholesterol-lowering drugs (statins) reduce the body's manufacture of CoQ10 by an average of 52%, and beta-blockers up to 40%, depending on dosage.

CoQ10 status was not tested for in the 2009 Nutrition Survey, but the daily intake of CoQ10 in NZ has been estimated at about 5 mg a day. There is no RDI set, but nutritionists recommend around 25 mg a day.

During the 1960's, Japanese researchers devised a fermentation process to produce CoQ10 from plant algae. Over 12 million Japanese are now reported to take CoQ10 as a daily supplement. This may partly explain their superior longevity.

Dr Emile Bliznakov, Scientific Director of the Lupus Research Institute of Connecticut spent years researching CoQ10 and then published his book *'The Miracle Nutrient Coenzyme Q10'*. From his research data he reports that 74% of heart attack patients recovered fully when given CoQ10. Also after two months of taking 60 mg of fermented CoQ10 a day, average high blood pressure readings dropped from 141/97 to 126/90, with a 20% increase in the heart's ability to pump blood.

Also in an experiment repeated three times, mice treated with CoQ10 lived 56% longer than average. Dr Bliznakov writes, *"Equally fascinating was the fact that the quality of youthful life was maintained well into the animals' extended life spans. They still had healthy glossy coats and little or none of the expected signs of ageing, like patchy loss of fur, organ degeneration and lack of mobility."* (Synthetic CoQ10 did not produce the same results, only the fermented variety.)

More recently, Dr Robert Atkins reported that some of his patients who were awaiting heart transplants and were given high doses of CoQ10 (100 mg a day) *"found that their old heart would do just fine."*

German researchers have found that taking extra CoQ10 can rebuild collagen and elastin in the skin of the aged and smokers, and reverse skin damage, especially eye wrinkles.

I myself have also seen a noticeable reduction in wrinkles (crow's feet) around my own eyes in recent years since taking a quality fermented CoQ10 supplement (75 mg a day) combined with fish oil in a capsule.

Researchers report wide variances in the quality of CoQ10 supplements, so it should be purchased from a reputable supplier and in a form that is infused in oil, for the best absorption.

Because taking a CoQ10 supplement normally increases energy, sometimes dramatically, the desire to exercise is normally also increased. This can help motivated dieters lose weight. In one study, those on a low calorie diet taking CoQ10 daily, lost an average of 14 kg compared to 6 kg for those not taking CoQ10.

CoQ10 (ubiquinone) is immediately converted to its usable form ubiquinol by the body. However, if you wish to take a high therapeutic dose of CoQ10 (over 200 mg a day) the already converted ubiquinol form should be used, as the body will not normally convert all of a heavy 200 mg dose of ubiquinone to ubiquinol. Ubiquinol can be expensive however, as it costs about four times as much to manufacture than ubiquinone and has a shorter effective shelf life.

Role of CoQ10 in our body
- Necessary for all body muscles to generate energy from food.
- An antioxidant, brain protector and blood regulator.
- Slows ageing of body cells.
- Assists the immune system to kill infections, especially in the gums.

Too little CoQ10
- Cardiovascular disease. Arrhythmia. Angina. High blood pressure.
- Blood clots. Heart attack. Stroke.
- Low energy. Shortness of breath.

- Memory loss. Dementia. Parkinson's disease. Alzheimer's symptoms.
- Lowered immunity to cancer and infections. Gum disease.
- Type 2 diabetes.
- Premature ageing, skin wrinkles and reduced life expectancy.
- Sore, weakened or wasted muscles.
- Numbness in hands and feet.

Too much CoQ10
- No known toxic effects.

Cooking losses
- Frying food can reduce native CoQ content about 20%.

RDI	COQ10 ENZYME		
Our body uses CoQ in fatty foods to make CoQ10 – the RDI's below are estimates from overseas studies but there is limited data available			
Child:	12 mg	Woman:	25 mg
Teenage boy:	25 mg	Pregnancy:	35 mg
Teenage girl:	20 mg	Breastfeeding:	35 mg
Man:	25 mg		

The figures below allow for conversion from CoQ in food to CoQ10 by the body

DAIRY / EGGS		mg
2 med	Eggs (cooked)	2.0

MEAT / FISH (cooked)		
100 g	Beef heart	11.5
100 g	Sardines	6.5
100 g	Pork	3.0

100 g	Beef	3.0
100 g	Chicken	2.0
100 g	Fish	2.0

OILS		
3 tbsp	Soy oil	2.0

"I am at a loss to explain why CoQ10 is not prescribed routinely to every heart patient."
Dr Robert Atkins MD

Vitamin H – Biotin

Biotin is a B vitamin made by our bodies in the intestines. Deficiencies have been found following severe dieting, or the long term use of antibiotics which kill the probiotic bacteria in our gut necessary to form the vitamin – babies are particularly vulnerable.

The balance of our gut probiotic bacteria is critical to health, especially in absorbing and manufacturing nutrients from food, also in avoiding food allergies and having a strong immune system. There's an old saying *'Health begins in the colon.'* It could also be said that *'Health ends in the colon'* – when it's not functioning properly.

Diabetic nerve damage has been halted or reversed with injections of 10 mg of biotin three times a week for six weeks, followed by 5 mg orally a day for two more months. Restless legs have also been cured with this regime.

Male baldness has been reported improved and female baldness cured with oral supplements of 10 mg of biotin a day.

Biotin can be obtained directly from our food, mainly eggs (cooked), peanuts, liver, malt extract and brewer's yeast.

Role of biotin in our body
- Helps maintain the health of our skin, hair and nerves.
- Helps manage blood sugar (glucose).
- Assists in the manufacture of body fats and acids.

Too little biotin
- Rash around the nose and mouth.
- Cradle cap in infants.
- Restless legs.
- Dry scaly skin. Greyish pallor.
- Stiff hair that is difficult to comb flat. General hair loss.
- Premature greying of hair.

Too much biotin
- No known toxic effects.

Cooking losses
- Low – about 10%. Biotin is mostly made by probiotics in our intestines.

RDI	VITAMIN H – BIOTIN
No RDI set and NO FOOD TABLE as biotin can be made by a healthy body	

112

How probiotics help us

Antibiotics (meaning 'anti-life') can be effective drugs for killing harmful bacteria, but when they are taken by mouth instead of the safer (and generally more effective) way of injecting them into the blood stream, they also kill vital food digesting bacteria in our intestines. It's like spraying an entire vegetable garden with weed-killer to destroy just a small patch of weeds.

We have trillions of these friendly digestive gut bacteria (weighing about a kilogram) living in the 7-metre (20 ft) length of our small intestine and our 1.5-metre (5 ft) long, large intestine. These bacteria are known as probiotics (meaning *'pro-life'*) and there are about 30 principal strains. Each strain has a role to play in the digestion of various types of food – dairy, wheat, eggs, nuts, etc. (Allergies, wind, IBS, etc, are generally signs of a deficiency.)

Our gut is originally colonised with probiotics at birth (before stomach acid forms) with probiotic bacteria from the birth canal of our mother and colostrum from her breast milk. When we develop a food allergy, it's usually because the bacteria required to pre-digest that type of food has been destroyed by an antibiotic. Our insoluble food is then no longer pre-digested (ie, converted to a liquid so it can seep through our intestinal walls into our blood-stream). As a result, many of the nutrients, are not absorbed into the bloodstream and food allergies, malnutrition, and health disorders like yeast infections follow.

When a strain of bacteria is wiped out, it can be difficult to recolonise it in our intestines, especially if the appendix (the body's probiotic storehouse) has been removed. This is because our powerful stomach acid destroys all but the most hardy strains of probiotics, which are normally only found in fermented foods.

Fermented foods can help our gut re-establish a few hardy strains of probiotics like acidophilus, but even these are mostly destroyed by stomach acid – around 70% of acidophilus from yoghurt for example.

Many dramatic cures of longstanding disorders have resulted from supplementing with a course of multi-strain probiotics (live friendly bacteria), using some form of protective capsule to safeguard them against stomach acid. The effect in our intestines can be like planting new seeds in a vegetable garden.

Vitamin H – Biotin

"Happy the man who has an excellent wife – his span of days is doubled."
Biblical proverb (Ecclesiasticus 26:1)

Vitamin K1 and K2

This oily yellow vitamin is in two distinct forms – K1 and K2. K1 helps clot our blood correctly and K2 helps retain calcium in our bones.

Vitamin K1 – for the healthy clotting of blood

The K1 form is called phylloquinone and plays a key role in the clotting of our blood. The letter K stands for *'koagulation'* a Danish word for blood clotting. Lack of K1 can cause excessive menstrual bleeding in women.

Newborn babies are occasionally deficient in vitamin K1, so in NZ it is routinely injected at birth to prevent internal brain bleeding problems, (the risk factor is 5 in 100,000 births). It can be given orally if a mother doesn't want her baby injected, as there is a slightly increased risk of leukemia later in childhood with injected K1.

Warfarin type anti-clotting drugs, or 'blood thinners' as they are commonly known (coumadin and marevan) work by hindering the action of vitamin K1. Aspirin has a similar effect, which is why too much aspirin can cause stomach bleeding.

Vitamin K1 can be made in our intestines if the correct probiotic is present. However antibiotics can destroy the bacteria necessary to form this vitamin.

Dark green vegetables such as silverbeet (chard), spinach and broccoli are food sources of vitamin K1.

Vitamin K2 – for healthy bones, arteries and prostate

Vitamin K2 is called menaquinone and is also made by probiotics in our intestines (by converting vitamin K1) or can be obtained from food, especially cheese and eggs. In recent years K2 has been recognised as a highly important vitamin, similar in its role to vitamin D.

K2 regulates the calcium in our body and keeps it in the bones where it's needed. Otherwise it can build up in our artery linings (athero-sclerosis) and heart valves, where it can be fatal – vitamin K2 helps prevent hardening of the arteries and osteoporosis at the same time.

In a Japanese study of 60 older women, 24 with vertebrae fractures and 36 free of fractures, the average blood level of vitamin K2 in the fracture free group was twice as high as in those in the fracture free group.

In 2004 the Rotterdam Study found that people who consumed 45 mcg of K2 daily lived seven years longer than those consuming only 12 mcg daily. Eating 25 g of firm cheese daily, plus one egg, can allow your gut probiotics to manufacture around 40 mcg of vitamin K2.

Dr Cees Vermeer of Germany, one of the world's top vitamin K researchers, reports that men with the highest amounts of K2 have around 50% less incidence of prostate cancer, and 50% fewer heart attacks than average, especially when their gut probiotics can make vitamin K2 from cheese. Dr Vermeer recommends at least 45 mcg daily of vitamin K2, up to an optimum of around 185 mcg.

A rich, ready-made source of vitamin K2 is a Japanese food made from fermented soybeans called natto. It has a cheesy smell, strong taste and a sticky mucous-like texture. Japanese love it but foreigners tend to loathe it (rather like the reaction of Americans to NZ Marmite (a dark brown yeast extract). Natto is thought to be another reason for Japanese longevity.

Role of vitamin K1 and K2 in our body

- Assists in the clotting of our blood (K1).
- Assists in maintaining calcium in our bones (K2).
- Helps prevent calcium being deposited in arteries and organs (K2).

Too little vitamin K1

- Slow blood clotting. Regular nose bleeds.
- Heavy menstrual bleeding.
- Internal bleeding. Easy bruising. Purplish patches under the skin.

Too little vitamin K2

- Osteoporosis. Easily fractured bones. Osteoarthritis.
- Atherosclerosis (hardened arteries and veins). High blood pressure.
- Calcium deposits in joints, and stones in body organs.
- Prostate cancer, lung cancer, liver cancer and leukemia.

Too much vitamin K1 or K2

- No known toxic effects of natural vitamin K1. However injected synthetic vitamin K1 given to newborn babies can slightly increase the risk of childhood leukemia.
- Supplements of vitamin K1 in adults can counteract prescribed warfarin type anticoagulant medication.
- No known toxic effects of vitamin K2.

Cooking losses

- No significant losses.
- K1 and K2 can be made by intestinal bacteria in a well nourished body.

"A full stomach does not like to think."   **German proverb**

| RDI | VITAMIN K1 and K2 |

RDI applies to both Vitamin K1 and Vitamin K2.
K2 can be made by intestinal bacteria in a healthy body from K1.

Infant:	5 mcg	Woman:	60 mcg
Child:	25 mcg	Pregnancy:	65 mcg
Teenager:	55 mcg	Breastfeeding:	65 mcg
Man:	75 mcg		

Vitamin K1 only

VEGETABLES (cooked)		mcg
½ cup	Spinach	440
½ cup	Silverbeet (chard)	290
1 cup	Broccoli	220
1 cup	Brussels sprouts	220
½ cup	Cabbage	80
1 tbsp	Parsley	60
1 cup	Lettuce	60
1 cup	Cauliflower	17
1 med	Tomato	7
FATS		
1 tbsp	Olive oil	8

Vitamin K2 only

DAIRY / EGGS		mcg
2 slices	Cheese 50 g (firm)*	38
2 slices	Cheese 50 g (soft)*	28
2	Eggs (yolk only)	32
2 tbsp	Butter	4
MEAT / FISH (cooked)		
100 g	Chicken	9
100 g	Beef	8
100 g	Pork	6
HEALTH FOOD		
100 g	Natto	1100
50 g	Goose liver paste	180

* Vitamin K2 from cheese requires
conversion in the body by
intestinal probiotics.

| HEALTH HINT | Avoiding headaches |

Headaches can be largely avoided by following these seven rules:
1. Sleep regular, consistent hours.
2. No food or beverages three hours before bed.
3. Arise from bed early.
4. Take a daily 2 km (1¼ mile) walk in the fresh air.
5. Avoid anxious thoughts and worry.
6. Get your full RDI of magnesium every day.
7. Avoid chemical sweeteners and MSG type flavour enhancers.

"Health is a state of complete physical, mental and social well being, not merely the absence of disease and infirmity." World Health Organisation

Aluminium

Aluminium is found in our bodies but is not believed to be a nutrient. It's included here as it's widely used as a food additive and also in other products that can be absorbed by our body.

Some of the uses of aluminium are –

- An ingredient in baking powder (aluminium phosphate – 541).
- An additive to table salt to promote free running.
- An additive to increase the whiteness of flour.
- An ingredient in stomach antacid preparations.
- An ingredient in under arm anti-perspirants.
- Added to municipal water supplies to clarify discoloured water.
- Added to some types of aspirin to counteract the acidity.

High aluminium levels are found in the brains of those suffering from Alzheimer's, and often in the blood of those with weak or defective memories (around 20 parts per billion). When magnesium, zinc and vitamin C levels are optimised, this high aluminium blood level decreases to normal (less than 10 parts per billion) and human memory improves.

The aluminium in stomach antacid preparations has been known to cause rapid osteoporosis and painful, weak muscles.

Chinese tests of dietary intake from using aluminium cookware revealed absorption of about 4 mg per person per day. The estimated average aluminium intake for US adults from all sources is 24 mg daily.

Eating a slice of a cake baked with a recipe using two teaspoons of baking powder will give you about 7 mg of aluminium.

(When baking you can substitute baking soda for baking powder, however baking soda is alkaline and needs an acid with which to react to create gas for rising. The sugar in a recipe normally supplies this, otherwise add 2 parts of cream of tartar to 1 part of baking soda.)

Role of aluminium in our body

- No known useful role.

Too little aluminium

- Research indicates the less the better.

Too much aluminium

- Inhibits dietary mineral action, especially magnesium and zinc.
- Linked to memory disorders and Alzheimer's.
- Can cause osteoporosis and painful, weak muscles.
- Hyperactivity and attention disorders in children (ADHD).

Boron

Boron is a mineral lacking in NZ soils, yet is highly important for our health, especially the health of our bones and joints. It's also needed for a healthy reproductive system in both sexes and a lively brain to help prevent dullness and poor co-ordination.

Only limited research has been done on boron, but it appears every bit as important to our body as other vital nutrients like vitamin D, magnesium and selenium.

A study released in 2001 found that men with an intake of 2 mg a day had at least a 62% lower chance of developing prostate cancer compared to those getting half that intake.

Three other studies of humans, temporarily deprived of boron, found symptoms of poor concentration, weak short term memory and lack of physical dexterity.

Research overseas has shown that the lower the level of boron in a nation's crop soils, the higher the incidence of osteoarthritis. Jamaican soils are reported to be chronically low (like the soils of NZ) and 70% of their population eventually suffer from osteoarthritis – the NZ percentage is similar.

The average daily food intake of boron in NZ is estimated to be about 2 mg, whereas the RDI to provide protection from osteoarthritis is believed to be 3 to 4 mg daily. One Australian doctor reported that 90% of his osteoarthritis patients improved with boron supplements, most obtaining complete relief from pain.

Boron also appears to be important in preventing osteoporosis (porous bones). In one study by the US Department of Agriculture, 12 older post-menopausal women were supplemented with an additional 3 mg daily of boron. After eight days all the women greatly reduced their excretion of calcium by an average of 44%, indicating far better calcium absorption and reduced risk of osteoporosis.

These same 12 women also, on average, doubled their body's production of estrogen, which is known to protect younger women from osteoporosis.

A later study showed that higher intakes of boron (about 10 mg daily from a supplement) can substitute for hormone replacement therapy in women and reduce menopausal problems.

As well as maintaining healthy estrogen and testosterone levels in women, boron is also known to help maintain DHEA levels – a major body youth hormone that begins to drop after age 30.

(Boron was not included in the NZ 2009 Nutrition Survey.)

Role of boron in our body

- Helps bones absorb and retain calcium and magnesium.
- Maintains health of bones and joints in old age.
- Helps maintain brain health.
- Helps regulate levels of sex hormones.

Too little boron

- Osteoarthritis. Osteoporosis. Kidney stones.
- Increased risk of prostate cancer.
- Weak short term memory. Poor concentration.
- Lack of estrogen in women. Vaginal dryness.
- Hot flushes during menopause.
- Low sex drive in both men and women.
- Low DHEA (youth hormone) levels.

Too much boron (over 100 mg day)

- Red skin rash with blistering.
- Vomiting and blue-green diarrhea.

Cooking losses

- No significant losses.

RDI	BORON	
The RDI's below are estimates from overseas studies – limited data available		
Child: 2 mg	Woman:	3 mg
Teenager: 3 mg	Pregnancy:	4 mg
Man: 3 mg	Breastfeeding:	4 mg

FRUIT		mg
1/3 cup	Raisins	2.4
½	Avocado	1.6
1/3 cup	Sultanas	.8
1 cup	Fruit juice	.6
1	Pear	.5
5	Prunes	.4
2	Plums	.4
5	Dates	.4
5	Apricots (dried halves)	.4
1	Orange	.3
1	Apple	.3
1	Kiwifruit	.3

GRAINS		
½ cup	Flour (soy)	1.9
½ cup	Oatmeal	.8

NUTS		
1/3 cup	Almond nuts	1.4
1/3 cup	Hazel nuts	1.3
5	Brazil nuts	.3
1 tbsp	Peanut butter	.3

FISH		
100 g	Fish (avg)	.3

VEGETABLES (cooked)		
¾ cup	Red kidney beans	2.8
2 cobs	Sweet corn	1.4
1 med	Kumara (sweet potato)	.3
2 med	Potatoes	.3

Calcium

Calcium is the most abundant mineral in our body and vital for every cell. Calcium is important for bone health, muscle action, maintaining optimum body pH, regulating our heartbeat, conducting nerve signals, clotting our blood and many hormone functions. Calcium is alkaline, and helps counteract the acid effects of sugar and phosphorus. One doctor claims 147 health disorders relate to calcium when this mineral is out of balance with other diet minerals.

Although calcium is the most abundant mineral in the body, there is not as much as we might think – we have on average only about 1.2 kg. Of this, approx 98% is found in our bones, 1% in our teeth and the rest in our blood and cells.

Calcium is a key ingredient of bone, but most of our bone is a collagen-like protein. If we took all the calcium out of a bone it would still look like a bone, but would be rubbery, like the kind of thing we give a dog to chew. This is why large amounts of gelatine (a collagen-protein) can be extracted from beef bones.

In osteoporosis however, both this collagen and calcium migrate from the bones, making them shrink and become porous and brittle. A healthy bone will bend rather than break, like the green branch of a tree compared to a dead one. When our magnesium intake is low, our bones absorb less calcium from food. When magnesium rises, our bones absorb more calcium and vitamin K2 helps keep it in the bones.

As most of our calcium is stored in our bones, if we are not getting enough from food, the body will use our bones as a bank and withdraw enough calcium to perform essential body functions.

Why such a high RDI for calcium (1000 mg)?

We only lose about 125 mg of calcium each day (through our skin, nails, hair, sweat and bowels) – you might then wonder why the RDI for calcium is set so high in NZ at 1000 mg.

That's a good question – in fact the non-profit World National Academy of Sciences, who advise nations on setting their RDI's, actually suggest that a daily intake of 300 mg of calcium should be sufficient. Women in poorer countries, even those on mainly vegetarian diets, get by on just 200 mg a day, with far less osteoporosis than the wealthier nations.

However it is absorption and retention of calcium in countries like NZ that is the problem – with our low magnesium intake and excess phosphorus from protein food (meat and grains) plus excessive sugar, we tend to acidify our bodies, which restricts the bone absorption of dietary calcium. This is because extra calcium is required to buffer (make more alkaline) the acidity of our body. A saliva pH reading below 6.0 can be an indication of excess acidity and low calcium intake.

Calcium's sister mineral magnesium is particularly important. Our magnesium intake as an adult should be in a ratio of about 1 part magnesium to 2 parts of calcium – so for every 100 mg of calcium in our diet, we should also take in about 50 mg of magnesium. (Milk, including human milk, has only a 1 part magnesium to 10 parts calcium, however a fast-growing newborn has a high need for calcium.)

Calcium works with numerous other nutrients

There are a huge number of other nutrients that work with calcium besides magnesium, in particular – boron, iron, sodium, vitamin D, vitamin K2, vitamin C, vitamin B6 and vitamin B12. Also to a lesser extent – phosphorus, silicon, manganese, copper, iodine, chromium, zinc and selenium.

Many of the health benefits attributed to increasing calcium intake, such as lowering high blood pressure, reducing anxiety, lowering the incidence of colon cancer, reducing kidney stones, eliminating PMT, etc, are now thought to be due to the high magnesium content of some calcium supplements – up to 33%.

The nursing home experiment mentioned earlier in the chapter on vitamin D, that reduced the number of hip fractures by 43% with daily supplements of vitamin D and calcium, used a calcium supplement containing 33% magnesium.

This makes sense, as the body normally has a big store of calcium in the bones to call upon if necessary, but often seriously lacks magnesium.

Vitamin D is especially important for calcium absorption and retention.

Avoiding osteoporosis

To prevent and reverse osteoporosis requires all the 16 nutrients listed above (boron, iron, etc,) all working in harmony with calcium. Take just one nutrient away and the beneficial effect can be lost – like leaving baking powder out of a cake recipe. It's highly unlikely that merely taking a calcium supplement will reverse a complex health disorder like osteoporosis – the other minerals and vitamins are also essential.

Sex hormones play a big role in bone formation and maintenance. Our peak bone mass is normally laid down between ages 14 and 30, when youth hormones are at their peak. However, in menopausal women (aged around 50) the hormone progesterone drops by about 75%, nature appears to have intended estrogen to drop by the same percentage, to maintain a balance. However, due to excess estrogen in the diet from modern processed foods, estrogen drops much less than progesterone (only about 35%). As a result of this imbalance, calcium begins to exit from the bones, bringing on a host of common health problems, including osteoporosis, broken bones and weight gain.

Raising progesterone levels with drug hormone replacement to balance estrogen levels can prevent this happening, but is known to increase cardiovascular risk. However, by supplementing boron intake to a maximum of 10 mg, avoiding high estrogen foods like soy, and ensuring the full RDI of all other nutrients, female hormones can normally be brought back in to balance without side effects.

Low testosterone levels in older men can also cause calcium to migrate from bones, but not so markedly as post-menopausal women. Testosterone is a bone density builder in both sexes. Strenuous, heavy exercise can increase testosterone levels in men.

Too much omega 6 from vegetable oils, and low iron levels can also cause bones to lose calcium at any age. Without sufficient vitamin K2, this calcium can become deposited in the arteries causing atherosclerosis.

This typical loss of calcium (and also bone collagen) makes bones brittle and easily broken. It also shrinks the height of the elderly – nearly everybody over the age of 50 loses height each year, men around 0.5mm and women about 1mm.

Exercise retains calcium in our bones

Lack of exercise can play a big role in osteoporosis. Astronauts have been found to lose significant amounts of calcium from their bones every day they spend floating in the weightlessness of space. Calcium migrates from bones that are not being stressed or flexed daily. Hours of sitting, or lying in bed without exercise can be similar to the effect of astronaut weightlessness.

Older men and women who remain fit and well nourished, and who do weight exercises for all muscle groups (legs, arms, back, shoulders, chest and stomach) generally do not develop osteoporosis. Another testimony to life's rule – *'Use it or lose it.'*

How to build our calcium reserves

Calcium is widespread in foods and also in drinking water – the content in NZ tap water is typically about 11 mg per litre, but can be as high as 200 mg per litre in hard water.

The NZ 2009 Nutrition survey estimated that calcium intake was deficient for 45% of European males, 76% of Maori male teenagers and a huge 88% of Pacific Island male teenagers. Women were estimated to be even more deficient, with 73% of European females, 90% of Maori and 95% of Pacific Island females.

These alarming figures are, however, based on the high NZ RDI for calcium of 1000 mg. As mentioned earlier, the National Academy of Sciences suggests that just 300 mg of calcium daily should be sufficient, provided other key nutrients, especially magnesium, vitamin D and vitamin K2 are present in the diet, and acidic phosphorus and sugar foods are not over supplied.

Milk was reported as the largest source of calcium (27%) followed by bread (10%). However, over 50% of Maori and Pacific Islanders and 9% of European adults have some difficulty digesting milk. Typical symptoms are diarrhea, stomach cramps and excess wind. This is normally due to missing friendly probiotics in the gut. (Children in all of these groups have much less of a problem.)

Milk is still the richest food source of calcium. Yoghurt has the same levels and is more easily digested for those who have a milk intolerance problem. Soy milk is 85% lower in calcium than cow's milk, but most manufacturers add extra calcium to increase this level. Low-fat milk has extra calcium added to improve colour and taste.

Soft drinks (sodas) contain little or no calcium (or any other nutrient for that matter) and some colas are high in phosphoric acid. Excess phosphorus increases our body's need for calcium. Racehorses have been known to develop osteoporosis and easily shatter leg bones when their fodder has been high in phosphorus and low in calcium for long periods.

Supplements of dolomite powder (limestone) or coral calcium are rich in calcium and usually also contain magnesium. For best absorption they should be taken along with foods high in calcium. Supplements should also ideally provide around a two to one ratio of calcium to magnesium and preferably some vitamin D.

Role of calcium in our body
- Combines with phosphorus, magnesium, boron, iron, vitamins D and K2 and many other vitamins and minerals to form and maintain the health of bones, teeth and nerves.
- Necessary for correct muscle and nerve action and also relaxation.
- Helps maintain the correct pH of our blood and body cells.
- Assists in the clotting of our blood.
- Helps regulate blood pressure by narrowing arteries.
- Helps form body hormones.
- Helps induce restful sleep.

Too little calcium

(Normally due to a lack of magnesium, boron, iron, vitamin D, vitamin K2 or vitamin C, or too much phosphorus).

- Shrinkage of our skeleton. Brittle, easily broken bones (osteoporosis).
- Increased risk of bone fractures.
- Pre-eclampsia (toxemia) during pregnancy.
- Weight gain in post menopausal women.
- Acid body cells (low pH). Arthritis.
- Increased risk of organ cancers.
- Increased risk of kidney stones.
- Increased risk of cataracts.
- Irregular heartbeat.
- PMT or PMS in women. ADHD in children. Anxiety.
- Poor sleep. Irritability. Nervous twitches. Psychiatric disorders.
- Frequent urination.
- Muscle cramps, numbness, tingling or trembling (especially legs).
- Malformed jaws and/or teeth in children.

Too much calcium

(Supplements of over 2400 mg of calcium a day, or over 1200 mg a day with insufficient magnesium, vitamin D or K2. No risk with natural, food-sourced calcium.)

- Increased risk of calcium deposits hardening the arteries.
- Increased risk of kidney stones.
- High blood pressure from atherosclerosis.
- Heart attack or stroke.
- Constipation.

Cooking losses

- No significant losses.

HEALTH HINT   **Stomach acid reducing drugs**

A proton pump inhibitor drug such as Losec, suppresses the strength of stomach acid for about 48 hours to avoid the discomfort of acid reflux. This however can hinder protein absorption and diet mineral breakdown, especially calcium and magnesium – it also reduces vitamin B12 absorption.

The following press release was issued by the American FDA, after a study of 80,000 women, using this type of drug, found a 35% higher incidence of bone fractures – *"Studies suggest a possible increased risk of bone fractures with the use of proton pump inhibitors for one year or longer."*

RDI · CALCIUM

One third of these RDI figures may be sufficient when magnesium, vitamin D, K2 and boron intake is adequate

Infant:	350 mg	Woman:	1000 mg
Child:	800 mg	Woman over 70:	1300 mg
Teenager:	1300 mg	Pregnancy:	1000 mg
Man:	1000 mg	Breastfeeding:	1000 mg
Man over 70:	1300 mg		

DAIRY / EGGS

		mg
2 cups	Milk (low-fat)	1100
2 cups	Milk (std)	600
2 cups	Milk (soy)*	600
4 tbsp	Milk powder (non-fat)	370
4 tbsp	Milk powder (whole)	310
100 g	Cheese omelette	280
25 g	Cheese	180
1 pot	Dairy food dessert	170
¾ cup	Ice cream	130
1 svg	Cheese cake	110

GRAIN / NUTS

1	Bran muffin (large)	140
1/3 cup	Almonds	130
4 slices	Bread white*	110

VEGETABLES (cooked)

1 cup	Taro leaves	230
½ cup	Spinach	130

FRUIT

½ cup	Rhubarb (stewed)	110

FISH

100 g	Sardines (canned)	460
100 g	Shrimp	320
100 g	Salmon (canned)	240
100 g	Mussels	160

FAST FOOD

1 svg	Pizza (large)	390
1	Milkshake (McDonalds)	210
1	Ice cream sundae	170
1	Eggburger (large)	160
1	Eggburger (std)	140
1	Cheeseburger (std)	120
1	Hamburger (Big Mac)	110

HEALTH FOOD

1 tsp	Dolomite powder	**1400
1 tsp	Coral calcium	**1600
1 cup	Soy milk (fortified)	250
2 tbsp	Sesame seeds	230

* Some calcium is normally added during manufacture.

** When taken with food or mixed with milk – calcium is not well absorbed when taken alone.

HEALTH HINT · Minimise long term bed rest

Long term bed rest can do more harm than good – if you are confined to bed for two or more days, you should still do your best to exercise as many muscles as possible, ideally with some weights in order to flex your bones and minimise calcium loss.

You should also get back on your feet as soon as you are able to prevent 'rubber knees', constipation and the overall weakness that comes from long term bed confinement.

Chloride (and Chlorine)

Chloride is typical of a number of body nutrients – harmful in some forms and dosages, but essential for life in others. When in chlorine gas form, at just 1% concentration in air, it is fatal to living organisms. (It was used as a chemical weapon in World War I.)

Yet when chlorine is combined with other elements, it changes to chloride form and is no longer harmful, but necessary for life. For example, chloride is part of the hydrochloric acid in our stomach that breaks down protein for digestion. Chloride can be obtained from common salt (sodium chloride) and is needed by every cell in our body.

Chloride as liquefied chlorine gas is added to domestic water supplies (and also swimming pools) to kill bacteria. This is normally in the form of concentrated sodium hypochlorite (household bleach) which creates chlorine gas in the water.

The chlorine gas slowly evaporates when the treated water is exposed to air. However, air concentrations of chlorine gas can reach dangerous levels in indoor swimming pools without good ventilation.

Although often criticised, the chlorination of domestic water supplies is regarded as a 'necessary evil' – it has helped to almost eliminate the often fatal water-borne diseases of typhoid and cholera which were common in the 19th century.

Chlorine gas, which is yellow/green in colour, still remains toxic to life. However, water filters using activated carbon cartridges remove the gas and its unpleasant smell and taste from drinking water.

There's no evidence that chlorinated water kills useful gut bacteria – chlorine is believed to be rapidly converted to useful chloride by hydrochloric stomach acid and other elements in our digestive system.

We need about 2300 mg a day of chloride and this is normally amply supplied by the salt in our diet, which is 60% chloride, 39% sodium and 1% other minerals and additives – provided our salt intake is sufficient, our chloride intake should also be sufficient.

No official NZ RDI has been set for chloride as deficiencies are rare, and are only found along with severe sodium deficiency.

Role of chloride in our body

- Assists in the digestion of our food.
- Part of our cell fluids (electrolytes).
- Helps maintain the health of our lymph system.
- Helps regulate the acidity/alkalinity of our blood.
- Helps maintain correct action and health of our liver.

Too little chloride
- Brain disorders. Poor co-ordination. Coma.

Too much chloride
- Mental confusion or coma.
- Miscarriage. Stillbirth. Malformed babies.
- Fatal suffocation by filling the lungs with fluid (in chlorine gas form).
- Bladder cancer (in chlorine gas form).

Cooking losses
- Boiling food in water can leach out the salt which contains chloride.

RDI CHLORIDE

Child:	2000 mg	Woman:	2300 mg
Teenager:	2300 mg	Woman over 50:	2000 mg
Man:	2300 mg	Pregnancy:	2300 mg
Man over 50:	2000 mg	Breastfeeding:	2300 mg

DAIRY / EGGS — mg

2 tbsp	Margarine	360
2 cups	Milk (std or low-fat)	260
2 tbsp	Butter	260
25 g	Cheese	250

GRAIN / NUTS

1 plate	Porridge (salt added)	2300
4 slices	Bread (all types)	1200
¾ cup	Spaghetti (canned)	1000
1 svg	Cheese cake	800
1 plate	Cereals (with milk avg)	570
1 plate	Muesli	350
1/3 cup	Nuts (salted)	330
2	Weetbix (with milk)	260

MEAT / FISH (cooked)

100 g	Bacon	4500
2	Sausages	2200
2	Fish cakes	1900
100 g	Corned beef	1700
100 g	Ham	1200
100 g	Processed meat (avg)	1100
2	Saveloys (boiled)	1000
100 g	Fish (canned)	900
5 g	Soup stock (Oxo cube)	800

FAST FOOD

1 svg	Pizza (large)	3200
1	Hot dog	2100
1 svg	Fish and chips	2000
2 cups	Chips (salted)	1900
1 svg	Potato salad	1600
1	Hamburger (large)	1500
1	Hamburger (avg)	1200
1	Meat pie	950
1 bag	Potato crisps (50 g)	650
1/3 cup	Gravy	650
2 pces	Chicken (fried)	440
½ cup	Coleslaw	370
1	Fruit pie	320

SALT

1 tsp	Salt (table)	3500

VEGETABLES (cooked)

1 cup	Soup (canned, avg)	1900
4 slices	Beetroot (canned)	630
½ cup	Peas (canned)	300

HEALTH FOOD

100 g	Kidney	520
1 tsp	Marmite (yeast extract)	510
100 g	Liver	110

HEALTH HINT **Rid drinking water of chlorine**

If your local drinking water is heavily treated and has an objectionable chlorine smell, put some aside overnight in an open container such as a jug. The chlorine will soon evaporate and the smell disappear. Stirring can speed up the process.

Water filters with activated carbon cartridges remove the gas and its unpleasant smell from drinking water.

"It's not what we don't know that harms us, it's what we do know, that ain't so."
Mark Twain

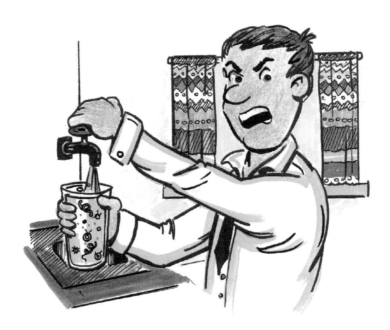

"Hell no! We haven't got that chlorine muck in our water!"

Chromium

Lack of chromium is believed to be the main cause of the common health problem of insulin/glucose resistance. This is a condition in which insulin becomes less effective at lowering our glucose levels.

The result is a high blood sugar level, which eventually leads to many of our modern chronic diseases – high blood fats (triglycerides), high blood pressure, obesity, type 2 diabetes, and artery inflammation leading to high LDL cholesterol and cardiovascular disease.

Lack of chromium can also cause hypoglycemia – a low blood sugar condition that causes mood swings and other related mental disorders.

Insulin/glucose resistance, hypoglycemia, type 2 diabetes and high LDL cholesterol are all on record as having been reversed by taking around 600 mcg of chromium a day in supplement form for a limited time. This should only be done under the guidance of a health professional. Results take about two months.

Generally, the more refined sugar we eat, the more chromium we require. Dr Robert Atkins writes, *"When your body exhibits low levels of the trace mineral (chromium), your craving for sugar grows. But the more sugar you eat, the more you deplete your chromium stores."*

Refined white sugar contains only traces of chromium – the original unrefined brown sugar does have sufficient chromium but this is lost during the refining process. It can be reclaimed by including a little molasses or treacle, the nutritious 'dregs' of refined sugar in your diet.

A huge 87% of chromium is also lost when wheat is refined to white flour. White flour is converted to glucose in our body, but requires chromium for the glucose to enter our body cells.

Most food grown in NZ crop soils test low in chromium, compared to overseas food. Surprisingly however, many of our NZ potato crisp brands test very high in chromium. This would appear likely due to a processing additive included during manufacture, as some brands contain barely a trace. A few other NZ processed foods are also surprisingly high in chromium, especially some heavy multigrain bread and Weetbix. However, these non-natural sources of chromium may possibly not be adequately absorbed. (The NZ 2009 Nutrition Survey did not include chromium, but similar American surveys have found widespread deficiencies – around 80% of the population. Pregnancy can halve body levels.)

Some nutritionists warn that chromium should be included with the intravenous glucose solution drips commonly given to patients in hospital after an operation.

In supplement form, both the polynicotinate and picolinate chelates of chromium appear to work well. Vanadium appears to play a similar role to chromium in the body, but has side effects, including mental instability.

Role of chromium in our body

- Assists in entry of glucose and fats to nourish our body cells.
- Helps maintain normal blood glucose levels.
- Helps prevent artery inflammation.

Too little chromium

- Insulin and glucose resistance. type 2 diabetes.
- High LDL cholesterol. High blood pressure. Heart attack. Stroke.
- Loss of effective blood sugar regulation. High homocysteine.
- Sugar craving.
- Hypoglycemia. Mood swing. Psychiatric disorders.

Too much chromium

- No known toxic effects.

Cooking losses

- No significant losses.

RDI	CHROMIUM			
Child:	15 mcg	Man:	35 mcg
Teenage boy:	25 mcg	Woman:	25 mcg
Teenage girl:	20 mcg	Pregnancy:	30 mcg

FRUIT		mcg
1	Kiwifruit (green organic)	7
1	Pear	6
100 g	Rhubarb	5
1	Apple	4

GRAIN / NUTS		
4 slices	Bread (heavy multigrain)	110
2	Weetbix	20
4 slices	Bread (wholemeal)	8
½ cup	Flour (wholemeal)	8

MEAT / FISH (cooked)		
100 g	Scallops	185
100 g	Paua	62
50 g	Oysters (rock)	31
100 g	Pork	28
100 g	Beef	25
100 g	Lamb	25
50 g	Oysters (dredged)	15
100 g	Chicken	6

VEGETABLES (cooked)		
1 bag	Potato crisps (50 g)	95
100 g	Yams	25
2 med	Potatoes	10
1 cup	Spaghetti	6
100 g	Most NZ vegetables	5

HEALTH FOOD		
1 tbsp	Brewers yeast	60
2 tsp	Molasses	35
1	Muesli bar	16
2 tbsp	Wheat germ	7
1 tsp	Marmite (yeast extract)	6

Chromium

HEALTH HINT   Use unrefined sugar

If we need to satisfy a sweet tooth it's better to do so using natural sugars such as fruit or honey, or less refined sugars such as raw sugar, brown sugar, golden syrup, treacle or molasses, all of which contain protective chromium, rather than foods made with nutrient-barren white sugar.

Molasses is especially rich in trace minerals, being the final remains of the sugar refining process.

HEALTH HINT   Test your own blood sugar

Home test kits are readily available to check your blood glucose levels using a drop of finger blood. They are quite cheap, only about $20 from online suppliers. You do however pay about 90c per test strip in NZ.

Normal fasting readings should be between 4.0 to 6.0 mmol/L (70 to 110 mg/dl). Higher readings up to 8.0 mmol/L (145 mg/dl) should only be seen while or after digesting a large meal.

Readings of 9.0 mmol/L (160 mg/dl) or over indicate insulin/glucose resistance and may require a diet change and/or more exercise.

HEALTH HINT   Pregnancy after using the pill

Major hormonal and cellular disturbances occur in a woman's body when she takes an oral contraceptive and it is generally best to avoid doing so if long term health is desired. Migraines and blood clots are among health issues linked to the contraceptive pill.

Women who are on the birth control pill and plan to eventually conceive, should use some other method of birth control at least three months before attempting conception.

The following nutrients should also be increased during that period – vitamins B1, B3, B6, B12, folate, vitamin C, selenium, zinc magnesium and iodine.

"The primitive diet was energy poor and nutrient rich, the modern diet is the opposite, which means we tend to be overweight yet malnourished."
Professor Robert Heaney, (calcium nutritionist for 50 years)

Copper

The right balance of copper in our body is essential – copper helps maintain collagen, to preserve the suppleness and depth of our skin, the flexibility of our bones and the strength and elasticity of our arteries and other body tissues.

Copper also helps slow our skin ageing and protect against stomach ulcers, bone fractures and most importantly, aneurisms and strokes. Some years ago in Canada, 32 young turkeys died suddenly from ruptured arteries and aneurisms. The cause was eventually traced to a commercial feed lacking in copper.

NZ farm animals are often deficient due to low copper levels in most of our soils.

Copper is required for the forming of our red and white blood cells and preventing oxidised LDL cholesterol from narrowing our arteries.

The correct copper balance is also essential to prevent the inflammation of rheumatoid arthritis – in one study of 1140 people with rheumatoid arthritis, 89% went into remission for three years following injections of copper (copper salicylate). Excess blood copper levels can likewise trigger this common disorder.

Excess copper, usually from water pipes can be fatal. The death of an Australian baby was traced to copper poisoning from the water pipes on the farm where the baby's family lived. The baby had been bottle-fed a milk formula using the farm water. A sure sign of high copper levels in tap water is a blue stain on white porcelain. NZ municipal water supplies are monitored to prevent excess copper levels.

An imbalance of copper can affect us mentally. Copper is a brain stimulant and can over enliven our brain at times. Young mammals, both animal and human, normally have higher copper levels than adults – this is believed by many nutritionists to explain the liveliness and high energy behaviour of most youngsters. It can also be a cause of the hyperactivity and short attention span of ADHD children. Supplementing with zinc, which helps regulate copper, has resulted in some ADHD children becoming normal.

A woman's blood level of copper normally doubles during pregnancy – this is to ensure her child retains sufficient copper for the early years when the infant's diet is low in this mineral. The excess copper in the mother's blood can take three months to return to normal and is thought to be a factor in the mental fragility of some women after pregnancy. Although an erratic sleep pattern (2 am feeds and night time crying) is generally accepted as the main cause. Other contributing factors during this time can be other mineral deficiencies, especially lack of molybdenum, zinc and the relaxing minerals, calcium, magnesium and selenium.

The birth control pill can also more than double copper levels in some women. (Temporary high copper levels are also believed to play a role in the onset of migraines.)

Zinc and vitamin C play key roles in regulating copper levels. Wherever an excess of copper is found, there is usually a deficiency of zinc and/or vitamin C.

Deficiencies of copper are commonly found in elderly women with osteoporosis, long term intravenously drip-fed hospital patients, and those with macular eye degeneration. In addition, whenever excessive zinc supplements (over 160 mg a day) have been taken without also taking extra copper.

Copper was not tested for in the NZ 2009 Nutrition Survey as it is widespread in food. Nevertheless, American surveys have revealed that 75% of the US population only get about half the recommended amount of copper, and the US RDA for copper is only about half that of the NZ RDI.

Shellfish, beans, nuts, whole wheat and liver are a rich food sources of copper.

A blood test can determine your copper status. The safe ranges for total copper are –

Men	11 – 22 umol/L	(64 –140 µg/dL)
Women	13 – 25 umol/L	(75 –160 µg/dL)
Women (pregnant)	19 – 47 umol/L	(110 –300 µg/dL)
Children	13 – 25 umol/L	(75 –160 µg/dL)

Role of copper in our body
- Assists in forming muscle, arteries, veins, collagen, skin and bone.
- Works with iron and zinc to form blood cells.
- Helps regulate and stimulate the brain.
- Helps protect the nervous system.
- Helps the body absorb iron.
- Assists in the pigmentation of hair and skin.

Too little copper
- Weak arteries and veins. Varicose veins. Stroke. Aneurism.
- Sagging muscles and early wrinkling of skin.
- Inflammation. Rheumatoid arthritis.
- Build up of oxidised LDL in arteries.
- Slow growth in children.

- Brittle bones. Osteoporosis.
- Macular degeneration.
- Weak red blood cells (anemia). Low white cells. Low energy.
- Lowered resistance to infections.
- Loss of hair and skin pigmentation.
- Nerve disorders. Loss of taste and smell. Sciatica.
- Depression.

Too much copper (often due to a lack of zinc)

- Hyperactivity. ADHD. Learning disabilities in children.
- Anxiety. Insomnia.
- Hallucinations. Autism. Schizophrenia.
- High blood pressure (anxiety based).
- PMT. Hair loss in women.
- Tinnitus (noise in the ears).

Cooking losses

- No significant losses.

HEALTH HINT   **Anxiety without obvious cause**

Anxiety without an obvious cause can be the result of mineral and/or vitamin deficiencies or imbalances and often affects sleep. High levels of copper or lead can bring about such symptoms. However, adequate vitamin C and zinc should flush these excesses from the body.

Lack of any of the B group vitamins, also vitamin C, and the minerals calcium, magnesium, manganese, zinc, selenium and potassium can produce similar symptoms.

Also taking a high dose of vitamin B6 (over 20 mg) or folate (over 4000 mcg) as a daily supplement.

HEALTH HINT   **Copper bracelets and arthritis**

On average, 78% of arthritics strongly maintain they feel less pain when they wear a copper bracelet. It's believed that a small amount of copper is absorbed through the skin.

"There is always a close connection between violent crime and severe mineral imbalances."   Dr Carl Pfeiffer, (Director Brain Bio Centre, USA)

RDI | COPPER

Infant:	220 mcg	Man:	1700 mcg
Child:	1000 mcg	Woman:	1200 mcg
Teenage boy:	1500 mcg	Pregnancy:	1300 mcg
Teenage girl:	1100 mcg	Breastfeeding:	1500 mcg

DAIRY / EGGS

		mcg
2	Eggs (med)	180

FRUIT

½	Avocado	270
1	Pear	220
10	Apricots (dried halves)	160
1 med	Banana	110

GRAIN / NUTS

4 slices	Bread (wholemeal)	930
1/3 cup	Cashew nuts	850
1/3 cup	Peanuts (roasted)	650
4 slices	Bread (white)	550
1/3 cup	Almond nuts	535
1/3 cup	Pistachio nuts	510
1/3 cup	Mixed nuts (avg)	500
1/3 cup	Pecan nuts	460
1 cup	Rice (brown cooked)	330
5	Walnuts	320
½ cup	Flour (wholemeal)	240
5	Brazil nuts	110
2	Weetbix	110
½ cup	Flour (white)	110
1 cup	Rice (white cooked)	100

VEGETABLES (cooked)

¾ cup	Baked beans	1700
2 cobs	Sweet corn	370
2 med	Potatoes (with skin)	340
½ cup	Green peas	260
1 cup	Vegetables (avg)	100

FISH (cooked)

5	Oysters (rock)	1800
50 g	Shrimp	1800
100 g	Crayfish	1300
50 g	Squid	1080
100 g	Paua	730
5	Oysters (dredged)	310
100 g	Fish (avg)	120

HEALTH FOOD

100 g	Liver (lamb)	9900
100 g	Liver (beef)	2300
100 g	Kidney (beef)	660
1 plate	Muesli cereal	534
2 tbsp	Pumpkin seeds	420
100 g	Kidney (lamb)	370
2 tbsp	Sesame seeds	390
1 tbsp	Molasses	100

"The greatest tragedy that comes to man is the emotional depression, the dulling of the intellect and the loss of initiative that comes from nutritive failure."

Dr James McLester, (former president of the American Medical Association)

135

Fluoride

Calcium fluoride, which is found naturally in the drinking water in some parts of the world, hardens teeth and slows down the rate of decay. However it is now believed that the calcium plays just as an important role as fluoride.

Other minerals also reduce tooth decay – magnesium, phosphorus, molybdenum and vitamins C and D. Sugar, with its high acidity is the arch enemy of tooth health, especially in chocolate and toffee.

The type of fluoride widely added to some domestic water supplies in New Zealand, Australia, the UK, Israel, Singapore and the US, is the toxic sodium fluoride. This chemical is far more easily absorbed by the body than calcium fluoride and is cumulative.

Signs of excess

Sodium fluoride does harden the teeth of growing children (up to the age of eight years) but too much can make their teeth more brittle and difficult to fill without breaking.

Staining of teeth is a reliable sign that a child's sodium fluoride intake is too high. This appears as a permanent white and yellowish-brown mottled effect. Surveys reveal that 25% of Auckland children in fluoridated areas have mild mottling and 3% serious mottling. Tooth mottling is linked with higher rates of bone fracture in people of all ages.

Sodium fluoride has also been found in 96 overseas studies to-date, to lower the IQ of children (and animals) by increasing the uptake of aluminium and lead into the brain. One Indian study found a 10% drop in average IQ. These effects start at a fluoride level of around 1.5 ppm.

Fluoride is rarely found above 0.01 ppm in breast milk, even when a mother's fluoride intake is high, which indicates it is harmful for infants. These side effects, along with serious doubts as to the effectiveness of fluoridated water in reducing decay, its accumulation in the body, and concern about lack of control over dosage in hot weather, fuel the emotionally charged debate that still continues.

Earlier studies challenged

An intake of 1500 mcg daily (1.5 ppm) of sodium fluoride was originally claimed on the basis of English and American studies in the 1950's to reduce child tooth decay an average of 55%. However in recent decades these studies have been widely challenged as being flawed.

Foremost among challengers was dentist John Colquhoun, once the Principal Dental Officer for NZ – when he learned that children drinking unfluoridated, but molybdenum-rich water in the city of Napier, had less tooth decay than those in the fluoridated city of Hastings, he travelled widely overseas to investigate the truth about fluoride.

It soon became apparent to him that the dramatic decrease in tooth decay worldwide was due more to the improved post-depression and wartime diet (which had been largely white bread and jam) rather than the effects of fluoride (see chart over the page).

Because of this evidence, he did an about turn from his former support of fluoridation and became a thorn in the side of his orthodox colleagues, who in his eyes appeared more anxious to preserve their reputations than accept the truth.

Tooth decay again on the increase

Nowadays, survey after survey both worldwide and here in New Zealand, clearly show no significant differences between non-fluoridated and fluoridated communities.

Some researchers believe this is due to the widespread availability of fluoridated toothpaste, which may well be the case. Fluoridated toothpaste has proven effective in providing growing children's teeth with the hardening effects of fluoride – it should not be swallowed however, but this is difficult to enforce with pre-schoolers.

Despite decades of dietary improvement, recent NZ studies have found tooth decay on the increase again among young children – this has been attributed to a reduced government school dental service.

Standard activated carbon water filters will not remove fluoride from drinking water – it requires an activated alumina filter, reverse osmosis system or a steam distiller. Fluoride is normally tasteless in water.

Role of fluoride in our body
- Increases mineral density in teeth and bones.
- Increases absorption of the toxic minerals aluminium and lead.

Too little fluoride
- Less resistance to acid tooth decay for children up to eight years old.

Too much fluoride (Over 1.5 ppm sodium fluoride in water)
- Mottled, brittle teeth.
- Lowered IQ from increased uptake of aluminium and lead.
- Hyperactivity and attention disorders in children (ADHD).
- Abnormally brittle bones. Osteoporosis.
- Increased risk of cataracts over the age of 60.

"The highest fluoride content in bone ash was observed in women with severe osteoporosis."   E.M. Alhava, Finland, (bone researcher)

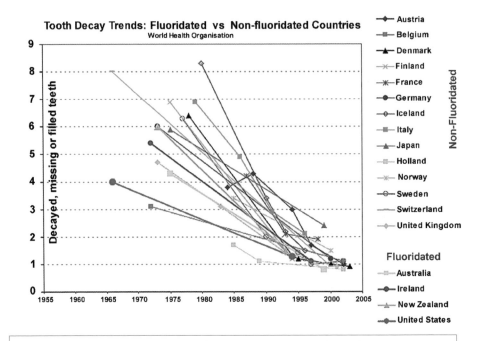

Tooth Decay Trends: Fluoridated vs Non-fluoridated Countries
World Health Organisation

Legend:
- Austria
- Belgium
- Denmark
- Finland
- France
- Germany
- Iceland
- Italy
- Japan
- Holland
- Norway
- Sweden
- Switzerland
- United Kingdom

Non-Fluoridated

Fluoridated
- Australia
- Ireland
- New Zealand
- United States

Y-axis: Fluoride / Decayed, missing or filled teeth (0–9)
X-axis: 1955 1960 1965 1970 1975 1980 1985 1990 1995 2000 2005

Fluoridated water supplies in New Zealand

If your town or city is not on this list, it is probably unfluoridated

Ashhurst	Milton
Auckland city (excl Onehunga & Huia)	Ngaruawahia
Buckland	North Shore City
Burnham Military Camp	Palmerston North
Clarks Beach	Papakura
Dunedin city	Paraparaumu
Feilding	Patamahoe
Flaxmere	Porirua
Gisborne city	Pukekohe
Hamilton city	Stratford
Hastings city	Tapanui
Havelock North	Taupo
Hawera	Thames
Hibiscus Coast (Orewa)	Timaru
Huntly	Tokoroa
Invercargill	Upper Hutt
Kaitangata	Waiau Pa
Linton	Waitakere
Lower Hutt (excl Korokoro & Petone)	Waikanae
Manukau	Wellington
Masterton	Whakatane
Methven Township	Waipukurau

Source FANNZ 2016

HEALTH HINT   Avoiding tooth decay

If you ever indulge in sticky sweet foods such as chocolate and toffee, which leave a residue in the hollows of your back teeth, you should immediately after eating, chew a dry crust of bread, or eat an apple. This should remove the sticky residue from your molars where most tooth decay occurs. But check in a mirror when possible, just to make sure it's all gone.

Sugar acid decay takes place during the first half hour after eating sticky sweets. Brushing our teeth later at night before bed is too late, the damage has already been done – immediate action is needed.

HEALTH HINT   Avoiding asthma

Two main causes of indoor asthma in NZ are –

1. Airborne dust-mite feces from bedding (especially wool blankets) and to a lesser extent wool carpets.
2. Ultra-fine airborne dried saliva from cat fur. (Surprisingly, a child's exposure to pet dogs is linked to reduced asthma sensitivity.)

Outdoors the main culprit in NZ is rye grass pollen.

To prevent indoor asthma, low humidity is essential – mites cannot survive below 50% humidity. The humidity of the average NZ home is high, typically between 60% and 80%.

An air conditioner or dehumidifier will lower indoor humidity, but window ventilation can also be an effective, lower cost approach. Cooking in a poorly ventilated kitchen is also a major source of moisture.

Bedrooms should be well ventilated, with ideally, a continually open window. Wash all bedding, even pillows, every two weeks in hot water over 54°C (130°F) – cold or warm water will not kill dust mites.

Vacuum carpets weekly with all exterior house doors wide open, to help remove the fine airborne dust, and afterwards wipe down dust-collecting surfaces with a damp cloth.

Nutrients from fruit and vegetables and the avoidance of sugary drinks and foods can greatly help in preventing over-sensitivity to airborne allergens, including rye grass pollen.

Increased sensitivity to asthma is linked to over-cleanliness when raising children (they need to be exposed to everyday bacterial germs to develop immunity), also excess sugar, excess phosphorus, MSG type flavour enhancers, nitrate preservatives in processed meat, sulphites in dried fruit, and lack of the minerals selenium, magnesium, manganese and zinc.

Iodine

A tiny but critical amount of this important mineral is essential for our body. Iodine is found in every one of our trillions of body cells. It helps regulate energy, produce numerous hormones and correctly forms a child in the mother's womb. It can also protect us to a degree from radioactive fallout.

Iodine is absorbed from our blood by the thyroid gland, located in the throat. If our diet lacks iodine, the thyroid gland will enlarge, sometimes hugely, in order to trap more particles. This condition is called goitre and was common in NZ before iodine was added to table salt.

Natural iodine is lost from sea salt during processing. An inorganic type, potassium iodate is added afterward to iodise table salt. Since 2009, iodised salt is also required to be used in NZ commercial bread making.

Goitre is beginning to appear again in NZ as iodised table salt usage drops and a previous 'contamination' source – iodine-based disinfectant in milk from processing plants has been reduced.

Iodine deficiency occurs at a staggering rate here in NZ (and many other countries also). The NZ 2009 Nutrition Survey, using urinary analysis which approximates the daily intake of iodine, incredibly did not find a single New Zealander even close to the RDI intake of 150 mcg per day (urine reading 150 mcg/L). One teenage Maori boy came close at 95 mcg/L, but the average level was only 53 mcg/L, with women at the critical childbearing ages the lowest of all at 42 - 55 mcg/L.

The average daily intake in the US is three times higher at 165 mcg. Japan's daily intake is an astonishing 57 times higher again, averaging around 9500 mcg. This is mostly due to their consumption of kelp (kombu) as a daily food.

This is a serious health concern, as iodine deficiency is one of the leading preventable causes of mental impairment (cretinism) in infants – IQ is typically reduced by 10 to 15 points. Other major problems are miscarriages, still-births, body malformations, stunted growth, ADHD and sometimes hearing and eyesight problems.

There is also evidence that this deficiency is responsible for the increase in some cancers. Dr David Brownstein, a specialist in iodine deficiencies states, *"I have no doubt that this deficiency is responsible (at least in-part) for the epidemic of cancers of the breast and prostate."*

Other health problems that afflict adults when iodine is deficient, (besides a swollen neck) are sluggish obesity, protruding eyes, a thick voice, painful lumps in the breasts of women, tremors, high LDL cholesterol levels and cardiovascular disease.

Although most NZ soils are low in iodine, kelp seaweed is an abundant source as it concentrates iodine from the minerals in seawater. NZ kelp powder is high in iodine and half a teaspoon provides more than enough for a week. It is also cheap at about $15 per 100 g. It can be added to home baking.

Unrefined rock salt is another source of quality iodine and one that can be recycled by the body. Rock salt is sea salt mined from ancient sea beds and is generally about seven times higher in iodine than unrefined sea salt.

Iodine can also be an effective disinfectant. In some tinctured forms it is used by trampers as a water purifier.

Role of iodine in our body
- Required to correctly form the body and brain of a fetus.
- Helps the body produce thyroid and other hormones.
- Assists in regulating our body temperature and energy levels.
- Helps control cholesterol levels.
- Can protect against radiation.

Too little iodine (less than 50 mcg daily)
- Enlarged thyroid gland (goitre).
- Painful breast lumps in women (fibrocystic breast). Infertility.
- Ovarian cysts. Uterine fibroids.
- Miscarriage. Still birth. Stunted growth of children.
- Over-sensitivity to cold. Reduced body temperature.
- Restless legs. Tremors.
- Underactive thyroid. Thick voice. Low energy. Apathy.
- Obesity. Dementia-like symptoms.
- Malformed, mentally slow or ADHD infants if the mother is deficient.
- Artery inflammation. High LDL cholesterol. Heart attack. Stroke.
- Cancer of breast, prostate, ovaries, thyroid and uterus.
- Dry skin and mouth.
- Macular degeneration (factor).

Too much iodine (Over 2,000,000 mcg daily inorganic)
- Overactive thyroid. Hyperactivity. Weight loss. Bulging eyes.
- No reported toxic effects from natural dietary iodine.

Cooking losses
- No significant losses.

"Hunger is good sauce."   Cervantes

RDI	IODINE		
Child:	100 mcg	Woman:	150 mcg
Teenager:	150 mcg	Pregnancy:	220 mcg
Man:	150 mcg	Breastfeeding:	270 mcg

ALL FOOD		mcg			
½ tsp	Kelp (powder)	1700	100 g	Fish (cooked, avg)	35
½ tsp	Salt (iodised table)	130	½ tsp	Salt (rock, unrefined)	30
5	Oysters	80	2 med	Eggs	13
2 cups	Milk (std or low-fat)	44	½ tsp	Salt (sea, unrefined)	4

More than 96% of doctor's patients had low iodine levels

Dr David Brownstein MD (who recommends 2000 mcg of iodine a day) writes, *"Iodine has consistently provided the most satisfying clinical results as compared to any other nutrient. To date (7 years) my partners and I have tested nearly 5000 patients for iodine levels. Our results show that more than 96 percent of patients tested have low iodine levels with the vast majority being severely iodine deficient. The consequences of iodine deficiency are severe – mental retardation, lowered IQ, attention deficit hyperactivity disorder (ADHD), infertility, thyroid problems, and cancer of the breast, prostate, ovaries, thyroid and uterus."*

HEALTH HINT   All trace minerals in unrefined salt

All the trace minerals required by our bodies are found in sea water, which contains 77 different minerals and elements – although mostly only in tiny amounts. However, they are in colloidal form (dissolvable in water) and therefore readily absorbed by our body. (Pygmy races are usually isolated from mineral-rich ocean foods and salt.)

Refined salt has had all but a few of the 77 minerals and elements removed, to cleanse it from sea pollutants, also to provide whiteness, long shelf life and free running characteristics.

Unrefined rock salt (rock salt is sea salt mined from ancient sea beds) is also a good source of colloidal sea minerals and is generally higher in iodine than unrefined sea salt.

Iron

Iron is used by our red blood cells to transport oxygen (using hemoglobin proteins) to every cell for energy, especially our muscles. Lack of iron reduces the number or size of these energy carrying red cells, or the amount of hemoglobin they can carry and they then become paler in colour. This is called anemia and is one of the most common nutritional disorders in the world among women.

Anemia (sometimes spelled anaemia) results in muscle weakness, low energy, easily broken bones, frequent infections and numerous other health problems. It can produce unnaturally pale skin and finger nails. Iron deficiency anemia is said to affect 25% of the world's population, mostly women of menstruating age. The average loss of iron per menstrual period is about 10 mg and can be as high as 30 mg.

Other persons commonly affected, are children going through growth spurts, elderly men over 70 with weak stomach acid, and athletes such as long distance runners and cyclists. Iron deficiency anemia develops slowly, and correcting it can also be a slow process.

In the NZ 2009 Nutritional Survey, 34% of girls aged 13 to 19 were deficient in iron – Maori/Pacific teenage girls were even worse at 49%. Women aged 20 to 50 fared better at 15% but again Maori/Pacific women were 27% deficient. All other groups had adequate levels.

Poor iron absorption a problem

Researchers have found there is nearly always enough iron in most diets, but poor absorption is the problem – this is allowed for in the RDI.

The absorption of iron from food ranges from a high of 50% in human breast milk (due to high amounts of lactoferrin in human milk), 25% from liver, shellfish and beef, and only 10% from grains. (However vitamin C enhances absorption from grains – just 25 mg of vitamin C with a grain meal can double the absorption of iron from 10% to about 20%.) Wheat is actually a good source of iron and our main source of the mineral in NZ, according to the above Nutrition Survey. It accounts for 40% of our total intake, with flesh protein foods next, accounting for 18%.

Healthy gut probiotics (friendly bacteria) are also critical for absorption. Researcher Dr Peter Rothschild says, *"Of the 750 million people on this planet who suffer from iron deficiency symptoms, less than half of them suffer from any actual lack of iron in their diet."* He then goes on to point out the vital role of probiotics in the digestive system, especially lactoferrin, which greatly enhances the absorbability of iron. Lactoferrin is found mostly in colostrum and whey protein.

Laboratory studies have found that tannin in tea and to a lesser extent in coffee, reduces iron absorption from food in some circumstances – however more recent studies have concluded that this is not significant in real life.

There is good evidence that a well nourished person can increase or decrease iron absorption according to their needs. Pregnant women commonly increase their absorption rate. Molybdenum also plays a role in regulating iron levels in the body.

The use of stomach acid lowering drugs such as Losec (Omeprazole) can hinder the absorption of iron and other minerals from protein foods, as they lower the amount of stomach acid produced.

Low iron levels can also be caused by internal blood loss from the stomach or intestines, which excessive aspirin can cause. High internal losses will normally darken the feces, whereas slow losses are hard to detect, but over a long period of time both can result in anemia.

Too much iron a serious problem

On the other hand, too much iron is just as serious as too little – even more so, and health problems can be severe.

Iron overload is typically due to cheap, inorganic forms of iron used in many pharmaceutical iron supplements and in fortified foods like breakfast cereals. When taking an iron supplement, or a food with added iron, we should ensure that the iron is organic and chelated (ie, combined with a digestible protein, like the iron found naturally in our food). This type of organic iron is called heme iron and is seldom if ever, over-absorbed by the body.

The inorganic, non-heme types of iron however (usually listed as ferrous sulphate, iron sulphate, gluconate or fumarate) can be absorbed up to 10 times more than organic heme iron, often far in excess of our body's needs – this promotes harmful, free radical oxidising activity.

Inorganic iron particularly affects people with hemochromatosis, which is a genetic inability to expel excess iron. Hemochromatosis affects about 20,000 New Zealanders, mostly of European descent.

Low energy can be a symptom of iron overload, just as it is a symptom of iron deficiency, but a more serious problem of non-heme iron overload is that it causes LDL cholesterol to oxidise and block arteries. Cholesterol normally only blocks arteries when it's been oxidised, and free radical activity from iron overload allows this to happen.

When a Finnish heart researcher first made this significant discovery regarding iron overload, Dr Robert Atkins astutely observed, *"Thus it turns out that iron, not estrogen, explains the low risk of coronary heart disease among women in their child bearing years."* Iron overload is rarely found in women of child bearing age, due to menstrual blood loss.

Iron overload is also found in approx 45% of arthritics, especially those with arthritis in their fingers.

Because of these important findings, inorganic iron has now been banned from food by France, Germany and other European nations.

Blood tests for iron deficiency or iron overload

Hemoglobin test One important iron test is the measuring of hemo-globin levels which determines the oxygen-carrying capacity of the red blood cells – the higher the better. Readings below 120 g/l (12 gm/dL) for women and 137 g/l (14 gm/dL) for men indicates anemia.

This test was also done as part of the NZ 2009 Nutritional Survey. Average levels were found to be quite low – 133 g/l (13 gm/dL) for women and 149 g/l (15 gm/dL) for men. Of concern were the 26% of men aged over 71 who were at or below the anemic level. This is normally due to weak stomach acid, often from medication to reduce stomach acid levels.

Serum Ferritin test This test was also done as part of the survey – it measures how much iron is stored in the body. The safe upper limit for women is around 200 mcg/L (ng/mL in USA) and for men 300 mcg/L. Readings below 12 mcg/L for women, or 24 mcg/L for men reveal seriously low iron stores. Readings above the 200/300 limits indicate iron overload and can seriously increase the risk of cardiovascular disease, arthritis and cancer. High readings can also indicate hemo-chromatosis.

The average for women was found to be 80 mcg/L, with 8% below the anemic level of 12 mcg/L. The average for men was 177 mcg/L with only 1% of men below the anemic level of 24. The highest reading was 287.

Role of iron in our body
- Assists in forming red blood cells.
- Transports oxygen energy to our muscles.
- Helps build and maintain bone and protein tissue.

Too little iron
- Weak red blood cells (anemia). Pale skin and nails
- Low energy. Muscle weakness. Depression. Chronic fatigue.
- Heart palpitations during physical exertion or stress.
- Soft, sometimes concave nails, especially thumbnails.
- Weak, easily broken bones.
- Dark circles under the eyes.
- Poor concentration. Easily distracted. Lowered intelligence.

- Lack of growth in children. Irritability. Fearfulness. Tantrums.
- Smooth shiny tongue. Difficulty in swallowing food.
- Low immunity to infection. Frequent colds and flu. Candida.
- Slow recovery from sickness or surgery.
- Redness and/or cracks at the corners of the mouth.
- Excessive PMT symptoms. Excessive bleeding. Low libido.
- Decreased fertility. Complications during pregnancy.
- Lowered thyroid function. Difficulty losing weight.
- Feel the cold unduly. Cold hands and feet.

Too much iron (over 70 mg daily of non-heme inorganic iron)

- Grey or black stools. Constipation. Diarrhea.
- Free radical damage. Greyish or bronze hue to the skin.
- Low energy. Lack of endurance. Muscle weakness.
- Reduced testosterone. Low libido. Impotence in men.
- Oxidised LDL cholesterol deposits. Narrowed arteries.
- Cardiovascular disease. Heart attack. Stroke.
- Increased risk of common cancers, especially breast cancer.
- Rheumatoid arthritis especially in the fingers.
- Risk of hemochromatosis. Cirrhosis of the liver.
- Ringing in the ears. Tinnitus.
- Dementia. Parkinsons disease. Alzheimer's.

Cooking losses

- No significant loss if cooking fluids are consumed.

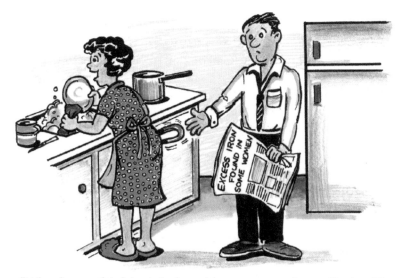

"Why do you think I might be taking too many iron pills dear?"

RDI IRON

Infant:	11 mg	Woman:	18 mg
Child:	10 mg	Woman over 50:	8 mg
Teenage boy:	11 mg	Pregnancy:	27 mg
Teenage girl:	15 mg	Breastfeeding:	9 mg
Man:	8 mg		

DAIRY / EGGS — mg

		mg
2 cups	Milo (all milk)	5.0
2 med	Eggs	2.2
1 cup	Soy milk	2.0

FRUIT

1/3 cup	Figs (dried)	2.0
1 cup	Cantaloupe	1.4
5	Prunes	1.2
½	Avocado	1.2

GRAIN / NUTS

4 slices	Bread (wholemeal)	6.0
½ cup	Soy flour (full fat)	5.1
1	Bran muffin (large)	5.0
2	Weetbix	4.3
1 plate	Breakfast cereal	3.0
4 slices	Bread (white)	2.6
½ cup	Flour (wholemeal)	2.5
1 plate	Corn/wheat cereal	2.2
1/3 cup	Almond/cashew nuts	2.0
1 tbsp	Cocoa	2.0
50 g	Chocolate	2.0
½ cup	Flour (white)	1.4
1 slice	Chocolate cake	1.2
1 plate	Muesli	1.2
1	Muesli bar	1.1
1 plate	Porridge	1.0
1/3 cup	Peanuts (roasted)	1.0

MEAT / FISH (cooked)

2	Paua (large shellfish)	12.6
100 g	Mussels	11.0
5	Oysters	7.5
100 g	Pipis (clams)	6.0
100 g	Shrimps/sardines	5.0
1	Eggburger	4.7
100 g	Beef	3.5
1	Hamburger	2.9
100 g	Lamb	2.7
100 g	Chicken	2.6
1	Pie meat	2.5
100 g	Pork	2.0
100 g	Fish (avg)	1.0
5 g	Soup stock (Oxo cube)	1.0

VEGETABLES (cooked)

¾ cup	Beans (boiled)	3.0
2 cobs	Sweet corn	2.4
¾ cup	Baked beans	2.0
1 cup	Broccoli	1.6
¾ cup	Peas	1.5
1 bag	Potato crisps (50 g)	1.3

HEALTH FOOD

100 g	Liver or kidney (lamb)	10.0
100 g	Liver or kidney (beef)	8.0
½ cup	Tofu	6.5
1 cup	Prune juice	5.0
2 tbsp	Pumpkin seeds	4.5
2 tbsp	Wheatgerm	3.0
1 tsp	Marmite (yeast extract)	2.3
1 tbsp	Brewers yeast	1 5
1 tsp	Curry powder	1.5
1 tsp	Turmeric	1.5
1 tsp	Cinnamon	1.5
2 tbsp	Sunflower seeds	1.0
1 tbsp	Molasses/treacle	1.0

"The most important crop is a race of healthy men and women. This is only possible if the soil is fertile."

Sir Albert Howard 1873 –1947 (English botanist, and organic farming pioneer)

Magnesium

Magnesium is the most seriously deficient bulk mineral in the NZ diet. Symptoms of too little magnesium include many common health problems. NZ soils tend to be low in magnesium and the mineral is not replenished by most commercial fertilisers.

Magnesium is also lost during the processing of food – about 80% is removed when wheat is milled into white flour and all the magnesium is lost during the refining of white sugar.

Also competing for the limited supplies of magnesium in our body is calcium, as it requires magnesium to enter our bones. This often leaves insufficient magnesium for the numerous other needs of the body.

Water-expelling diuretic drugs like frusemide and excessive sweating also deplete body supplies of magnesium.

Surprisingly, considering its huge importance to health and widespread deficiency, magnesium was not included in the NZ 2009 Nutrition Survey. However, a similar survey by the US Gallup Organization found 72% of adult Americans were short of their recommended RDA amount of magnesium, which is the same as the NZ and Australian RDI.

Magnesium is one of our body's seven bulk (macro) minerals – the other six are calcium, phosphorus, potassium, sulphur, sodium and chloride.

Keeps calcium in the bones, not the tissues

Magnesium has a huge effect on calcium absorption by our bones. Having the optimum amount of magnesium (about half our calcium intake) can cut our requirement for calcium to less than half the current NZ RDI of 1000 mg each day.

Magnesium deficiency is a common cause of calcium-hardened arteries, (also kidney and gallbladder stones). This is because magnesium helps retain calcium in our bones, and keep it out of our soft tissues and arteries where it can be harmful. Calcium hardened arteries are a major cause of high blood pressure in the elderly. (Vitamin K2 plays a protective role here also.)

Less cardiovascular disease

Men and women with diets high in magnesium have only half the rate of cardiovascular disease compared to those with low levels of magnesium in their diet. In areas of the world where the magnesium content of drinking water is high (around 150 mg per litre) ie, hard water, there is an average 13% lower incidence of heart disease. (Auckland tap water contains about 20 mg of magnesium per litre.)

Magnesium also helps protect against inflammation of our arteries, the main cause of cardiovascular disease. Our nerves depend on magnesium to avoid becoming overstimulated, which helps keep our arteries relaxed. This reduces stress related high blood pressure and the risk of fibrillation (erratic heartbeat).

Arteries contain muscles that cause them to tense and narrow under stress and anxiety. Blood pressure drugs work by relaxing these tense arteries, but sufficient magnesium can often do it naturally.

Other health benefits of magnesium

Frequent muscle cramps are generally caused by a lack of magnesium. Calcium is involved in muscle contracting (tensing) – magnesium balances this effect and afterwards relaxes the muscle.

Taking higher than normal amounts of magnesium, about 450 mg a day, has been found to relieve pre-eclampsia (toxemia) in women during late pregnancy. Many people also find relief from repetitive strain injury (RSI) by increasing their magnesium intake.

Epsom salts (magnesium sulphate) dissolved in bath water can be a relaxing way to supply magnesium to our body through the skin. Epsom salts is also a quick laxative remedy that's been used for centuries – just stir a tablespoon into warm water and drink it.

There are numerous other roles of magnesium in the body – researchers list over 300. They are so diverse there's hardly any body system unaffected by a magnesium deficiency. Our bones, blood, arteries, digestive system, nerves, kidneys, liver, hormonal glands and brain all rely on magnesium for proper function and protection. Even our tooth enamel is largely magnesium.

As magnesium helps relax muscles, nerves, brain and mind, people who are deficient can be tense and irritable – they often report difficulty in relaxing and sleeping. Magnesium administered intravenously has given rapid relief from migraines and stopped asthma attacks instantly. Up to 600 mg a day has cured cases of chronic fatigue.

Low levels of magnesium are commonly found among depressed adults, autistic children and those with Alzheimer's. Magnesium is critically important in protecting our brain and eyes from MSG-aspartate excitotoxin damage. More about this later in the book.

Blood tests to detect magnesium deficiency are virtually useless, as only about 1% of our body's magnesium circulates in the blood – 99% is held inside the cells.

Role of magnesium in our body

- Protects and relaxes muscles, arteries and our nervous system.

- Promotes a calm mind and lessens the effects of stress.
- Helps regulate movement of potassium in and out of the cells.
- Builds and maintains strength of our muscles and bones.
- Helps regulate bone growth in children.
- Helps absorb and retain calcium in our bones and teeth.
- Forms and maintains tooth enamel.
- Helps prevent fibrillation (erratic heartbeat).
- Helps regulate blood pressure by relaxing the arteries.
- Helps optimise HDL and LDL cholesterol levels.
- Helps prevent internal blood clots.
- Assists blood sugar regulation and energy production.
- Helps maintain the correct pH of blood and body cells.
- Promotes healthy and restful sleep.
- Protects brain and nerve neurons from MSG/aspartate damage.
- Promotes bowel regularity and healthy digestion.
- Reduces symptoms of PMS.

Too little magnesium

- Poor absorption and regulation of calcium from food.
- Low levels of potassium in the blood and cells.
- Calcium build up in arteries (atherosclerosis) and other tissues.
- Calcium build up in the kidneys, gallbladder or bladder (stones).
- Weak bones. Osteoporosis. Bunions.
- Easily decayed teeth. Porous enamel.
- Abnormal heart rhythms. Heart valve damage. Angina.
- High blood pressure. Rapid pulse. Water retention.
- Artery inflammation. High LDL cholesterol. Heart attack. Stroke.
- Migraines. Nervousness. Irritability. Jumpiness. Frequent urination.
- Low tolerance to stress. Headaches. Cold hands and feet.
- Poor sleep and relaxation. Anxiety disorders. Panic attacks.
- Oversensitivity to loud sounds. Tinnitus.
- Prostate enlargement in men. Difficult urination.
- Hyperactivity. Attention disorders in children (ADHD).
- Depression. Confusion. Autism. Convulsions. Parkinsons. Alzheimer's.
- Repetitive Strain Injury (RSI). Poor co-ordination.
- Numbness. Tingling. Trembling hands. Multiple Sclerosis (MS).
- Muscle weakness. Tremors. Spasms. Restless legs.
- Low energy. Weak muscles. Apathy. Chronic fatigue.
- Muscle cramps. Facial twitches.
- Fibromyalgia. Polymyalgia. Back and neck muscle pain.
- Chest tightness. Difficulty in breathing. Asthma.
- Fluctuating blood sugar levels. Hypoglycemia. Type 2 diabetes.
- Excessively wrinkled skin for age.
- Macular degeneration. Blurry vision. Light sensitivity. Glaucoma.

- Pre-menstrual tension (PMT). Menopausal difficulties.
- Pre-eclampsia (toxemia) during pregnancy.
- Breast tenderness.
- Stomach ulcers. Constipation. Body odour.
- Loss of appetite. Nausea. Anorexia nervosa. Crohn's disease.
- Sugar, chocolate, salt craving. Alcohol addiction.

Too much magnesium
(Over 450 mg a day from supplements)
- Stomach upset. Diarrhea.
- Light headedness. Low blood pressure.

Cooking losses
- No significant loss if cooking fluids are consumed.

RDI	MAGNESIUM			
Child:	100 mg	Woman:	320 mg	
Teenage boy:	410 mg	Pregnancy:	360 mg	
Teenage girl:	360 mg	Breastfeeding:	320 mg	
Man:	420 mg			

DAIRY   mg

		mg
4 tbsp	Whey protein powder	55

FRUIT

1 med	Banana	45

GRAIN / NUTS

1/3 cup	Almonds	135
1 plate	Wheat bran cereal	115
1/3 cup	Other nuts (avg)	90
1 plate	Muesli (with milk)	85
½ cup	Flour (soy)	80
1 plate	Porridge (with milk)	60
5	Brazil nuts	55
50 g	Chocolate (dark)	55
4 slices	Bread (wholemeal)	55
½ cup	Flour (wholemeal)	50
2	Weetbix (with milk)	45
½ cup	Rice (brown)	45

MEAT / FISH (cooked)

100 g	Pipis (clams)	140
100 g	Shrimp	110
2	Paua	95
100 g	Oysters	55
100 g	Fish (avg)	45

VEGETABLES (cooked)

1 cup	Taro leaves	210
1 cup	Taro root	110
2 cobs	Sweet corn	110
¾ cup	Chick peas	85
¾ cup	Baked beans	60
2 med	Potatoes	40
½ cup	Silverbeet (chard)	35

HEALTH FOOD

1 tsp	Dolomite powder	450
2 tbsp	Pumpkin seeds	160
2 tbsp	Sunflower seeds	105
2 tbsp	Wheat bran	60
1 tbsp	Molasses	50
2 tbsp	Wheat germ	40

"For every drug that benefits a patient, there is a natural substance that can achieve the same effect."   Dr Carl C. Pfeiffer MD, PhD

HEALTH HINT Healing tinnitus

Ringing, buzzing or hissing in the ears, known as tinnitus can be caused by a magnesium and/or potassium deficiency, aggravated by stress. There is no known medical drug cure.

Taking high dosages of aspirin too frequently can cause tinnitus, as can the anti-depressant drug citalopram.

There have been reports of the problem going away when ceasing the excessive drinking of diet soft drinks (sodas) containing the chemical sweetener aspartame.

All of the above indicates a link with glutamate/aspartate brain damage. (See chapter on **Avoiding Alzheimer's.**)

German researchers have found that the herbal extract ginkgo biloba at 180 mg a day (half in the morning and half at night) can sometimes provide relief.

Tinnitus can be a cruel affliction – if dietary changes fail to bring relief, numerous dramatic cures, or at least a great reduction in noise, have been reported by Christian faith healers.

HEALTH HINT Stress and health problems

Tenseness from anger, resentment, racing the clock or prolonged worry, can cause narrowed arteries and heart disease just as surely as smoking, poor diet and a lack of exercise.

Tenseness also causes numerous other health disorders – this is mostly due to stress hormones such as adrenalin and cortisol being constantly released into the bloodstream.

To counteract this, three minerals act as natural relaxants to our body and mind – these are magnesium, calcium and selenium.

Some foods also help – milk, chicken, tuna, bananas, oranges and pears. These foods have a relaxing and sleep-inducing effect on the body due to their tryptophan content.

Also three principles that minimise emotional stress can be found in the Health Hint on page 82 – **Three rules to minimise stress.**

"As a cardiologist, I see more people for heart related ailments than for any other problem. About 98% I'd guess, need magnesium, and all of them benefit from it."   Dr Robert Atkins MD

HEALTH HINT   Chronic fatigue or CFS/ME cures

A common factor preceding chronic fatigue syndrome (CFS or ME), is a stressful incident – commonly hospitalisation, or the death of a loved one, usually followed by prolonged lack of restful sleep. CFS is notoriously difficult to cure medically as there is usually no apparent physical cause, however, the combination of a nutritious diet, a peaceful lifestyle and patience seem to eventually work in most cases.

Interestingly, an American psychologist Dr Edith Fiore reports that she has immediately cured thousands of CFS patients, by releasing under hypnosis, the spirits of deceased relatives or friends, who have attached to them and are draining their energy. Her fascinating book on this topic (for the open minded) is called *"The Unquiet Dead"*. Psychiatrists worldwide are adopting her methods with equal success.

In a 1995 study of 23 CFS sufferers at Johns Hopkins University, it was found that 22 of them had lower than normal blood pressure. So 19 of them agreed to try a high salt diet. The result was that 9 were completely cured and the 10 others improved in varying degrees.

HEALTH HINT   Breaking an addiction

Most NZ adults will at some stage be prescribed a sleeping pill or tranquilliser to help them through a stressful period.

Medical practitioners are generally reluctant to take this course as many patients rapidly become seriously addicted to these drugs and their lives can be seriously shortened with continual use.

Manufacturers of these drugs (such as zopiclone and temazepam) generally warn strongly against taking them for periods longer than 10 days, but this appears to be widely ignored.

For those who are addicted and need to give them up, the following guidelines have been found to work:

1. Choose a settled time in which to break the addiction.

2. Be prepared for a temporary increase in anxiety, insomnia and forgetfulness – these are withdrawal symptoms and will pass.

3. Cut down your total weekly dosage by approx 25% for the first two weeks, by taking only a section of the pill. Then cut back a further 25% again for another two weeks. Keep reducing the weekly dosage 25% at two weekly intervals until only the equivalent of one pill a week is taken. Then stop completely.

Withdrawal symptoms should end three weeks after the final dose.

Manganese

Manganese has numerous roles in our body – many of them similar to magnesium. Manganese works hand-in-hand with zinc and is involved in creating enzymes for thousands of chemical processes in the body. These processes range from maximising brain efficiency to retaining the youthfulness of our skin, joint and bone collagen and also our arteries and nerves.

Manganese is also required for the correct formation of a child in its mother's womb – it helps form all the baby's bones correctly and to avoid body tissue defects such as cleft palate.

The NZ intake of manganese has generally been thought satisfactory, especially for farm animals, so it wasn't tested for in the 2009 Nutritional Survey. It may not be all that satisfactory for humans however – wheat is our main source of manganese and the milling of wheat into white flour removes half the manganese.

100% whole wheat products are rare in NZ – we should perhaps be grateful that Weetbix, bran flakes, muesli and similar wholegrain cereals are still popular. We may never have produced sports teams of the calibre of the All Blacks without such mineral-rich whole breakfast foods.

Soy is rich in manganese, but is also high in plant estrogens which have been linked with estrogen/progesterone hormonal imbalances in post-menopausal women and breast growth in older men.

Mineral content of our food continues to fall

Manganese is one of many trace minerals not often replenished by fertilisers in our crop-growing soils. The mineral content of food crops has shown a steady decline worldwide in developed countries over the past 150 years. As I mentioned in the introduction to this book, even during the 28 years I have been publishing updated editions of this book, with every major update I've had to drop plant foods off various food charts, as their mineral content no longer reached the cut off point set at 10% of the RDI.

Exceptions to this trend are phosphorus and potassium, which remain high as they are part of common crop fertilisers.

Modern health disorders linked to low manganese

Manganese deficiencies are firmly linked with modern health disorders, especially insulin resistance, diabetes and cardiovascular disease, which are usually all found together.

An American study of 122 diabetics found their average body levels of manganese to be only half those of healthy people.

Asthma, MS, epilepsy, balance problems and noises in the ears are other common disorders linked with lack of manganese. Asthma sufferers sometimes have only a quarter as much manganese in their blood as those without asthma.

MS and epilepsy have been reportedly cured by manganese and zinc supplements.

As manganese is used extensively for nerve and brain functions, in gross amounts it can become a neurotoxin (nerve poison). Some hard drinking water from underground bores in rural areas overseas contains so much manganese that it lowers the IQ of children who drink it, along with causing other psychiatric disorders. Public water suppliers in NZ monitor the manganese content of our water. High manganese in farm or bore water supplies can make water look blackish and create a grey stain in toilets, baths, showers and clothes.

You can have a blood test done to determine your manganese status – the normal range in whole blood is between 185–210 nmol/L (10–12 mcg/L). Over 300 nmol/L (17 mcg/L) is dangerous and under 150 nmol/L (8 mcg/L) indicates a deficiency.

Role of manganese in our body
- Helps maintain healthy collagen in bones, joints and skin.
- Helps strengthen artery walls.
- Helps manufacture insulin to regulate blood sugar.
- Helps body utilise carbs and fats from food.
- Important for health of the brain and nervous system.
- Works with vitamin K1 to regulate blood clotting.
- Assists in sex hormone production.
- Regulates bone and tissue development in the unborn child.
- Assists in forming mother's breast milk.
- Antioxidant protecting against free radicals from excess iron.
- Promotes normal hair growth.

Too little manganese
- Osteoarthritis. Sore joints. Bone fractures.
- Spinal disc problems.
- Insulin resistance. High blood sugar. Diabetes. Hypoglycemia.
- High blood pressure. Heart attack.
- Aneurism. Stroke.
- Birth defects. Cleft palate. Convulsions in infants.
- Nervousness. Insomnia. Depression. Psychiatric disorders.
- Epilepsy. Schizophrenia.

- Multiple Sclerosis (MS).
- Noises in ears. Tinnitus. Balance problems.
- Repetitive Strain Injury (RSI).
- Hair loss in women.
- Premature ageing of skin. Excessive wrinkling.

Too much manganese (over 11,000 mcg daily)

- Only toxic in continual high doses from bore water or industrial fumes (usually mining). Can cause impaired brain function resulting in tremors and other Parkinson's like symptoms.

Cooking losses

- No significant losses.

RDI MANGANESE

Child:	2500 mcg	Woman:	5000 mcg
Teenage boy:	3500 mcg	Pregnancy:	5000 mcg
Teenage girl:	3000 mcg	Breastfeeding:	5000 mcg
Man:	5500 mcg		

BEVERAGES		mcg
4 cups	Tea	2000
1 cup	Pineapple juice	1400

FRUIT		
½ cup	Pineapple	1700
1/3 cup	Blackberries	650

SWEETS		
1	Muesli bar (med)	700
50 g	Chocolate	650
1 tbsp	Maple syrup	650

GRAIN / NUTS		
½ cup	Flour (soy)	4300
2	Wheat bran biscuits	3900
1 plate	Bran cereal	3700
½ cup	Flour (wholemeal)	2400
1 plate	Muesli cereal	2200
1	Bran muffin (large)	1800
4 slices	Bread (wholemeal)	1600
1 plate	Porridge	1200

½ cup	Rice (brown cooked)	900
2	Weetbix	850
1/3 cup	Nuts (avg)	800
4 slices	Bread (white)	800
½ cup	Flour (white)	750

MEAT / FISH (cooked)		
100 g	Mussels	900
2	Saveloys	800
1	Meat pie (med)	750

VEGETABLES (cooked)		
½ cup	Silverbeet (chard)	1200
¾ cup	Baked beans	1000
1 med	Kumara (sweet potato)	800
½ cup	Tofu	800
1 cup	Taro root	550

HEALTH FOOD		
2 tbsp	Wheat germ	4800
2 tbsp	Wheat bran	2800
1 tsp	Ginger powder	550

"Organic lettuce is 170 times higher in manganese and organic tomatoes 68 times higher."   Jon Barron, (author of "Lessons From the Miracle Doctors")

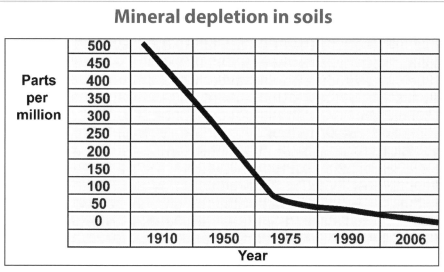

Mineral depletion in soils

Parts per million	1910	1950	1975	1990	2006
500					
450					
400					
350					
300					
250					
200					
150					
100					
50					
0					

Year

Manganese

Above is a worrying graph from the US Department of Agriculture showing the decline in minerals in American food crops over the past 100 years.

The United Nations Earth Summit in 1992 reported an average depletion of 85% in the useful mineral content of American crop soils in the past 100 years. The Australian figure was 55%. New Zealand was not reported on, but due to extensive cropping and heavy rainfall could well be similar to the US figures.

HEALTH HINT   Exercise can be enjoyable

An enjoyable way to exercise indoors at home is to use well designed exercise equipment such as a treadmill, elliptical cross trainer, exercycle, stepper or rowing machine. These allow you to watch TV, listen to music or even read while you're exercising. (However buy quality gear, as cheap equipment is seldom satisfying. If cost is an issue, there's always a good selection of quality brands available for hire, or to buy second hand.)

When exercising outdoors you can use ear bud headphones and an iPod type player to listen to music or radio programs to help pass the time more quickly, by taking your mind off the effort – boredom is the enemy of fitness.

For an exercise method that will give you good results in just 16 minutes a day, see the Health Hint on page 240 – **'Super 8' exercise method.**

"The veterinary profession is decades ahead of human health doctors."
Vaughan Jones, (NZ farmer, researcher and consultant, age 86)

Molybdenum

Molybdenum protects teeth against decay – it was the high level of molybdenum in the water supply, and also in home-grown vegetables of Napier city that protected the teeth of Napier's children in the controversial 1950's NZ study of the effects of fluoride in drinking water. (The fluoridated water of Hastings was compared with the unfluoridated water of Napier – it turned out that Napier's children had significantly less decay than the fluoridated Hastings children.)

With hindsight, it may have been better over the intervening years to have added molybdenum to our drinking water, rather than toxic sodium fluoride.

While a high intake is desirable for better teeth, deficiencies are not generally reported in NZ (although they are seldom tested). One indication of a deficiency is a low level of uric acid in the blood – men below 0.20 mmol/L (3.36 mg/dl) and women below 0.14 (2.35).

Molybdenum is found mostly in plant foods, provided the soil is not deficient. Whole wheat products and beans are good sources.

Molybdenum (like vitamin C) is used by our body to rid our cells and intestines of chemical toxins and yeasts. It's also been used in relatively high doses of 500 mcg a day to clear up brain fog caused by excessive yeast overgrowth in the intestines. Molybdenum has also been used medically to restore appetite after a long convalescence.

A high dose of molybdenum at 500 mcg a day is also reputed to heal obscure aches and pains, especially in the body joints. This may be linked with molybdenum's role in helping the body absorb and regulate iron and copper.

If we have an excess of sugar and protein in our diet, we need more than the normal amount of molybdenum.

Dr Robert Atkins had a lot of success with this mineral and believed the American RDA of 75 mcg was too low. He wrote – *"A daily dosage of 200-500 mcg of molybdenum is probably the minimum necessary for most people."* Taking high doses of molybdenum in supplement form can raise uric acid levels and the risk of gout, but this is rare.

Role of molybdenum in our body

- Helps rid toxins from cells and the digestive system.
- Helps the body utilise and regulate iron and copper.
- Helps regulate uric acid levels.
- Assists in sex hormone production.
- Strengthens tooth enamel and helps prevent tooth decay.

Too little molybdenum

- Easily decayed teeth.
- Foggy brain.
- Osteoarthritis. Obscure joint aches.
- Possible copper and iron deficiency anemia.
- Cancers of bowel system (factor).

Too much molybdenum (over 1000 mcg a day)

- Higher uric acid levels.
- Can hinder uptake of copper if over 1,000,000 mcg ingested daily.

Cooking losses

- No significant losses.

RDI	MOLYBDENUM		
Limited data available and figures vary according to soil content			
Child:	30 mcg	Woman:	45 mcg
Teenager:	43 mcg	Pregnancy:	50 mcg
Man:	45 mcg	Breastfeeding:	50 mcg

SWEETS		mcg
50 g	Chocolate dark	5
GRAINS		
1	Bran muffin (large)	29
4 slices	Bread (wholemeal)	28
4 slices	Bread (white)	18
½ cup	Flour (wholemeal)	12
1	Pizza svg	12
¾ cup	Spaghetti (canned)	8
5	Walnuts	7
½ cup	Flour (white)	7
½ cup	Flour (soy)	5
2	Weetbix	5
MEAT / FISH (cooked)		
2	Saveloys	22

1	Meat pie (med)	17
2	Sausages	10
100 g	Chicken	8
100 g	Oysters	5
VEGETABLES (cooked)		
¾ cup	Baked beans	55
2 cobs	Sweet corn	18
¾ cup	Cabbage	15
2 med	Potatoes	12
½ cup	Mung bean sprouts	12
¾ cup	Pumpkin	11
HEALTH FOOD		
100 g	Liver	125
2 tbsp	Wheat germ	17
2 tbsp	Wheat bran	7

"The greater our knowledge increases, the more our ignorance unfolds."

John F. Kennedy

Phosphorus

Phosphorus is found in protein foods and is the most abundant macro (or bulk) mineral found in our body after calcium – it's found in every cell, but mostly in our bones and teeth.

Phosphorus is also acidic – the other macro minerals (potassium, calcium, magnesium, sodium and chloride, with the exception of sulphur) are all alkaline. You will see below why this is important to note.

Too much phosphorus can be harmful

A dietary deficiency in phosphorus was common in NZ during the poverty of the 1930's Great Depression and the two World Wars. This was due to a restricted, low-protein diet and resulted in widespread tooth decay and weak bones.

Nowadays most people in NZ consume too much phosphorus, at least in relation to calcium. For calcium being alkaline, reduces the harmful acidity of too much phosphorus. Phosphorus works hand in hand with all the alkaline minerals, especially calcium, to maintain the correct pH (acid/alkalinity) balance of our blood and cells. Too much acid phosphorus, and too little balancing alkaline minerals like calcium, can eventually result in harmful acidity.

To avoid modern acidic diseases such as cancer, osteoporosis and inflammatory disorders, our phosphorus intake should be about half our calcium intake.

However, at present in NZ, our phosphorus intake is about four times our calcium intake. In fact, intakes of more than 2000 mg of phosphorus a day are common. This requires our body to continually draw calcium from the bones in order to buffer the acidity of phosphorus. The ultimate result is weak bones and shrinkage of the skeleton, especially in later life, when our bone-building sex hormones – DHEA, progesterone and testosterone have diminished.

The safe ratio of phosphorus to calcium appears to be one to two, ie, one part phosphorus to two parts calcium. This is also the ratio found in human breast milk and strong healthy bone.

Dairy food is high in phosphorus, but has the advantage of being equally high in calcium. Grains and eggs fall somewhere in the middle. The danger food is meat, which is high in phosphorus and has virtually no calcium at all.

Phosphorus (as phosphoric acid) is also increasingly being used as an acidifier in cola drinks and other processed food.

However, provided we can maintain a one to two ratio of phosphorus to calcium in our diet (or one to one maximum) there appears to be no great harm done. However, this is also dependent on us getting enough magnesium to absorb the extra calcium into our bones – the ratio of magnesium should be about half of our calcium intake, the same one to two ratio as phosphorus to calcium.

As always, good nutrition relies on a complex inter-dependence of minerals – so the ideal ratio that would appear to apply here is 1–1–2, ie, 1 part phosphorus, I part magnesium, 2 parts calcium.

Free booklet on NZ phosphorus and calcium foods

To help in this important matter, I've put together a 17 page booklet called **'Is Your pH Healthy?'** It shows you how to raise or maintain your saliva pH to a healthy 6.8 (which can protect you from serious health disorders). It also gives you the phosphorus and calcium content and ratios of 500 common NZ foods, and has a list of acid and alkaline foods.

The booklet is provided free from Health House, Tauranga (who also market this **'Stay Healthy'** book). If you would like a copy of the booklet, just phone Health House on 0800 140 141 and they'll be happy to post you a copy for free, or order it online using their website www.healthhouse.co.nz.

Linked to arthritis, asthma, gout and ADHD

The right phosphorus-calcium balance is also important for the correct balance of zinc and niacin in our body, and to help prevent arthritis, asthma and gout.

The late German researcher, Hertha Hafer in her book **'The Hidden Drug – Dietary Phosphate'** reports on experiments which showed that asthma and ADHD symptoms in children worsened as the phosphorus content of their food increased, especially the inorganic phosphorus added to processed meat and soft drinks (sodas).

A cause of the modern cancer epidemic

Phosphorus and sugar, without sufficient alkaline calcium and other alkaline macro minerals to buffer their acidity, will eventually lower the pH level of our body cells.

This in turn seriously drops the amount of oxygen that can enter the cells and as a result, greatly increases our cancer risk. Cancer cells thrive in low oxygen conditions, but will die in a high oxygen cell environment. This is one of the leading reasons for the cancer epidemic we are now experiencing. (See also the chapter on **Avoiding Cancer**.)

The acidity of our body cells can be quickly and cheaply measured using a saliva pH test strip – just soak the tip with your saliva and then

Phosphorus

compare the colour change to the colour ranges on the packet. If your saliva pH consistently reads less than the healthy norm of 6.8 - 7.0 it is a sign of cell acidity. These strips can generally be purchased at low cost from a health shop or pharmacy and Health House in Tauranga also stock them. I've yet to come across a cancer sufferer (apart from skin and colon cancer cases) whose saliva is above pH 6.0.

Role of phosphorus in our body

- Combines with calcium and magnesium, also sodium, potassium, zinc, vitamin D and niacin, to form and maintain the health of blood, bones, teeth, muscles and tissues.
- Helps balance the correct pH level of our blood and cells.
- Helps absorb nutrients from food and produce energy.
- Necessary for correct nerve and muscle action.

Too little phosphorus

- Malformed bones and teeth. Stunted growth in children.
- Weak bones. Easily decayed teeth. Gum disease.
- Low energy. Muscle weakness.
- Low appetite.

Too much phosphorus (ie, exceeding calcium intake)

- Calcium, magnesium or zinc deficiency.
- Loss of calcium from bones.
- Brittle easily fractured bones. Osteoporosis.
- Greatly increased risk of organ cancer.
- Eczema. Rough skin.
- Asthma.
- Arthritis. Gout.
- ADHD in children.
- Sinus and ear infections.

Cooking losses

- No significant losses.

"All truth goes through three stages. First it is ridiculed. Then it is violently opposed. Finally, it is accepted as self-evident."
Arthur Schopenhauer 1788–1860 (German writer)

RDI PHOSPHORUS

Should not exceed daily calcium intake

Infant:	300 mg	Woman:	1000 mg
Child:	500 mg	Pregnancy:	1000 mg
Teenager:	1250 mg	Breastfeeding:	1000 mg
Man:	1000 mg		

DAIRY / EGGS — mg

2 cups	Milk (trim)	600
2 cups	Milk (std)	480
100 g	Cheese omelette	290
4 tbsp	Whey protein powder	280
2 med	Eggs	230
1 svg	Cheese cake	220
25 g	Cheese	120
100 g	Ice cream	120

SWEETS

50 g	Milk chocolate	150

GRAIN / NUTS

1 plate	Muesli (with milk)	430
1 tsp	Baking powder	420
1 plate	Bran cereal (with milk)	400
1	Bran muffin (large)	360
2	Weetbix (with milk)	280
1	Filled roll	250
2	Wheat bran biscuits	250
1 plate	Porridge (with milk)	240
1/3 cup	Nuts (avg)	210
1	Lamington	200
½ cup	Flour (wholemeal)	200
4 slices	Bread (wholemeal)	170
1 svg	Carrot cake	160
½ cup	Rice (cooked)	120
5	Brazil nuts	115
4 slices	Bread (white)	100

MEAT / FISH (cooked)

100 g	Prawns	450
100 g	Sardines (canned)	430
100 g	Pork	370
2	Sausages	330
100 g	Fish/shellfish (avg)	270
100 g	Chicken	190
100 g	Beef	170
100 g	Lamb	160

FAST FOOD

1	Eggburger (large)	600
1 svg	Pizza (large)	500
1	Hamburger (Big Mac)	330
1	Milkshake (McDonalds)	320
1	Ice cream sundae	260
1	Cheeseburger (std)	250
1	Eggburger (std)	250
1	Fish burger	180
1	Toasted cheese s/wich	150
1	Hamburger (std)	130
2 cans	Cola drinks	110
1 svg	Potato fries	100

VEGETABLES (cooked)

2 cobs	Sweet corn	310
¾ cup	Baked beans	200
1 cup	Broccoli	130
¾ cup	Peas	100
1 cup	Taro root	100

HEALTH FOOD

2 tbsp	Pumpkin seeds	350
2 tbsp	Sunflower seeds	170
2 tbsp	Wheat bran	130
2 tbsp	Wheat germ	150

"Disease is the censor pointing out the humans, animals and plants who are imperfectly nourished."

Dr G. T. Wrench, (author of "'The Wheel of Health")

Phosphorus

163

Potassium

We require more potassium daily than any other mineral in our diet – huge quantities compared to other nutrients. Fortunately, potassium is found in most carb foods, even when processed or cooked. However, if you ever go on a low carb diet and begin to lack energy or lose muscle, it would probably be due to lack of potassium.

Potassium is mainly responsible, along with other macro (bulk) minerals, (especially sodium and chloride from salt) for maintaining our electrolyte balance (cell fluids). Virtually all our body's potassium (98%) is held inside the cells.

Electrolytes is a scientific term for the macro minerals potassium, sodium, chloride, calcium and magnesium which are required to operate our body cells. They are called electrolytes as they are able to hold an electrical charge and can be controlled accordingly.

Potassium works closely with sodium to help regulate the constant flow of nutrient fluids into and out of the trillions of cells in our body. Each body cell is a marvellously intricate, miniature world. If the fluid-electrolyte balance is not kept within strict limits, the cell quickly dies, and so will our entire body if enough cells are affected. This sometimes occurs due to shock following a serious accident – the potassium-sodium balance in our heart muscle cells are thrown out of electrical balance by the extreme emotion and our heart can go into fibrillation and cease to pump properly. Blood pressure then drops drastically and our life is at serious risk. The same thing can happen to animals during capture, especially wild deer.

Incredibly, about a third of our body/brain energy is used in maintaining this critical potassium/sodium balance – it plays a huge role in controlling all of our muscle action and nerve impulse transmission.

High blood pressure can be due to lack of potassium

If heart disease or high blood pressure problems run in your family, potassium is one mineral you must be certain not to lack.

Too much sodium from salt in the diet is often blamed for high blood pressure – however it is not the excess salt itself in our diet that raises blood pressure, but the effect of the excess sodium in the salt depleting our potassium reserves. Too much salt results in excessive thirst – this is to allow our body to flush the excess sodium from our body in the urine. However, when we do flush the excess sodium from our body, a large amount of potassium goes with it, as the sodium quickly links with potassium during digestion.

Excess salt will not normally cause high blood pressure, provided our potassium intake matches our sodium intake, in a one to one balance.

In fact, just increasing our potassium intake, along with magnesium can be a very effective way to lower high blood pressure and also prevent a cardiac arrest or a stroke.

Salt intake is so high in most NZ diets, that potassium deficiency is common. Generally speaking it's more important to obtain enough potassium in our diet to achieve the ideal 1 to 1 potassium – sodium balance, than it is to worry about the harm of excess sodium from salt.

Other ways potassium is lost from our body

Potassium is also lost through excessive sweating. If we are often in situations where we perspire heavily, we should consume extra potassium. Raw fruit is ideal. Sugar, especially in soft drinks (sodas) worsens the situation, as does alcohol.

Diuretic drugs can dangerously deplete potassium body reserves. A salt substitute containing potassium chloride can help when on this kind of medication, but obtain medical guidance first. Fluid retention is one of the symptoms of potassium deficiency, so it may be wise to try extra potassium before taking a diuretic.

Other signs of potassium deficiency include muscle cramps and irregular heartbeat. (Type 2 diabetics often lack potassium.)

Potassium necessary for energy

A combined lack of both potassium and magnesium can lead to severely low energy levels, even chronic fatigue (ME).

To reverse all kinds of fatigue, Dr Robert Atkins recommended a daily supplement of 350 mg of potassium and 350 mg of magnesium until body levels are back to optimum balance and energy returns. He writes, *"The reversal can often occur within a week."*

Potassium intake was not included in the NZ 2009 Nutrition Survey. I feel it should have been – in 2012 The *'American Journal of Clinical Nutrition'* reported 97% of Americans fail to obtain the American RDA of potassium which is 4700 mg. (The NZ RDI is lower at 3800 mg for men.)

I've normally tried to maintain my potassium – sodium balance by avoiding high salt foods and eating plenty of fruit, vegetables, dairy and grains, all of which are high in potassium. However of late, I have begun mixing potassium chloride powder 50/50 with my unrefined table salt.

The maximum potassium level permitted in supplements is only 100 mg, which appears far too low and I feel needs to be reconsidered.

Role of potassium in our body

- Helps regulate the fluid-electrolyte balance in our cells.
- Assists our body in using other minerals, especially sodium.
- Helps maintain the correct acidity (pH) of our blood and cells.
- Helps regulate our heartbeat and blood pressure.
- Helps convert blood glucose to energy.
- Helps our body cells absorb minerals from food.
- Assists in nerve impulse transmission and retaining muscle.
- Helps regulate growth in children.
- Helps our kidneys eliminate toxins.

Too little potassium
(often due to excess salt or diuretic drugs)

- Body cell pH too acidic.
- Low energy. Listlessness. Type 2 diabetes.
- Chronic fatigue (when also low in magnesium).
- Flabby, weak or wasted muscles.
- Too high or too low blood pressure. Rapid or irregular pulse (fibrillation).
- Heart failure (cardiac arrest). Stroke.
- Swelling of legs and other parts of the body (fluid retention).
- Paralysis or heaviness of the arms and legs.
- Leg, foot, stomach or hand muscle cramps.
- Numb/tingling hands or feet.
- Headaches. Mental apathy, confusion or depression.

Too much potassium

- No known toxic effects from food sources, or up to 18,000 mg daily from supplements when kidney function is normal. When kidney function is suspect, only take a potassium supplement under medical guidance as excess build up can trigger heart fibrillation.

Cooking losses

- Boiling food in water can leach out up to 50% of the potassium, but this can be recovered if the cooking water is consumed.

HEALTH HINT   **Lowering your risk of stroke**

A 12 year American study of 850 men and women found that just one serving each day of fresh fruit or vegetables (ie high potassium foods) lowered their stroke risk by 40%.

"Some men eat and drink anything put before them, but are very careful about the oil they put in their car."   **Anonymous**

RDI POTASSIUM

Should equal or exceed sodium intake
(The USA RDA is 4700 mg for adults)

Infant:	1000 mg	Man:	3800 mg
Child:	2500 mg	Woman:	2800 mg
Teenage boy:	3600 mg	Pregnancy:	2800 mg
Teenage girl:	2600 mg	Breastfeeding:	3200 mg

DAIRY / EGGS

		mg
2 cups	Milk (trim)	1060
2 cups	Milk (std)	860
4 tbsp	Whey protein powder	625
1 cup	Soy milk	320

SWEETS

50 g	Chocolate	310

FRUIT

1 cup	Honeydew	750
1 cup	Rock melon	620
1 cup	Cantaloupe	540
½ cup	Rhubarb (stewed/sugar)	510
1 cup	Pawpaw	495
1 cup	Orange juice (pure)	460
1 med	Banana	430
½	Avocado	420
5	Prunes	360
¼ cup	Raisins/sultanas	340
1	Peach	310
5	Dates	300
1	Nectarine	300
1 cup	Grape juice (pure)	290
½ cup	Grapes	275
1	Kiwifruit	240
1/8	Water melon	200

GRAIN / NUTS

1 plate	Bran flakes (with milk)	810
½ cup	Flour (soy)	700
1 plate	Muesli (with milk)	690
¾ cup	Christmas pudding	625
2	Weetbix (with milk)	500
1/3 cup	Nuts (avg)	350
½ cup	Flour (wholemeal)	270
4 slices	Bread (wholemeal)	250

MEAT / FISH (cooked)

100 g	Pork	590
100 g	Fish/shellfish (avg)	440
100 g	Beef	420
100 g	Chicken	320
100 g	Lamb	275

FAST FOOD

1 svg	Potato fries	410

VEGETABLES (cooked)

1 cup	Taro leaves	920
2 med	Potatoes	760
2 cobs	Sweet corn	720
¾ cup	Baked beans	600
1 cup	Taro root	600
1 med	Kumara (sweet potato)	590
1 bag	Potato crisps (50 g)	580
1 cup	Broccoli	560
¾ cup	Chick peas	520
¾ cup	Parsnips	480
1 cup	Brussels sprouts	390
¾ cup	Pumpkin	380
½ cup	Silverbeet (chard)	350
1 med	Tomato (raw)	340
6 med	Mushrooms	310
1/3 cup	Beetroot slices	260

HEALTH FOOD

1 tbsp	Molasses/treacle	290

"One grandmother is worth two MD's." Dr Robert Mendelsohn MD

167

Selenium

Throughout the world, in every community noted for longevity, the intake of selenium is high. Cancer levels are also much lower than normal – six times lower in one Finnish study of 12,155 people with a high selenium intake. This dropped further to an astonishing 11 times less cancer when vitamin E levels from food were also high.

This same Finnish study found heart disease and asthma to be much lower and there were fewer birth defects in newborn babies.

Another 10-year study of 1312 people (mostly men) by the California Cancer Centre found that when blood levels of selenium were increased by an average of 67%, the following reductions in cancer were found – colon cancer 58%, lung cancer 46% and prostate cancer 63%. Selenium did not however reduce basal and squamous cell skin cancers to the same extent as other cancers.

These remarkable results have been repeated in animal studies, especially with higher selenium intakes, equivalent to 400 mcg a day for humans.

One exception was a major seven-year study of men, supplementing with 200 mcg of organic selenium daily and a very high 400 iu dose of synthetic vitamin E. They found no decrease in prostate cancer rates. However these men were mostly Americans, who generally have a very good selenium intake – three or more times higher than men in NZ. One alarming finding of this study was a 17% increase in prostate cancer rates in the men taking the 400 iu of synthetic vitamin E only. This dosage is 12 times higher than the RDI for natural vitamin E and appears to reduce the protective effects of selenium.

Other protective effects of selenium

As well as boosting our body's cancer immunity, selenium is believed to provide antioxidant protection against the ageing effects of free radical damage and inflammation, which helps preserve the elasticity of our arteries and skin.

The topical application of selenium to skin can heal skin infections such as psoriasis, inflammation and dandruff of the scalp – selenium is commonly used in anti-dandruff shampoos.

Studies also report impressive results using selenium to treat major inflammation disorders like rheumatoid arthritis. Even 'wear and tear' osteoarthritis generally shows improvement after six months of selenium supplementation.

Overseas studies have found that men with low levels of selenium have a 70% greater risk for coronary heart disease. This ties in with an unexpected major benefit of selenium reported by participants in an English health magazine test – a notable reduction in anxiety.

Asthma is another problem – New Zealanders with our very low levels of selenium are five times more likely to suffer asthma attacks than Americans, and flu virus symptoms tend to be more virulent.

Selenium also helps neutralise the effects of toxic minerals in our body. In one study, refinery workers were found to have abnormally low blood levels of selenium, despite an adequate intake from their diet. It was discovered that most of the selenium in their diet was being used by their immune systems to neutralise the high levels of toxic minerals from their work environment. An accumulation of toxic minerals in the body is a known cause of multiple sclerosis.

In a study of 35,000 American cot deaths, 9000 were found to have a selenium or vitamin E deficiency. Almost all of the 9000 babies had been bottle fed. Human milk has on average six times as much selenium and twice as much vitamin E as cow's milk.

New Zealand soils low in selenium

Many NZ soils are low in selenium – sheep and dairy farmers are aware of this and to ensure fertility, health and rapid growth of their livestock, apply selenium - containing fertilisers to their pastures when necessary, or inject it directly into their animals.

Unfortunately NZ crop growers do not have the same profit incentive – food crops appear to grow equally well, with or without selenium.

Australian crop growing soils are mostly adequate in selenium and intake there is reported to be higher than in NZ, although the Australian cancer rate is as horrific as our own. (Only Denmark and Ireland have higher rates of cancer than Australia and NZ.)

Senegal in West Africa has the world's lowest cancer rate – their population is almost entirely dependent on underground water which is the world's hardest. It contains high levels of calcium, magnesium and selenium.

Finland, like New Zealand, has low levels of selenium in most of its crop-growing soils. The Finns are now required by law to add selenium to crop fertilisers – their average daily selenium intake has increased from a low 26 mcg to 56 mcg.

The NZ 2009 Nutrition Survey showed that the average intake of selenium here had increased from 52 mcg at the last survey, to 67 mcg this time. (It was a very low 28 mcg during a previous survey.) This surprisingly large increase seems mostly due to imported higher selenium Australian wheat, as bread was reported as the main food source. However South Island bread flour is still milled from low-selenium, locally grown wheat. South Island selenium intake was not however separated out in this survey.

There is nevertheless still a widespread selenium deficiency in NZ – 45% of the NZ population overall. The worst group are older men who are 64% deficient and older women, 78%. According to the World Cancer Research Fund, NZ women have the world's second highest rate of cancer, after Denmark, which also has selenium-poor soils.

There would appear then, to be a sound case for requiring that selenium be added to fertiliser on all deficient meat and crop growing soils in our country. It has also been suggested from time to time that selenium be added to table salt, along with iodine.

The NZ selenium RDI for men is 70 mcg, however most nutrition researchers recommend a higher RDI of about 175 mcg, with a temporary increase to 400 mcg whenever there is a need to fight a viral infection, inflammation or heavy metal build up.

Intake of iodine, chromium and natural vitamin E from food also need to be adequate as selenium works hand in hand with these nutrients.

Fish flesh can be an excellent source of selenium, but not fish oils.

Blood testing for selenium

If you decide to have your blood levels of selenium tested, the typical NZ range is 0.5 to 1.4 µmol/L (40 to 110 ug/L). The American Journal of Clinical Nutrition recommends a minimum of 1.3 µmol/L (100 ug/L) for full immune system effectiveness – this normally requires a daily intake of at least 150 mcg of organic selenium each day.

Blood levels do not necessarily confirm that selenium is being absorbed by our cells – adequate iodine, chromium and vitamin E from food is required for good absorption. It may seem bizarre, but analysis of the selenium content of a person's toenails is regarded as the most reliable test of absorption.

Selenium in inorganic form (selenate or selenite) is used for farm animals. These forms appear to work well, but are quickly expelled from the body, whereas the organic forms, found in food and quality health supplements (mostly selenomethionine) are recycled by the body.

Role of selenium in our body

- Assists the immune system to kill cancerous cells and infections.
- Assists the immune system to eliminate toxins.
- Helps the brain mood function remain positive and alert.
- Helps maintain health of male and female reproductive systems.
- Helps maintain elasticity of arteries and skin.

- Helps prevent cell and skin inflammation.
- Antioxidant activator and booster.
- Protects unborn children from spinal malformities.
- Helps regulate blood pressure and clotting.
- Assists thyroid function.
- Works hand in hand with iodine, chromium and vitamin E.

Too little selenium
- Low immunity to infections and most cancers. Hepatitis.
- Build up of toxic heavy minerals.
- Increased levels of anxiety and depression. Frequent urination.
- Prostate enlargement. Difficult urination.
- Low fertility (sperm count) in men. Impotence.
- Muscle aches, wasting and weakness (dystrophy).
- Hardened arteries (atherosclerosis). Cardiovascular disease.
- Abnormal heartbeat (arrhythmia).
- Increased risk of heart attack and stroke. Heart muscle failure.
- Birth defects, especially spinal (neural tube). Miscarriage.
- Increased risk of cot death among infants.
- Stunted growth in children.
- Cystic fibrosis (clogging of lungs with mucous).
- Increased risk of asthma.
- Pancreatitis (inflammation of pancreas).
- Skin inflammation or roughness. Psoriasis. Dandruff. Eczema. Acne.
- Premature ageing of skin and tissues. Brown old age spots.
- Multiple sclerosis (due to accumulation of toxic minerals).
- Free radical damage. Eye cataracts.
- Decreased thyroid function.
- Rheumatoid arthritis. Osteoarthritis.
- Macular degeneration (factor).

Too much selenium
(over 1200 mcg inorganic, or 2400 mcg organic daily)
- Numb or tingly hands and feet.
- Bad breath (garlic-like odour). Metallic taste in mouth.
- Brittle nails, especially thumb nails. Easily decayed teeth.
- Brittle hair and hair loss.

Cooking losses
- No significant losses.

"A substance (selenium) that can decrease the cancer death rate by 50% should be heralded as our greatest medical breakthrough and dispensed to every person in the world."   Dr Robert Atkins MD

Selenium

RDI SELENIUM

Child:	35 mcg		Woman:	60 mcg
Teenage boy: 70 mcg		Teenage girl: 60 mcg	Pregnancy:	65 mcg
Man:	70 mcg		Breastfeeding:	75 mcg

DAIRY / EGGS   mcg

		mcg
2 med	Eggs	15
2 cups	Milk (trim)	10
4 tbsp	Whey protein powder	7
2 cups	Milk (std or non-fat)	5

GRAIN / NUTS

5	Brazil nuts*	210
5	Walnuts	14
4 slices	Bread (multigrain)**	13
1/3 cup	Cashew nuts	10
4 slices	Bread (white)**	10
4 slices	Bread (wholemeal)	10
1/3 cup	All other nuts	3

MEAT / FISH (cooked)

100 g	Oysters (raw)	140
100 g	Crayfish	130
100 g	Snapper	120
100 g	Orange roughy	100

100 g	Tuna (canned)	90
100 g	Flounder	80
100 g	Hoki	75
100 g	Salmon (canned)	75
100 g	Oysters (canned)	75
100 g	All other fish (avg)	50
100 g	Pipis (clams)	35
100 g	All other shellfish (avg)	25
100 g	Chicken	14
100 g	Pork	15
100 g	Beef	15
100 g	Lamb	6

HEALTH FOOD

100 g	Kidney (cooked)	65
2 tbsp	Sunflower seeds	10
100 g	Liver (cooked)	9

*   Brazil nuts can vary in selenium content as much as 10 fold according to soil content – the above figure is a NZ average.

** North Island bread only – South Island figures are about 50% lower.

HEALTH HINT   Five laws of longevity

An extensive study of longevity came to the conclusion that ideally:

1. We should live in a slow paced society
2. In a mild climate
3. About 1.5 kms above sea level (1500m or 5000 feet)
4. In a region with selenium - rich soil
5. Do a lot of walking

"In the average unfarmed topsoil (down to seven inches) there exists only enough minerals to take off 40 good crops or 100 poor crops."
Dr Weston Price DDS (1870 – 1948)

Sodium (from common salt)

Sodium is obtained by our body from common salt (sodium chloride) which is 40% sodium and 60% chloride. Sodium works hand in hand with potassium and is essential for every cell in our body.

Assuming that we consume about six cups of liquid daily, our NZ RDI for sodium is set at 700 mg a day (about a fifth of a teaspoon). This increases to 920 mg with a high fluid intake. (A litre of perspiration will cause the loss of about 950 mg of sodium.)

However, our average intake of sodium is about 4000 mg a day, over five times the RDI. This may seem excessive, but the average Japanese adult is reported to consume 11,000 mg a day – 15 times our RDI. Yet Japanese life expectancy surpasses ours by four years, so obviously other dietary factors are compensating. Perhaps their high potassium intake, superior omega 3 to 6 balance, high levels of vitamin B12 and K2, and superior iodine and CoQ10 status. Tibetan people who are renowned for their longevity, are also said to consume extraordinary amounts of raw rock salt by stirring it into their tea.

Most of our salt is concealed in processed foods – natural foods are very low in salt. Fast takeaway foods and processed meats (including bacon) can contain huge amounts of salt. Another unexpected source is baking powder and self-raising flours, which contain sodium bicarbonate (baking soda). Also numerous other food additives such as MSG contain sodium (look for sodium in the **Food Additives** chapter).

Health benefits of unrefined salt

Most table salt is refined to remove decaying organic matter from the sea and thereby increase shelf life and also to enhance pouring qualities and whiteness. NZ table salt has iodine added as a health measure to compensate for our soil deficiencies in this mineral, and to replace iodine lost during refining.

Salt refining, which includes heating to around 600°C, is another example of man damaging a natural, healthy food for the sake of convenience. During the refining of raw salt, 16% of it is lost – this 16% comprising over 70 trace minerals and elements, including every mineral our body requires for optimum health. These minerals are also in colloidal form (meaning fully dissolvable) and as such, are highly bioavailable to our body. About 2% of new chemicals are also added, to prevent caking and improve flow – normally sodium aluminosilicate or magnesium carbonate.

Refined salt is regarded by many nutritionists as one of the *'three deadly white foods'* – white sugar, white flour and white salt.

Unrefined salt on the other hand, retains the lost 70-plus trace minerals and elements – this salt can be either evaporated sea salt or rock salt. Rock salt is sea salt mined from an ancient sea bed deposit.

Unrefined salt has traditionally been grey, chunky, slightly damp, and needing to be ground at home before use. However finely ground, free-pouring varieties of unrefined rock salt are now available.

Health enthusiasts swear by the benefits of unrefined salt – some even consume a tablespoon of raw sea water every day. However there would appear to be no additional benefits from sea water over unrefined salt.

So for optimum health we should use unrefined salt when possible and match our sodium intake with our potassium intake 50-50.

Can excess salt raise blood pressure?

Excess sodium triggers thirst, in order to expel the surplus sodium from our bodies, but does take valuable potassium along with it as the two minerals link together in the body. This frequently results in a potassium deficiency which can cause high or erratic blood pressure. Provided potassium intake is increased also, excess salt itself should not normally raise blood pressure unduly.

Salty tasting potassium chloride powder (52% potassium) can be used as a salt substitute, but tastes better mixed half and half with rock salt.

For a fuller understanding of the importance of the sodium-potassium balance for our cardiovascular health, the chapter on potassium should be read along with this one.

Sodium deficiency

Because salt is found in almost every food, sodium deficiencies are uncommon in normal diets, unless diuretics are being taken or heavy sweating has occurred over several days. The NZ army formerly issued salt tablets for soldiers to take during long hot marches.

Drinking large amounts of water unnecessarily, can dilute our sodium balance as sodium is mostly stored in our blood.

Symptoms of sodium imbalance or deficiency can be salt cravings, leg cramps at night, low energy, aching joints and muscles, dizziness, fainting, mental confusion and vomiting. Serious harm can result if the situation is not quickly rectified.

Diuretics

Diuretic (water expelling) drugs can severely deplete the body of sodium (and other important minerals). My elderly mother nearly died from a severe sodium deficiency after taking a moderately high dose of the common diuretic frusemide for a year or more. It caused symptoms of mental confusion and severe weakness which were fortunately

Sodium

detected in time when one of my sisters who is a registered nurse, happened to visit her and recognised the symptoms.

Role of sodium in our body

- Helps regulate the fluid/electrolyte balance in our cells.
- Assists our body to utilise other minerals, especially potassium.
- Helps maintain the correct acidity (pH) of our blood.
- Helps regulate our heartbeat and blood pressure.
- Assists in muscle action and nerve impulse transmission.

Too little sodium

(Normally from diuretics, diarrhea or excess sweating)

- Apathy and low energy. Chronic fatigue (factor).
- Mental confusion. Impaired vision. Dizziness. Fainting.
- Low blood pressure.
- Nerve pains, aching joints and muscles.
- Muscle cramps after heavy sweating (especially in legs).
- Constipation. Vomiting.

Too much sodium (over 2300 mg daily)

- High blood pressure (due to loss of potassium).
- Stroke (also due to loss of potassium).
- Swelling of tissues (fluid retention).

Cooking losses

- No significant loss if cooking fluids are consumed.

HEALTH HINT **Why salt and sugar cravings?**

One of the proof readers of this book queried why sugar and salt cravings are so widespread.

There is no clear answer to this question, however, the fact that pregnant women experience cravings, would indicate they are urgently needing nutrients found in the type of food craved.

I too had both sugar and salt cravings when I was younger. However I no longer got sugar cravings when I began taking a teaspoon of unrefined molasses in a Milo drink each day – nor salt cravings since I began using unrefined rock salt.

"Contrary to conventional medical advice, salt has little effect on blood pressure in most people. Iodine's impact throughout the body is far greater. By avoiding salt we throw the baby out with the bathwater."
Dr Robert Atkins MD

RDI SODIUM

The RDI is set to vary 50% up or down from the averages below, according to daily fluid intake.

Infant:	170 mg	Woman:	700 mg
Child:	450 mg	Pregnancy:	700 mg
Teenager:	700 mg	Breastfeeding:	700 mg
Man:	700 mg		

BEVERAGES

		mg
1 can	Soft drink (soda avg)	60
1 can	Beer	6
2 glasses	Wine	6

DAIRY / EGGS

4 tbsp	Whey protein powder	325
2 tbsp	Margarine	220
2 cups	Milk (std or low-fat)	220
2 med	Eggs	160
25 g	Cheese	160
2 tbsp	Butter	140

FRUIT

1 cup	Melons (avg)	25
¼ cup	Dried fruit (avg)	20
1 svg	All other fruit (avg)	3

GRAIN / NUTS

1 plate	Porridge (salt added)	1500
¾ cup	Spaghetti (canned)	900
4 slices	Bread (all types)	560
1 plate	Noodles (instant)	550
1 svg	Cheese cake	500
½ cup	Flour (self-raising)	450
1 tsp	Baking powder	400
1 plate	Cereals (milk avg)	370
1 plate	Muesli	210
1/3 cup	Nuts (salted)	210
2	Weetbix (with milk)	170
1/3 cup	Nuts (salted)	170
2 med	Biscuits (avg)	60
1/3 cup	Nuts (unsalted)	2
½ cup	Rice (cooked)	1
½ cup	Flour (white std)	1

MEAT / FISH (cooked)

100 g	Bacon	2900
2	Sausages	1400
2	Fish cakes	1400
100 g	Ham	1300
2	Saveloys (boiled)	1100
100 g	Corned beef	950
100 g	Processed meat (avg)	900
100 g	Fish (canned)	600
5 g	Soup stock (Oxo cube)	520
100 g	Chicken	80
100 g	Lamb	80
100 g	Pork (unsalted)	80
100 g	Fish (avg)	70
100 g	Beef	50

FAST FOOD

1 svg	Pizza (large)	2200
1 svg	Potato salad	1500
2 pces	Chicken (fried)	1500
1	Hot dog	1400
1 svg	Fish and chips	1400
1	Hamburger (large)	1100
1 bag	Potato crisps (50 g)	950
1	Hamburger (avg)	900
2 cups	Chips (salted)	600
1	Meat pie	590
1/3 cup	Gravy	400
½ cup	Coleslaw	270
1	Fruit pie	250

SALT

1 tsp	Salt (table)	2300
1 tsp	Baking soda	930

VEGETABLES (cooked)

1 cup	Soup (canned avg)	460
¾ cup	Sweet corn (canned)	410
½ cup	Peas (canned)	200
4 slices	Beetroot (canned)	410
1 svg	Vegetables (avg)	20

HEALTH FOOD

100 g	Kidney	400
1 tsp	Marmite (yeast extract)	290
100 g	Liver	110

HEALTH HINT Curing frequent urination

An enlarged prostate is often blamed for the problem of frequent urination in men, especially during the night, which is called nocturia.

Enlarging of the prostate can make urination slow, or difficult, but it has little to do with the urge to urinate frequently, provided the bladder is fully emptied, which is normally the case.

The main cause of a frequent urge to urinate is anxiety – the traditional 'nervous wee' which applies to both men and women, and anxiety can also cause the male prostate to enlarge temporarily.

When we fall asleep normally, our body passes quickly into a deep stage of sleep, due to the effect of the sleep hormone melatonin – at the same time our kidneys receive the message to slow down the amount of urine they process to send to the bladder.

If we go to bed stressed, worried, hyped up by caffeine, lively conversation or arguing, stimulating reading, late night computer activity or traumatic TV, we override the effect of melatonin and fail to enter this deep sleep stage – instead we enter a restless, lighter stage.

This restless, lighter stage of sleep can also be caused by too much light in the bedroom, a restless partner, eating food too close to bedtime (ie, after 7pm), a dietary deficiency of niacin (vitamin B3), magnesium, selenium, and sometimes calcium, or taking a daily high dose of vitamin B6 (over 20 mg a day).

Unless we reach a deep, melatonin-induced stage of sleep, our kidneys fail to get the signal to slow down, and continue to operate at normal daytime rates. So within a few hours, our bladder is full and the discomfort awakens us, and up we get. When we get back to bed, it's even more difficult to relax into deep sleep, due to a diminished supply of melatonin.

The best solution is to reach a deep stage of sleep as soon as possible after turning the lights out, when our melatonin is at its peak. Melatonin is made by the body from the hormone serotonin. The supplement 5-HTP can help if your body is lacking serotonin.

In a nutshell, anxiety in all its many forms is the main cause of frequent urination.

"Up to 90 percent of the doctor visits in the USA may be triggered by a stress-related illness." USA Government ('Centers for Disease Control and Prevention' Atlanta City.)

Sodium

HEALTH HINT   PMT and a woman's blood pH

The pH of the venous blood in our veins (venous is the used blood returning from our body cells to the lungs, not the fresh oxygen-rich arterial blood coming from our lungs and heart) is an indication of the pH level of our cells. Normally this venous blood should be pH 7.46. (Fresh arterial blood from the lungs and heart is pH 7.40).

Small variations in the pH of venous blood, from the norm of 7.46 can have a profound negative effect on the body and brain. Extremes are a low of 7.40 (too acid) or a high of 7.50 (too alkaline).

Smaller variations than these often occur in a woman's blood during the week prior to menstruation – these give rise to symptoms of PMT such as irritability, mood swings and fluid retention.

Dr Rudolf Wiley in his book *'BioBalance'* reports that PMT symptoms can generally be eliminated each month if a woman corrects this imbalance in the pH of her blood by temporarily changing her diet to either more acid, or more alkaline foods during her PMT week, depending on in which direction the pH imbalance lies – usually acidic.

This means eating extra fruit and vegetables for more alkaline blood, or consuming more acidic foods like sugar, meat, coffee, etc, for more acidic blood.

A woman needs to experiment to know which direction to go, but more often the diet needs to be more alkaline. My free booklet *'Is Your pH Healthy?'* (see page 161) contains a list of acid and alkaline NZ foods.

HEALTH HINT   Avoiding leg cramps

The causes of leg and other muscle cramps can be complex, but they usually have to do with an imbalance of magnesium, sodium, calcium, water or potassium. The most common causes are lack of magnesium or potassium, too much sodium at one meal, or too little sodium after heavy perspiration during the day.

A well-balanced diet and/or magnesium supplement should largely overcome this problem.

However, if you have been sweating continuously in hot conditions, and have already drunk four litres of water, to avoid leg cramps you should increase both your potassium and sodium intake by 900 mg for every litre of water you drink.

"These results do not support a general recommendation to reduce sodium intake." American Medical Association, (after reviewing 114 separate trials on the effects of reduced salt intake on high blood pressure)

Sulphur

Sulphur is important for the health and appearance of our skin as it is required to make collagen. It's also necessary for the health of our joints and the gloss of our hair. A sulphur deficiency is known to cause early greying. Some nutritionists refer to sulphur as *'Nature's beauty mineral.'*

Sulphur is one of the least-studied minerals, yet there's more sulphur in our body than sodium – it's found in every cell and works closely with protein.

Eggs are a high quality source of sulphur. Other food sources vary in quality. A respected American nutritionist, Dr Carl Pfeiffer has stated – *"Rheumatoid arthritis patients seem, as a rule to dislike eggs, at present our only good source of sulphur. All patients with rheumatoid arthritis would do well to eat at least two eggs per day to provide adequate sulphur for their needs."*

Foods high in sulphur tend to be smelly when they decompose or burn, ie, fish, meat and eggs.

Some people are allergic to sulphur compounds, especially those used in medicines and inorganic supplements. MSM is an organic, safer form of sulphur found in better quality supplements and is similar to the sulphur found in food. Soaking in geothermal sulphur baths can help the skin.

No RDI for sulphur has been set – it's assumed that as long as our RDI for protein is met, we should be obtaining enough for our needs, although numerous nutritionists question this

Role of sulphur in our body
- Helps form and maintain the health/appearance of our skin and hair.
- Helps form and maintain the health of our joints and nervous system.
- Assists in multiplying useful bacteria in our intestines.
- Helps our body cells absorb and utilise nutrients including vitamin D.
- Assists the body to rid itself of wastes and toxins.

Too little sulphur
- Dry or prematurely wrinkled skin. Brittle nails.
- Dull or prematurely grey hair.
- Eczema. Psoriasis. Constipation. Imbalanced gut probiotics.
- Rheumatoid arthritis.

Too much sulphur
- No known toxic effects of dietary sulphur.

Cooking losses
- Up to 50% in vegetables when boiled.

RDI SULPHUR

The RDI's below are estimates from overseas studies – limited data available			
Child:	350 mg	Woman:	450 mg
Teenage boy:	550 mg	Pregnancy:	550 mg
Teenage girl:	450 mg	Breastfeeding:	550 mg
Man:	550 mg		

DAIRY / EGGS

		mg
2 med	Eggs	220
2 cups	Milk (trim)	190
2 cups	Milk (std)	140

GRAIN / NUTS

1/3 cup	Peanuts/Macadamia	190
½ cup	Flour (soy)	150
1 plate	Muesli cereal (with milk)	135
1 plate	Porridge (with milk)	130
4 slices	Bread (all types)	100
2	Weetbix (with milk)	100
½ cup	Flour (all types)	70
5	Brazil/Cashew	60
1/3 cup	Almonds	50

MEAT / FISH (cooked)

100 g	Shellfish	470
100 g	Beef	270

100 g	Chicken	270
100 g	Pork	270
100 g	Lamb	230
100 g	Fish	220

VEGETABLES (cooked)

¾ cup	Baked beans	130
1 cup	Brussels sprouts	80
1 cup	Cabbage	80
2 med	Potatoes	80
1 cup	Cauliflower	70
¾ cup	Split peas	75
2 cobs	Sweet corn	75
½ cup	Asparagus	45
¾ cup	Peas	55

HEALTH FOOD

2 tbsp	Pumpkin seeds	85
1 tbsp	Mustard powder	75

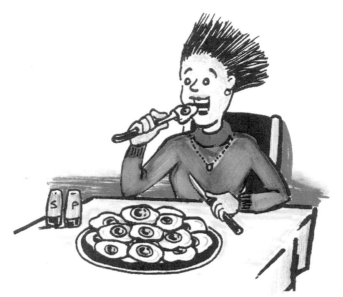

Sulphur, found in eggs may help curl your hair….

90-day Arthritis Cure

Dr Joel Wallach is a veterinary pathologist, turned naturopath who lectures worldwide on nutritional healing, usually in an outspoken and humourous manner. He is critical of most orthodox medical drug treatment and surgery.

He claims that all types of arthritis, even serious bedridden cases can be permanently cured in 90 days by taking gelatine and colloidal (liquid) minerals, which he sells. Earlier editions of my book included this 90-day cure and I requested feedback from readers. Some miraculous cures were reported, but a number of failures also. I did more research and the problem appears to be that insufficient amounts of key minerals (boron, selenium, zinc, sulphur and calcium) are obtainable from colloidal solutions.

So here is a modified version of the 90-day cure that appears to work well. You can take the minerals in chelated powder form in capsules. Absorption from chelated minerals is satisfactory at approx 50%. When or how you take the gelatine is not critical.

The Cure

1. Each day for 90 days, consume two heaped teaspoons of unflavoured gelatine (which is made from beef bone and cartilage collagen and contains building material for bone cartilage and joints). It's best stirred into wet food like stews, beans, spaghetti, mashed veges, etc, or blended in smoothies. Consume as soon as mixed or it will turn the food into a jelly. The taste is bland and not noticeable in most foods. Gelatine can be bought through bulk food sellers in 500 g or 2.5 kg packs, or 8 oz and 1 lb packs overseas. Alternatively, you can substitute with capsules providing approx 1500 mg of glucosamine and 1500 mg of chondroitin daily.

2. Restrict your overall food intake during the evenings of each day of the cure, so that you go to bed a little hungry every night (very important).

3. Settle any long standing disputes that can still stir up anger or resentment (even when you're in the right) – stress hormones are strongly linked with inflamed joints.

4. Soon after your evening meal, throughout the 90 days, take the following dietary minerals and vitamins as a supplement. These should be obtainable from any health shop. If taking a multi, avoid any that contain more than 10 mg (10,000 mcg) of vitamin B6 and ensure that the magnesium and calcium are in fine powder form (ie, in a capsule, not a tablet). You can omit any of

the minerals or the folate below if you're confident your regular diet is supplying them in the required amounts.

3	mg	Boron (essential)
600	mg	Sulphur (MSM type) or two eggs (essential)
15	mg	Zinc
2	mg	Copper
500	mg	Calcium (not in hard tablet form)
500	mg	Magnesium (essential) (not in hard tablet form)
100	mcg	Selenium (essential)
10	mcg	Vitamin D (or summer sunshine from sunbathing)
600	mg	Vitamin C (divide 3 x 200 mg during the day)
400	mcg	Folate (also known as folic acid)

(Some readers have reported success just taking these minerals and vitamins alone, without the gelatine.)

"The enemy of man is his stomach."   Syrian proverb

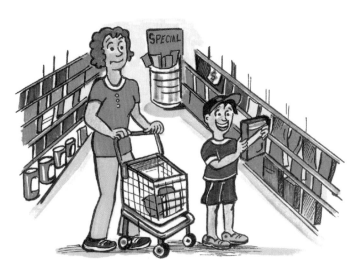

"Contains nothing remotely nutritious. Wow, Mum, can we buy these?"

Zinc

There are more roles in the body for zinc than any other nutrient – over 2000 known processes. Zinc is therefore one of the most important minerals for our health, yet one of the most deficient in our diet. According to the NZ 2009 Nutrition Survey, 52% of middle-aged men don't get enough zinc each day, increasing to 90% for men over 71. Overseas figures are similar.

According to the survey, grains are the main source of zinc in our diet, yet 66% of zinc is lost from wheat during milling and refining to white flour. The next best source is beef – however neither NZ grains nor meats are high in zinc. The only rich natural source is rock oysters. Although surprisingly, some fast foods (due to huge serving sizes) are reasonably good sources of zinc in NZ.

Low zinc content in soils

One of the reasons for a low zinc content in our foods is that, unless crop soils are replenished by fertiliser, as few as ten crops in succession can seriously deplete the soil of available zinc. There is normally no zinc in the NPK (nitrogen-phosphorus-potassium) fertilisers commonly used today. Fortunately, fertiliser companies are now more aware of the importance of trace minerals and have soil and plant analysis services for crop growers and farmers to test for trace mineral deficiencies.

Plants cannot make minerals (neither can our bodies), they can only extract them from the soil. If minerals are lacking in the soil, they will be lacking or absent in the plant, or animal product. I see this frequently in our food and crop research figures – often they will report an adequate level of a mineral in one sample of food, but only a trace of the same mineral in another sample of the same food, from a different grower.

Swedish studies have found an average 60% higher zinc content in food from certified organic growers. Regrettably however, the emphasis in organic growing appears to be mainly the avoidance of toxic chemicals. I believe an equal high emphasis should be put on high mineral content – a well-nourished body can be highly efficient at ridding itself of toxins, just as a well-nourished plant can resist pests and diseases.

Zinc and magnesium protect the brain and eyes

Health disorders of every description, including psychiatric disorders are linked with low body levels of zinc. The symptom list of '**Too Little**' in this chapter is the longest in the entire book. (The next longest list is for magnesium.) Deficiencies in both zinc and magnesium are very common. These two minerals are critically important in protecting our brain and eyes from excitotoxin additives common in our food today, (excitotoxins are covered in the chapter **on Avoiding Alzheimer's**).

Test yourself for a zinc deficiency

Blood tests are not reliable for detecting zinc deficiency, as around 85% of our zinc is held inside our body cells rather than in our blood.

There is a simple, cheap test for a zinc deficiency – you will need a small amount of zinc sulphate heptahydrate. This can normally be obtained from a farming supplies outlet as a green crystal. (Some health shops also stock it, and some will provide the test free of charge.)

Dissolve a tiny amount of the crystal in water to a 0.1% solution. This is 1 g (or ¼ teaspoon) in 1 litre of water. Take a dessertspoon of the liquid into your mouth, swish it around – then swallow or spit it out.

If you instantly notice a bitter, unpleasant taste, you are not zinc deficient.

If you have a delayed (1 to 10 second reaction) followed by a bitter taste, you need more zinc in your diet. If it takes over 10 seconds to taste the bitterness, or continues to taste like water, you have a severe zinc deficiency.

This test works because zinc is required for our taste buds to work fully, but you must ensure it is correctly diluted before tasting.

Generally, when you test deficient in zinc, you are also deficient in magnesium, and sometimes in vitamin B6. Zinc has limited storage in our body, so a deficiency can develop quickly when our diet is lacking.

Restore your lost energy

Zinc is important for absorbing and regulating other minerals and vitamins for optimum health and to promote antioxidant activity.

Lethargic teenagers going through growth spurts have been known to miraculously spring back to energetic life when given a zinc and magnesium supplement. So called 'growing pains' often disappear also.

Many years ago, I saw this happen with one of my sons – he was aged 17 at the time. A supplier sent me some sample cans of a pleasant tasting vitamin protein powder with zinc and magnesium added. My listless teenage son visited me, tried some, liked it and took two tins home with him to his flat. Within a week he had transformed into a human dynamo. Next time he visited, he literally ran into our house and then ran back out again to his car. My daughter phoned later and said, *"What on earth's happened to Jared?"* Other experiences like this over the years have continued to confirm to me that we are seriously lacking minerals in our diet.

Numerous health disorders disappear with zinc

Other symptoms of zinc deficiency are repeated colds and infections, glue ear (otitis media) slow wound healing, a weak sense of smell, early greying hair, easily split fingernails with white specks, yellow fungus growth on toenails and abdominal stretch marks in women after childbirth. Many skin disorders are related to insufficient zinc.

Zinc is also important for avoiding type 2 diabetes and heart disease – it helps balance blood sugar levels, also to protect against or reduce oxidised LDL cholesterol in the arteries.

Deficiencies of zinc are common among young children, older men, women taking the birth control pill and pregnant women. Lack of zinc can also be a factor in post-natal depression.

Zinc supplements have been used to successfully treat many common health disorders, including dementia. Macular degeneration eyesight problems have also been slowed, or even reversed in the elderly.

Heart disease patients have recovered well, and even dwarfism has responded if caught during the early growth years. Many psychiatric disorders respond to zinc, especially when its supporting mineral manganese is also supplemented.

In one overseas study, zinc supplements doubled testosterone levels in men aged over 60, in six months. Interestingly, during treatment with zinc supplements, red headed people have found their hair turn a rich brown, and blonde haired people have become brunette.

Zinc helps our body repair DNA genes and is believed to protect against the early stages of cancer damage. Fighting cancer, or any inflammation disorder, quickly exhausts the body's supply of zinc – so does pregnancy, or the healing of a serious injury or surgery.

With the help of vitamin C, zinc helps our body expel harmful minerals and poisons. Liquid zinc in spray form can knock out a developing cold virus when sprayed and breathed into the nose and throat passages. (The 0.1% zinc sulphate heptahydrate liquid test solution, mentioned on the previous page can be used for this.)

Role of zinc in our body
- Necessary for over 2000 bodily processes.
- Helps our body absorb and utilise nutrients from food.
- Helps convert omega 3 from plants to usable DHA and EPA forms.
- Helps retain accuracy of the body's DNA.
- Necessary for health and correct development of unborn children.
- Necessary for optimum growth of children.
- Regulates sexual development in adolescents.

Zinc

- Helps maintain sexual fertility and libido in adults.
- Helps maintain health of the prostate gland in men.
- Helps maintain our sense of taste, smell and vision.
- Helps maintain health of our hair, gums and elasticity of our skin.
- Assists in healing inflammation, wounds and surgery.
- Helps maintain health of the liver.
- Helps regulate copper levels.
- Promotes calmness of mind and mental health of the brain.
- Protects brain and nerve neurons from MSG/aspartate damage.
- Assists in the regulation of sugar and alcohol.
- Assists in forming and employing insulin in the body.
- Helps regulate blood cholesterol levels.
- Helps maintain bone density and muscle bulk.
- Helps the immune system overcome viral and bacterial infections.
- Assists our body to eliminate toxins – along with vitamin C.

Too little zinc

- Damage to cell DNA. Free radical damage to nerves and the brain.
- Suppressed immune system. Increased risk of cancer.
- Fetal autism, dwarfism and Down's syndrome. (Pregnancy)
- Post natal depression in women.
- Stretch marks in abdominal skin after childbirth.
- Lack of growth in children. Poor muscle development.
- Frequent colds and infections. Yeast and ear infections (glue ear).
- Lethargy in teenagers during growth spurts. Growing pains. Acne.
- Delayed sexual development in adolescents.
- Impotency and low sperm count in males. Infertility in females.
- Low libido in both men and women.
- Enlarged prostate in men. Difficulty in urination.
- Enlarged male breasts.
- Inflammation. Rheumatoid arthritis. Eventual osteoporosis.
- High blood pressure and LDL cholesterol. Heart attack. Stroke.
- High blood sugar. Hypoglycemia. Diabetes.
- Weak sense of smell and taste. Gum disease (gingivitis).
- Brittle thin nails with white spots and horizontal lines.
- Yellow toenails and/or fungus growth.
- Stiff or prematurely grey hair and ageing of the skin. Psoriasis.
- Dandruff. Hair loss in women.
- Slow wound healing. Skin disorders. Bed sores.
- Liver disorders. Unpleasant body odours.
- Chest tightness. Difficulty in breathing. Asthma.
- Crohn's disease. Parasites in intestines. Toxin buildup in the body.
- Depression. Confusion. Anorexia nervosa. Bulimia nervosa.

- Poor memory and attention span. Dementia. Alzheimer's.
- Convulsions. Epilepsy. Schizophrenia.
- Dirt eating (observed among seriously deficient children).
- Hyperactivity and attention disorders in children (ADHD).
- Cataracts. Poor night vision. Macular degeneration.
- Weak red blood cells. Low energy. Paleness (anemia).

Too much zinc (over 200 mg daily for long periods)
- Nausea, headache and digestive upsets.
- Copper deficiency.

Cooking losses
- No significant losses.

RDI	ZINC		
Child:	5 mg	Woman:	8 mg
Teenage boy:	13 mg	Pregnancy:	11 mg
Teenage girl:	7 mg	Breastfeeding:	12 mg
Man:	14 mg		

DAIRY / EGGS		mg
2 cups	Milk (trim)	3.1
2 cups	Milk (std)	1.5
2 med	Eggs	1.3
25 g	Cheese	0.8

GRAIN / NUTS		
1/3 cup	Peanuts	3.5
4 slices	Bread (wholemeal)	2.2
1/3 cup	Pecan nuts	2.1
½ cup	Flour (wholemeal)	1.9
1	Bran muffin	1.8

MEAT / FISH (cooked)		
100 g	Oysters (rock)	28.0
100 g	Oysters (dredged)	10.0
100 g	Beef	4.0
100 g	Lamb	4.1
100 g	Pork	3.5
100 g	Crayfish	3.4
100 g	Sardines (canned)	2.5
100 g	Chicken	1.6
100 g	Shellfish (excluding oysters)	1.5
100 g	Salmon (canned)	1.0

VEGETABLES (cooked)		
2 cobs	Sweet corn	2.8
½ cup	Split peas	1.8
¾ cup	Baked beans	0.9

HEALTH FOOD		
100 g	Liver (cooked)	4.3
2 tbsp	Wheat germ	4.0
2 tbsp	Pumpkin seeds	2.2
2 tbsp	Sesame seeds	1.7
2 tbsp	Wheat bran	1.0

FAST FOOD		
1	Eggburger (large)	7.0
1 svg	Pizza (large)	5.5
1	Eggburger (std)	5.4
1	Fish burger	4.8
1	Cheeseburger (std)	4.7
1	Hamburger (Big Mac)	4.5
1	Hamburger (std)	3.4
1	Milkshake (McDonalds)	1.2
1	Ice cream sundae	1.2
1 svg	Potato salad	1.2
1	Toasted cheese sandwich	1.1

"Just about all skin disorders improve if you build up your zinc stores."
Dr Robert Atkins MD

Avoiding common health disorders

This second part of this book shares the latest research on how you can avoid some common diseases, also types of treatments available – and how you can permanently remove unwanted weight.

"If God made it, eat it. If man made it, don't eat it."
Jack LaLanne 1914–2011, (body builder and nutritional expert)

"When in doubt, try nutrition first."
Dr Bea Rogers, age 92, (Director of Friedman School of Nutrition, Boston)

Avoiding a heart attack or stroke

While cancer is currently the leading cause of death in NZ, heart attack, stroke and general heart failure still remain major killers.

In simple terms, a heart attack or stroke is caused by a blockage to the flow of blood (and therefore oxygen) to the heart, brain or lungs. This is almost always due to a blood clot. If we are aged over 65 and living a typical NZ lifestyle, the odds are quite high that a blood clot in an artery will be the cause of our exit from this life.

About 10% of strokes (and an occasional circulation failure) are caused by the swelling or rupturing of a weak artery, again denying the brain or lungs oxygen – however, by far the greater risk is a blood clot.

A clot causes a problem when it glides along inside our arteries to a place where it becomes stuck, and then blocks part, or all of the blood flow to one of the heart muscles, lungs or brain.

Common symptoms of a heart attack

1. Breathlessness
2. Nausea, dizziness or disorientation
3. Sweating and/or abnormally pale face
4. Crushing sensation in the chest (feels like an elephant's foot)
5. Pain in the chest, arms, jaw, or neck

In one third of heart attacks, symptom number five is absent, ie, there is no pain – but if any of the other symptoms occur, with no obvious cause, seek medical help immediately.

While waiting for help, loosen your clothing, lie down and put your feet up (this allows the heart to pump with greater ease). Coughing also helps pump blood through your lungs – this simple act of coughing has saved many lives.

The five common cardiovascular problems
In all, there are five common cardiovascular disorders. These are –

1. A blood clot
2. An aneurysm (a swollen or ruptured artery)
3. Arrhythmia (an abnormal heartbeat)
4. A leaky heart valve
5. Artery inflammation

We look first at the common causes of these cardiovascular disorders, and then what we can do to avoid them.

Causes of a blood clot

The most common cause of a blood clot is recent surgery, especially in the leg area. The first seven days following surgery are critical and it's best to begin walking as soon as possible.

The next most common cause of a fatal clot is arrhythmia or fibrillation, which is an abnormal and inefficient beating or racing of the heart. This can hinder the heart from pumping all the blood out of the chambers. After a few minutes of fibrillation, stale blood remaining in the heart begins to clot. When the heartbeat returns to normal, this clotted blood passes out into the arteries, normally up the neck arteries into the brain, where it can block one of the numerous brain arteries and cause a stroke. About 90% of strokes are caused by blood clots originating from inside the heart. This is why blood anticoagulants are prescribed for those at risk of fibrillation – they greatly extend the time before stale blood in the heart clots.

When a clot blocks a lung artery, it is called a pulmonary embolism. These clots normally come from stale, clotted blood in the legs after sitting for too long (especially on long air flights), or from breakaways of congealed blood and other debris from cholesterol repairs to inflamed arteries. (Smoking increases the tendency of blood to clot.)

These same clots also frequently block the coronary arteries that feed the heart muscles – this is called a myocardial infarction, or heart attack. The heart muscle it feeds will normally be damaged, or die, and cause fibrillation.

Arteries don't need to be narrowed by plaque for a clot to get stuck. A natural fork in an artery can trap a clot. In fact most clot blockages occur in arteries that are still 80% or more of normal width.

Causes of fibrillation (abnormal heartbeat)

Arrhythmia is a term for any abnormal heartbeat. The most serious kind is called fibrillation. In fibrillation the heartbeat is erratic, or racing at over 100 beats a minute with no apparent reason. Defibrillator machines are designed to restore a normal heartbeat with an electric shock.

Any fibrillation should be taken seriously, but some kinds are more serious than others. The two main kinds are the rarer, but often fatal ventricular fibrillation, and the very common atrial fibrillation. If consciousness is retained during fibrillation, it's usually the less critical atrial fibrillation.

Ventricular fibrillation This involves fibrillation of the lower heart (ventricle) chambers and is serious – it disrupts the main blood supply to the lungs and brain. This is your classic heart attack and unconsciousness can happen within 30 seconds. Normally, for this fibrillation to occur, there are underlying cardiovascular problems, usually a blocked coronary artery, a faulty heart valve, or a damaged heart muscle. Help needs to be obtained quickly and every second counts to avoid brain damage or death.

Atrial fibrillation This is much more common and is caused when the upper heart (atria) chambers pump erratically, usually racing and not pumping the blood properly. Although common, it is still the main cause of strokes, due to stale clotted blood from the upper heart passing up into the brain.

Atrial fibrillation usually results in weakness, shortness of breath, light headedness, fainting, chest pain (angina), and sometimes sudden death. It can be caused by a sudden emotional shock, which upsets the sodium–potassium balance in the body cells and overwhelm the heart's self-generating electrical signal. The heart has a natural pacemaker (rather like a miniature brain) located within the heart itself.

Atrial fibrillation is also commonly caused by exertion when not fit. The risk is even greater when there is a dietary deficiency of magnesium or omega 3 fat. Other causes can be surgery, drug withdrawal, excess alcohol, or even a spike in blood sugar.

Highly strung wild animals like deer, captured in traumatic circumstances, easily go into shock and die quickly from atrial fibrillation – usually from a stroke, or fluid filled lungs from lowered blood pressure.

Causes of aneurysm (a swollen or ruptured artery)

If an artery in the body weakens and swells up, or ruptures (splits) under normal or high blood pressure, it's called an aneurysm. When this happens to an artery located in the brain, the brain cells that the artery feeds die, causing a stroke.

If a rupture-type aneurysm occurs in the high pressure, exit artery of the heart (the aorta), it is medically difficult to treat and normally fatal 50% of the time. However, if a person initially survives for a few days, an aneurysm has a better recovery rate than a stroke.

High blood pressure is often blamed for aneurysms, and it can increase the risk, but is not the principal cause. The main cause is weak collagen, the base material from which arteries are formed.

Healthy collagen requires copper, vitamin C, organic silica, CoQ10, vitamin B12 and folate. When any of these are lacking, especially copper, arteries become weak and flabby. People who die of an aneurysm have been found to have copper levels as low as 26% of those in a normal healthy person. Copper helps strengthen arteries, just as criss-crossed nylon cords strengthen a garden hose.

Causes of a leaky heart valve

Leaky heart valves are usually the aortic and mitral valves on the left hand side of the heart. A leaky aortic valve can cause fluid build up in the lungs, which can be fatal, whereas a leaky mitral valve can cause a fluid build up in the legs.

A leaky aortic valve is normally due to hardening of the valve by a build-up of mineral deposits, especially calcium. This mineral build up appears linked to the same problem that causes hardening of arteries (atherosclerosis) – a failure to absorb and retain dietary calcium in the bones, due to a lack of magnesium or vitamin K2.

A leaky mitral valve is usually due to loss of shape and firmness, because of weak collagen – similar to weak, flabby arteries, due perhaps mostly to a lack of copper (see above) – or from bacterial inflammation.

Fluid build up in the chest or legs from a defective heart valve is very common, and is normally treated with diuretic (water shedding) drugs like frusemide. However, diuretic drugs can seriously deplete the body of important electrolyte minerals such as sodium, potassium and magnesium. These minerals may need to be supplemented when taking a diuretic.

Artery inflammation – the major problem

Dr Dwight Lundell, a heart surgeon with 25 years experience writes – *"We physicians with all our training, knowledge and authority often acquire a rather large ego, that tends to make it difficult to admit we are wrong. So, here it is. I freely admit to being wrong. The discovery a few years ago that inflammation in the artery wall is the real cause of heart disease is slowly leading to a paradigm shift in how heart disease and other chronic ailments will be treated."*

Inflammation of the arteries is now recognised as the leading cause of cardiovascular disease, and the main reason for high levels of LDL cholesterol – a LDL blood cholesterol level over 3.0 mmol/L (120 mg/dl) is a sign (but not the cause) of arterial inflammation, unless oxidised.

Inflammation is usually in response to an attack by harmful bacteria in any part of the body – it normally involves redness, heat, swelling, itching or pain (a boil is an example of inflammation and so is eczema).

As far as our arteries are concerned, the harmful bacteria is most often chlamydia pneumoniae (not the venereal disease bacteria chlamydia trachomatis). Chlamydia pneumoniae is nearly always present in our bodies (about 95% of humans) and is the same bacteria that causes pneumonia, a major cause of death among the sick and elderly. It is normally kept suppressed by our immune system, but acid foods, damaged omega 6 vegetable fats, old age, or smoking weaken our immune system and can allow it to thrive.

Artery inflammation can also be caused by oxidised LDL cholesterol called oxysterol. These oxidised particles are small enough to enter our artery walls. Once lodged there, they are seen as harmful by our immune system and are attacked, resulting in inflammation. The damage is afterwards healed by fresh, non-oxidised LDL cholesterol. This fresh LDL is what causes high readings in cholesterol blood tests.

Vitamin C plays an important role in preventing the oxidation of LDL cholesterol, but smoking reduces this protective effect.

What is angina pain?

Angina pain is a warning that one of our heart muscles is not getting enough blood from the heart's coronary arteries. This is normally due to the twin problem of an artery being narrowed with plaque build up, plus being temporarily constricted (squeezed) by stress hormones (more about this shortly). A blockage from a clot can also cause the same pain.

Nitroglycerin vasodilator medication, in the form of an 'under the tongue' spray or pill, normally rapidly relieves angina pain by counter-acting the artery-squeezing effects of stress hormones (such as adrenaline). It releases nitrous oxide in the body tissues which causes coronary arteries to relax and dilate (widen) again, passing more blood and allowing the heart muscle to work normally again. Sunshine on our skin can have a similar effect.

What are triglycerides?

Triglycerides are fats travelling in the blood, prior to being stored as body fat. They are formed from surplus blood glucose, normally as the result of eating more calories than we need, especially from refined grains and sugars. In other words, energy from our food is entering our bloodstream faster than we are burning it off and is being converted to fat by insulin.

High triglycerides are strongly linked to heart disease and diabetes. A healthy level is 2.0 mmol/L (175 mg/dl) or lower.

So now let us look at what else we can do to avoid a heart attack or stroke.

Eight steps to avoid a heart attack or stroke

The best solution, as with almost every health problem, is to strengthen our natural defence and immune systems. We can do this by following the eight steps below:

Step 1: Avoid long term stress – A major cause of heart attacks or stroke is long term stress. This stress is usually caused by one or more of the three F's – family, finances, and fellow workers.

Stress results in the release of the hormones adrenalin and cortisol into our blood. We can feel this effect vividly when we have a sudden fright, such as a near collision when driving. However, the same thing happens on a slower scale with other anxieties in life.

Adrenalin and cortisol work by temporarily increasing our heart rate and narrowing our main arteries to increase blood pressure, and therefore energy, to our leg and arm muscles. This can be useful in handling temporary 'fight or flight' emergencies, which is exactly what these stimulating hormones are designed to do.

This is the reason our blood pressure rises when we are stressed – the stress hormone adrenalin is able to narrow our large, main arteries (these arteries are made from muscle-like material).

Adrenalin and cortisol can be worked off by some immediate vigorous action or exercise. However, in the absence of vigorous exertion, or with continual stress, these hormone levels can remain high for a long time, in some cases semi-permanently. This seriously increases the risk of a heart attack or stroke.

For example, an English study of 1600 workers whose jobs were seriously at risk over a four year period (a long term stress factor) found a 50% increase in cardiovascular disease. Such long term stress can also lead to depression which is known to increase the risk of heart disease by nearly 100%.

Step 2: Diet – We must obtain the RDI of all health promoting minerals and vitamins, as outlined in the pages of this book. This is so important, especially with regard to minerals, which tend to work in groups. A deficiency of just one mineral in a group will hinder the other minerals from doing their work.

We should try to obtain our RDI with only just enough daily calorie intake, ie, we should stop eating when we are about 80% full. Adequate protein and ample fibre will help restrict our appetite. Sugar intake needs to be kept to a minimum. If we have a sweet tooth we can substitute natural stevia as it has virtually zero calories – I use it myself.

We also need ample good fats, especially omega 3, which protects against dangerous blood clots. A 2001 study found that women who ate at least 225 g of fish each week cut their risk of a stroke by 47%.

Step 3: Avoid harmful trans fat from processed oils – There is some trans fat in dairy foods and animal fats, but this is a natural, non-heat damaged form and is not harmful – in fact it's believed to be beneficial.

Toxic trans fat is created during the manufacturing process of partial hydrogenation of seed oils to make them solid or increase the shelf life – this involves the oils being held at extreme heat for hours at a time.

Studies have shown that the risk of a heart attack doubles for every 2% increase in calories from processed trans fat, although any overheated fat is harmful to the body.

Because of its bad image in the press, trans fat has been largely removed from labelled supermarket margarines, but it is still found in unlabelled commercial baking and frying fats. This is because partial hydrogenation provides a longer shelf life and other significant benefits for commercial users, especially for fried takeaway foods. These fast foods are not subject to labelling, so it's almost impossible to know when trans fat is being used, however it is reported to be widespread in NZ.

Step 4: Vegetables, fruit and dairy lower your risk – A Swedish insurance company and several public health organisations sponsored a 12-year study of cardiovascular disease among 1752 rural Swedish men aged around 50. The results, published in 2009 state – *"Daily intake of fruit and vegetables, combined with a medium-high intake of dairy fat was associated with a lower risk of coronary heart disease in this prospective population-based cohort of 1,752 rural men."* (Sweden has A1 type milk, the same type as New Zealand, rather that claimed, healthier A2 type.)

Also in 2008 the Journal of the American College of Nutrition reported – *"A recent review of 15 studies of vascular disease and milk and dairy consumption found lower relative risks of stroke and/or heart disease in subjects with a high milk and dairy consumption relative to the risk in subjects with low consumption."*

In 1920, the average annual NZ intake of animal fat, particularly dairy was 12 kg per person, and for vegetable fat 5 kg. Cardiovascular disease did not become a nation-wide problem until the 1980's. By that time animal fat intake had fallen to 5 kg per person, and vegetable fat (mostly processed oils and margarine) had risen to 23 kg per person.

Therefore, dairy does not appear to be the villain it's commonly made out to be, but does require the right probiotics in the gut in order to be digested well.

Step 5: Probiotics – Taking a course of high quality probiotics (live friendly intestinal bacteria) from time to time can work wonders in assisting our gut to absorb important dietary minerals, especially following a course of antibiotics or alcohol abuse. Food preservatives can also damage our gut flora. Probiotics need to be protected from stomach acid as it kills most of them. Probiotics live, work and multiply in the non-acid environment of the small and large intestines.

Step 6: Exercise, fitness, weight control and no smoking – It's of major importance to exercise regularly if we want good cardiovascular health. Being moderately fit is highly protective – we should move around actively on our feet at least every two hours during the day to avoid the risk of blood clots forming in our legs from too much sitting.

Being male, obese and unfit increases the risk of death from a heart attack or stroke by a massive 60%. Smoking raises the risk even higher – it increases the tendency of blood to clot and encourages the oxidation of LDL cholesterol by destroying vitamin C in the body.

Step 7: Monitor your blood homocysteine – A high homocysteine level is a clear indicator of artery inflammation and therefore increased cardiovascular risk. Blood homocysteine levels usually range from a safe 5 to 6 µmol/L up to a dangerous 15 µmol/L. If your level is over 6 µmol, it indicates inflamed artery walls and therefore an increased risk of blood clots from damaged arteries, or their repair (see below).

One study found that for each 3 µmol/L increase in homocysteine above 6 µmol, there is a 35% increase in the chance of a middle-aged man dying of a heart attack.

Homocysteine's purpose in the body is unclear, but when chromium, folate and vitamin B12 are lacking in the diet, inflammation and homocysteine levels become high. Medically lowering homocysteine levels does not stop artery inflammation, so it is not believed to be the cause. Perhaps like LDL cholesterol, homocysteine is part of the cure.

Step 8: Keep your HDL cholesterol level high – Inflammation erodes the smooth inner linings of your arteries, especially around the forks – these are repaired by our immune system using LDL cholesterol to rebuild the linings and to help protect against further attacks. It is the job of HDL cholesterol to clear away the debris afterwards. When there is a lack of HDL cholesterol, excess congealed blood and other debris can build up on the repairs and break away. This debris can then block an artery – often one of the heart's coronary arteries.

A HDL blood level of 2.0 mmol/l (80 mg/dl) or higher is generally safe, provided it is at least 60% or more of our LDL cholesterol reading (there's more about this in the earlier chapter on **Cholesterol**).

How to test your risk of a heart attack or stroke

The three main tests are –

Blood homocysteine test: An important blood test for inflammation of the arteries (see **Step 7** above – **Monitor your blood homocysteine**)

5 - 6 µmol/L	No inflammation of arteries
7 - 8 µmol/L	Inflammation – minor increased risk of heart attack
9 - 12 µmol/L	Inflammation – 35% increased risk of heart attack
13 - 15 µmol/L	Inflammation – 70% increased risk of heart attack

CRP (C-Reactive protein high sensitivity artery inflammation) test: This is also a check to see if you have inflammation of the arteries.

0 - 1 mg/l	Low risk of heart attack
2 - 3 mg/l	Intermediate risk of heart attack
Above 3 mg/l	High risk of heart attack

Cholesterol and Triglycerides test: (for more detail, see the earlier chapter on **Cholesterol**) – The optimum levels to look for are:

HDL cholesterol 2.0 mmol/l or higher (80 mg/dl USA)
LDL cholesterol 2.0 mmol/L or lower (80 mg/dl USA)
Total cholesterol to HDL ratio (TC /HDL ratio) 2.5 or lower
Triglycerides   1.7 mmol/L or lower (150 mg/dl USA)

Bear in mind that the nutritional status of your blood is more important than the condition of your arteries, or your blood pressure. Healthy blood will protect you against the problems of inflammation, clotting, weak arteries, damaged heart valves and high triglycerides.

However, healthy blood will not necessarily protect you against the long term effects of the anxiety hormones like adrenalin and cortisol – narrowed arteries, high blood pressure and high blood sugar levels. Our relationships with other people largely determine that.

Proven heart medications

Nitroglycerin vasodilators – Nitroglycerin is the active ingredient in under-the-tongue sprays, gel pills and skin patches prescribed for angina sufferers. It releases nitrous oxide in the body which opposes the stress hormone adrenalin, which temporarily narrows our arteries. This allows them to relax, widen and carry more blood. Nitroglycerin has saved countless lives since it was first introduced in 1879. It can have temporary side effects – mostly migraine-like headaches or light-headedness from suddenly lowered blood pressure.

Anti-coagulants – Anti-coagulants reduce the likelihood of blood clots, the principal killer in cardiovascular disease. They are often referred to as blood thinners, but they do not thin the blood, nor dissolve clots, just slow down the clotting time. These medications, which include aspirin, have side effects like internal bleeding and unsightly red blood patches under the skin, but they do save lives. In the past, warfarin (coumadin) was commonly used, but nowadays safer anti-coagulants which do not block the activity of vitamin K are available.

Other heart medications

ACE inhibitors, Angiotensin blockers and Vasodilators – These medications block the actions of the stress hormones adrenalin and cortisol which narrow arteries and increase blood pressure.

Beta-blockers and Calcium Channel blockers – These calm anxiety and slow the heart rate and reduce blood pressure by blocking the stress hormone adrenalin and restricting calcium (the effect on the body is similar to a sedative). However, beta-blockers, like statins, hinder CoQ10 production in the body, so CoQ10 should be supplemented.

Statins – These restrict the liver from making LDL cholesterol, but also CoQ10 – see important information in the **Cholesterol** chapter.

Diuretics – These increase the activity of the kidneys to expel more fluid as urine, and are used to reduce fluid retention in the small veins of the body, especially in the lungs or legs, however mineral losses can be high.

Digitalis – This drug strengthens the heartbeat and helps minimise arrhythmia problems.

Can I avoid these drugs?

A well-nourished and physically active lifestyle should largely avoid the need for cardiovascular drugs and their inevitable side effects – promoting such a healthy lifestyle is the main purpose of this book. The basics of good nutrition, sound sleep, a useful, anxiety free life and regular exercise are the foundation of lifelong cardiovascular health.

Conclusion on cardiovascular disease

It's clear that the main causes for the upsurge in cardiovascular disease back in the 1950's are still with us – lack of omega 3 fat, excess sugar, white flour, insufficient exercise, long term stress, and lack of important nutrients like folate, vitamins C and D, selenium and magnesium.

The 1950's assumption that animal fats were the cause of cardio-vascular disease, has now been proven false. At that time it led to the blanket recommendation of a low-fat diet and changing to vegetable fats like margarine instead of butter and other animal fats.

Those recommendations made matters worse – for as well as the above factors, we now have a toxic mix of large amounts of polyunsaturated vegetable fats and oils, which are high in heat damaged omega 6, yet still low in omega 3. This has led to inflamed arteries, suppressed immune systems and increased cardiovascular disease. Fortunately we now have better diagnostic methods and life-saving anti-clotting heart medications available, so the cardiovascular death rate is not increasing.

We will finish with the words of Dr Dwight Lundell, a heart surgeon with 25 years experience – *"The discovery a few years ago that inflammation in the artery wall is the real cause of heart disease is slowly leading to a paradigm shift in how heart disease and other chronic ailments will be treated. The injury and inflammation in our blood vessels is caused by the low-fat diet recommended for years by mainstream medicine."*

"What are the biggest culprits of chronic inflammation? Quite simply, they are the overload of simple, highly processed carbohydrates (sugar, flour and all the products made from them) and the excess consumption of omega-6 vegetable oils like soybean, corn and sunflower that are found in many processed foods."

"While you may not be able to see it, rest assured it is there. I saw it in over 5,000 surgical patients spanning 25 years, who all shared one common denominator – inflammation in their arteries."

"Animal fats contain less than 20% omega-6 and are much less likely to cause inflammation than the supposedly healthy oils labelled poly-unsaturated. Forget the 'science' that has been drummed into your head for decades. The science that saturated fat alone causes heart disease is non-existent. The science that saturated fat raises blood cholesterol is also very weak. Since we now know that cholesterol is not the cause of heart disease, the concern about saturated fat is even more absurd today."

"The cholesterol theory led to the no-fat, low-fat recommendations that in turn created the very foods now causing an epidemic of inflammation. Mainstream medicine made a terrible mistake when it advised people to avoid saturated fat in favour of foods high in omega-6 fats. We now have an epidemic of arterial inflammation leading to heart disease and other silent killers."   Dr Dwight Lundell, author of 'The Cure for Heart Disease'.

HEALTH HINT   Smoking and heart disease

Smokers over the age of 40 are twelve times more likely to have high levels of LDL blood cholesterol than non-smokers of the same age, and three times more likely to develop a blood clot.

However, after quitting for 10 years, the risk of heart disease or stroke drops to that of a non-smoker. Smoking is frequently a sign of ongoing stress – it may be that the stress is contributing as much harm as the nicotine.

"A man is as old as his arteries." Traditional proverb

High blood pressure

Our blood pressure should ideally not increase as we get older – in long-lived societies it remains stable, but in affluent, well-fed, under-exercising and stress laden societies like ours, blood pressure steadily increases with age, largely due to hardened arteries.

Pumping (systolic) blood pressure (the higher of the two) is normally around 120 in a 20-year old healthy male, and the lower resting (diastolic) pressure about 70. This is normally shown as 120/70. The average for a 40-year old NZ male is 130/80, and for a 40-year old female 117/75.

Blood pressure is measured in mm/Hg and is comparatively quite gentle – the water pressure of a household tap (faucet) is normally around 60 psi, whereas a blood pressure reading of 80 (mm/Hg) is only 1.5 psi.

Blood pressure guidelines

For purposes of measuring longevity, the lower diastolic (or resting blood pressure), typically around 80 is the important figure. It's important that blood pressure be measured only after being relaxed for at least 5 minutes, and under conditions totally free of anxiety.

Below are the typical number of years said to be lost from a man's life by higher diastolic (resting) blood pressure at age 45 – usually from anxiety related diseases, not the high blood pressure itself.

Diastolic pressure	Average years lost at age 45
70	Ideal for a long life
80	Average in NZ
90	3 years lost
95	6 years lost
100	12 years lost

A resting pressure over 90 is regarded medically as a warning symptom that all is not well with our lifestyle – it's normally the result of anxiety, obesity, lack of exercise, or poor diet.

High blood pressure is not in itself the major danger – it is the stress or anxiety causing it (people rarely die of high blood pressure). Sound arteries can withstand huge pressure (during a leg press, the pumping pressure of a body builder averages around 400). Blood clots are many times more dangerous than high blood pressure.

However, a diastolic pressure consistently around 90 or above, and taken after sitting still for 5 minutes and being totally relaxed, is a warning that we should be looking seriously at our current lifestyle.

Abnormally high pressure during a doctor's check up is common due to anxiety (even the discomfort of the cuff tightening on our arm can trigger this effect). If the pressure is sufficiently high for a doctor to be concerned, we should recheck it ourselves at home under more relaxed conditions before considering medications (which numerous studies show do not increase lifespan). Reliable home blood pressure monitors can be purchased online for as little as $20.

Blood pressure medications do lower blood pressure, but like cholesterol-lowering medications, they have side effects and have not been found to extend lives or improve health. This is because the underlying cause (usually stress) is not addressed – ie, treating the symptom not the disease.

How anxiety can raise blood pressure

During 2016 (in my 70th year) I decided to visit a respected Auckland naturopath for a long overdue health check-up. I was stressed when I arrived, as I was 20 minutes late after a 2 hour drive from Tauranga and then being held up in Auckland's diabolical traffic. When he checked my blood pressure, my diastolic or resting pressure was over 100. I was concerned about this and the following week purchased a home blood pressure monitor and began checking my own blood pressure under a variety of conditions. I was amazed at the massive difference under varying conditions.

When warm and relaxed and sitting in the sunshine, in a parked car, or watching TV my diastolic pressure (the lower of the two) could be below 70. Yet if I was anxious, slightly irritated, or anticipating a demanding event, it could be as high as 126. When deeply engaged in a difficult mental task it could soar as high as 140. Most of the time it was between 81 and 91.

Our brain's high demand for energy

My home monitor is a wrist type, which needs to be held at heart level for a reading comparative to an upper arm monitor. By alternatively holding the monitor up at brain level, or down at thigh level I found a huge 60 point variation in resting diastolic blood pressure – much lower at brain level than thigh level – no doubt the effect of gravity.

Blood pressure is increased by the 'stress hormone' adrenalin which narrows our arteries by muscular action (assisted by cortisol which increases our blood sugar). Both combine to boost energy to our muscles and brain when required. As a result of my experiments, It appears that a similar reaction occurs to supply extra blood to our brain for demanding mental tasks – it could be revealing to measure the blood pressure of a TV quiz contestant struggling to answer difficult questions.

Lack of increased blood flow to the brain could be why many hypertensive drug users report memory problems and brain fog – medications such as ACE inhibitors, angiotensin, beta-blockers and vasodilator drugs like nitroglycerin, block the adrenalin artery-narrowing effect and are in effect artery and nerve tranquillisers.

'Stress Confronters' and 'Stress Avoiders'

In handling life's stresses, we can be divided into two basic types – 'Confronters' and 'Avoiders'. 'Confronters' face up to life's problems, 'Avoiders' ignore them, hoping they will go away.

As an experiment to demonstrate anxiety induced high blood pressure, a large group of volunteers were given periodic electric shocks at timed intervals. The 'Confronters' in the group watched the clock, braced for the shock, then relaxed again. The 'Avoiders' did not watch the clock, not wanting to know when the shock was coming. The results – due to their constant anxiety, the 'Avoiders' blood pressure was continually an average of 30% higher than the 'Confronters'. Whereas, the blood pressure of all the 'Confronters' remained normal for their age.

Other causes of high blood pressure

High blood pressure can also be caused by thick blood, due to dehydration (lack of water), inflexible arteries hardened by calcium, arteries narrowed by plaque, or sheer body bulk from obesity.

HEALTH HINT   **Minimise colds and flu**

Oxygen is our most essential nutrient – we die in just four minutes without it. Our daily RDI of oxygen would need to be measured in kgs (lbs), not mgs. Oxygen is vital for our immune system – as the oxygen level in our blood drops, so does the efficiency of our immune system.

Colds are more prevalent in winter because we seal our houses against cold, fresh outside air and breathe oxygen-reduced stale, damp air. Native Americans claim they never got colds when they lived in their well ventilated tepee tents, also, the health giving qualities of the low lying Dead Sea region are due to the higher density of oxygen.

So to minimise colds by avoiding stale, damp air, have windows open sufficiently to provide a change of air (but not a draught) about every 20 minutes or so in all rooms, including bedrooms. Even better is a fan-assisted, fresh air ventilation system which can greatly improve winter health (the effects on home heating can be surprisingly minimal).

"Stress has the ability to worsen just about every disease we encounter."

Dr Joseph Mercola

Avoiding cancer

Three generations ago, about 3% of New Zealanders died from cancer. Since then, the cancer death rate has increased 10-fold, to 30% of all deaths. It's now the leading cause of death in NZ and is a very unpleasant way to go. However, there is hope when we understand the causes.

The three main causes of cancer

Cause 1: Too much omega 6 fat – A major cause of cancer is now recognised as an excess of omega 6 vegetable fat in our diet, and not enough omega 3. Evidence for this is increasing daily worldwide. Excess omega 6 suppresses our immune system, which is responsible for destroying cancer cells.

Omega 6 is necessary for health, but the optimum ratio is 3 parts of omega 6 to 1 part omega 3. (In our typical NZ diet we consume around 18 parts of omega 6 to 1 part omega 3 – six times too much.) This also causes other health issues, which are covered in the chapter on **Fats**.

Cause 2: Acidic body cells – A second major cause of cancer is body acidity from acid-forming foods. These usually contain the acidic mineral phosphorus (found in protein foods and some cola drinks) and/or too much sugar (especially sweet drinks) which is also acidic.

As both phosphorus and sugar are acid-forming in the body, too much will lower the pH balance of our body cells. The pH scale is an acid–alkaline measurement between 0 and 14. Zero is very acid and 14 is highly alkaline. The ideal range for our body cells (best measured in our saliva) is a neutral pH of 6.8 to 7.0. Below 6.0 the body is said to be acidic.

Cancer thrives in an acidic body – this is because acidity seriously limits the amount of oxygen that can enter our cells. Cancer cells multiply in low-oxygen conditions, yet die in a high oxygen environment.

You can check your general cell pH by measuring your saliva with litmus paper pH test strips – it should be 6.8 or higher. A reading consistently below 6.0 indicates cell acidity and vulnerability to organ cancers (but not to colon or sun skin cancers which have other causes).

It's reported that just a tiny increase in cell pH – from 6.3 to 6.4, can make 10 times more cell oxygen available.

Cause 3: Not enough vitamin D – In over 800 studies, the over-whelming majority of them have found that vitamin D provides protection against a wide variety of cancers. In one study, the number of people who reduced their risk of cancer by taking a vitamin D supplement was so high, at 60%, that the figure was thought to be a typo error.

Dr M. F. Holick, a vitamin D expert states – *"We estimate that vitamin D deficiency is the most common medical condition in the world."*

Medical treatment of cancer

Chemotherapy, only about 2% effective – According to a 2004 study by the Royal North Shore Hospital in Sydney, the average 5-year cancer survival rate of adults treated with chemotherapy is only 2.3%.

The US Journal of Clinical Oncology also reports that chemotherapy has an average five-year survival success rate of just over 2% for all cancers. Outspoken American MD, Dr William Douglass says, *"I'm a doctor – and if I were suddenly diagnosed with the 'Big C' just about the last thing I'd do is take chemo drugs."*

Radiation – Radiation kills cancer cells, but also causes genetic mutation to healthy cells, which often leads to more cancer a few years later.

Surgery – Surgery can be the best medical treatment for some tumours, but it heavily exhausts the reserves of the body at a time when every ounce of vitality is needed. It should always be combined with massive nutritional support.

After billions spent researching drug cures, people are still dying from cancer at almost the same rates as years past, and at younger ages. Cancer treatment is a lucrative, billion dollar industry and it takes a brave medical professional to announce that he or she may have found a cure. (Severe persecution and defamation inevitably appear to follow.) However, there are some treatments that report effective results.

Alternative cancer treatments

Raising pH with baking soda – Dr Simoncini is a gentle Italian oncologist who has pioneered a cheap sodium bicarbonate (baking soda) cure. (Baking soda is alkaline – typically pH 8.4.)

He simply intravenously introduces baking soda (dissolved in purified water) using a small catheter, into the artery that feeds the tumour. This solution hits the cancer cells with a shock of alkalinity, allowing more oxygen into the cancer cells than they can tolerate. (Cancer cells die in the presence of high levels of oxygen.)

Dr Simoncini says, *"In the cases of cancers caught early, lumps smaller than 3 cm, with minimal incidence of metastasis, 90% of patients have made a recovery."*

There is both support for, and mockery of Dr Simoncini's treatment. Some oncologists firmly believe that cancer is genetic and are scathing of his theory that cancer is a fungal infection. However none of these oncologists appear to have tested his method, which is independent of the fungus theory.

To this scorn (much of it surprisingly arrogant) Dr Simoncini replies – *"There is a selfishness and lack of spirituality within the medical ruling class. It prevents them from looking beyond their acquired ignorance. The fundamental theory behind cancer is based on the hypothesis that it is caused by a genetic disorder, resulting in an over-reproduction of the cancerous cells. This theory is simply wrong and has never been demonstrated. Many doctors agree with my methods and have used the sodium bicarbonate treatment. Over-acidification of the body leads to the development of chronic yeast and fungal infections and ultimately cancer. Cancer is fundamentally, a relatively simple oxygen deficiency disease and the use of bicarbonate increases oxygen carrying and reaching capacity."*

Dr Simoncini's methods are being adopted by other doctors worldwide with great success, provided the blood supply to the tumour is accessible. Even taking one teaspoon of baking soda daily, dissolved in a warm drink with a teaspoon of molasses, has proven effective.

Like other doctors worldwide claiming to heal cancer, Dr Simoncini has been persecuted, struck off the Italian medical register and sentenced on fraud and manslaughter charges, due to the death of a cancer patient from a medical mishap with a catheter.

For more information type 'Simoncini baking soda' into an online search engine.

Alkaline foods plus digestive enzymes – At the age of 37, Dr William Kelley, an American dentist was suffering from multiple tumours in his liver, pancreas and other organs and had been given one month to live. Nevertheless, he managed to cure himself with an alkaline, vegetarian, raw food diet. He also took various supplements, high doses of the digestive enzyme pancreatin and had coffee enemas.

In the years following, he wrote his famous book '**Cancer: Curing the Incurable'**. He also helped thousands of cancer patients by supplying information to their doctors.

He maintained that cancer can usually be cured if there is at least a month of life expectancy when starting his program. His methods are designed to boost the patient's immune system and have a reported cure rate of over 90% for newly diagnosed, untreated cancer. (Dr William Kelley died in 2005 at age 79 of a heart attack.)

Starving cancer with a ketogenic diet – Many cancer sufferers are now overcoming the disease by eating a strict ketogenic diet. This means eliminating all glucose producing carb foods and replacing them with proteins and fats. Normal body cells which rely on glucose for energy can adapt to this diet and use non-glucose energy sources such as ketones as a fuel supply. But cancer cells lack this ability. They rely entirely on glucose and die without it. So when you totally eliminate carbs, you effectively starve the cancer.

Water only fasting for long periods can be even more effective. For more information on this treatment, try a Google search for Dr. Dominic D'Agostino who appears to be a leading pioneer in this approach.

Bogus cures – There are of course many bogus cures for cancer – a high treatment price is generally a reliable reason for suspicion.

Prevention of cancer

Cancer is far more easily prevented than treated. The latest research gives rise to the following 13 recommendations:

Get enough omega 3 – A deficiency of omega 3 seriously limits our immune system.

Reduce omega 6 fat intake – Omega 6 polyunsaturated fat, mostly from margarine, shortening and vegetable fats/oils seriously suppress the human immune system when not balanced correctly with omega 3. We should keep our ratio of omega 6 to omega 3 to below 9 to 1. The optimum is 3 to 1. (See the chapter on **Fats** for more detail on this.)

Greatly reducing the intake of polyunsaturated vegetable oils, vegetable shortening and margarine should dramatically reduce or eliminate our risk of internal cancer and melanoma. These oils are all high in omega 6 fats and are nearly all heat damaged. Consumption of omega 6 has increased about 80-fold since 1920 and appears to be causing numerous other health problems besides cancer.

Avoid excess acidity of body cells – Of the top five bulk minerals in the human diet – potassium, sodium, chloride, calcium and phosphorus – only phosphorus is acidic – the other four are alkaline.

Nature designed the acidic mineral phosphorus to be buffered (neutralised) with alkaline calcium. The ideal ratio in our diet to achieve this, should be 1 part phosphorus to 2 parts calcium.

The typical NZ diet is around six times worse than this ideal – about 3 parts phosphorus to only 1 part calcium. Our body therefore needs to rob available calcium from the bones to maintain the correct pH balance.

If our phosphorus intake continues to remain higher than our calcium intake, our available bone calcium begins to become restricted, especially as we age and the body is less able to lay down new bone.

The result is that the pH of our body cells becomes lower than normal. (This is revealed by a saliva pH reading of less than 6.8.) This condition greatly restricts the availability of oxygen to our body's cells, allowing them to become vulnerable to cancer – bone strength is also weakened.

The RDI of phosphorus is loosely set at 1000 mg a day, the same as calcium. However many experienced nutritionists set the optimum amount at 500 mg for women and 600 mg for men, or about half our current calcium RDI, giving a healthy ratio of 1 part phosphorus to 2 parts calcium. So for cancer resistance, our long term phosphorus intake should never exceed our calcium intake. (Phosphorus alone is used as a rabbit poison.)

Phosphorus is found mostly in high protein foods like meats, grains, nuts and dairy. (See the separate chapter on **Phosphorus**.)

Two interesting books explore the strong link between excess phosphorus and cancer risk. They are *'The Hidden Drug - Dietary Phosphate'* by German researcher Hertha Hafer, and *'Cancer: Cause and Cure'* by a 97-year old Australian farmer, Percy Weston.

To help keep our cell pH high, we should eat fruit, vegetables and other foods high in the alkaline minerals of potassium, calcium and magnesium.

Cut down sugar intake – When our body cells are deprived of oxygen through acidity, high blood sugar levels worsen the situation and create ideal conditions for cancer to thrive through fermentation. Dr Otto H. Warburg, a German biochemist and Nobel Prize winner wrote, *"Cancer has countless secondary causes, but there is only one prime cause, the replacement of the respiration of oxygen in normal body cells by a fermentation of sugar."*

High blood sugar levels are most commonly caused by sweet beverages and white flour products.

Obtain enough vitamin D – Obtaining a high amount of around 70 mcg (2800 iu) a day of vitamin D reduces our cancer risk up to 50%. Blood tests can easily be obtained (see chapter on **Vitamin D**). Ideally our blood level should average at least 150 nmol/L (48 ng/mL). Most people have a level far below this.

Higher blood levels of around 200 nmol/L (80 ng/mL) can reduce our cancer risk even more. To obtain these high levels generally requires exposure of large areas of our skin to the sun during summer, while avoiding sunburn, and also not washing the oils off our skin until the vitamin D has had time to form (see the chapter on **Vitamin D**).

Avoid processed meat – In 2007, after extensive investigation of cancer causes, the World Cancer Research Fund (WCRF) strongly recommended avoiding processed meat. These typically include sausages, hot dogs, hamburger, bacon, luncheon, etc.

Nearly all processed meat contains powerful preservatives such as nitrites which are known carcinogens (cancer causing), especially when exposed to high temperatures during cooking.

These meat products can also contain MSG type flavour enhancers and sulphites, often in large amounts – so can tofu, a soy-based meat substitute.

Other studies have found that eating processed meat increases our risk of colon cancer by 50%, bladder cancer by 59%, stomach cancer by 38% and pancreatic cancer by 67%. The WCRF study mentioned above, reported that eating just one sausage a day raises our risk of developing colon cancer by 20%.

Freshly made sausages, supposedly without additives are often advertised by local butchers, however, ask if you can have a quick glance at your butcher's preparation area. Look for bags of chemical additives – you might be unpleasantly surprised.

Plain, unprocessed meat does not carry the same risk.

Avoid burning protein foods – Charring, or burning protein food creates potent cancer-causing compounds, such as acrylamide and heterocyclic amine. So rather than barbequing, grilling or frying protein foods, it is safer to steam, boil, poach or bake them, and at no higher temperature than 200°C (390°F).

Exercise five days a week – Half an hour of exercise, five days a week, drives down your insulin level and is a powerful way to reduce your cancer risk. Your fasting insulin level (not blood sugar level) taken after 12 hours without food should be below 35 pmol/L (5.0 µIU/mL) and ideally around 17 pmol/L (2.5 µIU/mL). Above 105 pmol/L (15.0 µIU/mL) is regarded as risky and a sign of diabetes. This test is quite common and can be arranged by your doctor or a nurse at little cost.

A healthy insulin level reduces high blood sugar that feeds the growth of cancer cells. Some studies put the reduction in risk at around 40% in men. Diabetes raises overall cancer risk by 25%.

Get enough oxygen – Ensure a constant change of fresh air from partly opened windows on two sides of your home, even in mid-winter. As the percentage of oxygen in our breathing air drops, so does the efficiency of our immune system. NZ homes are generally badly ventilated with stale air and water condensation. Stale air and dampness are huge contributors to numerous human diseases. If you can afford it, install a constant fresh air ventilation system.

Learn to relax and sleep well – Nearly all disease has an underlying stress component among its causes. When we are stressed for long periods by strained relationships, shift work, overworking, or money problems our body steadily releases the stress hormones adrenalin and cortisol. Long term, this can weaken our immune system, allowing cancer, arthritis, cardiovascular disease and other chronic disorders to afflict us.

It is nearly always beneficial to have a loved one or a pet in your life. Stress reduction is probably the most important factor of all in avoiding cancer. There is truth in the old saying, *'Happy people rarely get cancer'*.

Take 200 mcg of selenium daily – In a seven year study of 1300 older people, the overall incidence of cancer among those who took 200 mcg of selenium daily was 42% lower than those given a placebo. The men in the study who took the selenium had 63% less prostate cancer, 58% less colon cancer and 46% less lung cancer.

Take 400 mcg of folate daily – A large similar study found 400 mcg a day of folate reduced the incidence of colon cancer by a massive 75%.

Eat predominantly alkaline foods – Cancer withers and dies in an alkaline environment. A list of alkaline foods can be found in my free booklet '**Is Your pH Healthy?**' available from Health House in Tauranga www.healthhouse.co.nz (see page 161 of this book for details).

Melanoma (skin cancer)

6% of skin cancer is melanoma and it causes 2% of all cancer deaths. The reason melanoma is so serious is that the tumour is seated below the skin and can therefore metastasise (spread via the lymph system or bloodstream) causing cancer tumours to grow anywhere inside the body.

Common belief is that sun exposure causes melanoma. The media continue to fuel this false belief, despite the obvious fact that melanomas usually occur on parts of the body mostly shielded from the sun – commonly on the upper back for men and lower legs for women.

Melanoma continues to increase at 11% a year worldwide, despite record use of sunscreen. The number of melanoma cases in NZ have doubled in the past 30 years.

The unexpected truth is that exposure to the sun (but not sunbeds) actually protects us against melanoma. Swedish researchers have found that people who spend long hours outdoors in summer have 20% less melanoma than those who work indoors. Australian researchers have found the same. Australian beach lifeguards have a low incidence of melanoma, while indoor office workers (under fluorescent lights) have the highest.

The melanoma rate in Iceland (with its weak sunshine) is 90 per 100,000 people a year. Yet in sunny tropical regions of the world the rate is typically only around 25 people per 100,000.

Swedish researchers have however found that three or more bouts of sunburn every year, from age 20 onward, can double melanoma risk. They found no link between melanoma and occasional childhood sunburn.

A deeply tanned, distinguished dermatologist, Dr B. Ackerman has published 625 research papers in his field and agrees that the sun is not the cause of melanoma. He says, *"The field is just replete with nonsense."*

The reason why sunshine on bare skin (without sunscreen) can protect against melanoma is due to the higher levels of vitamin D generated. For this reason, over-use of sunscreen is believed to increase the risk of melanoma.

Australian researchers found a strong link between margarine eating (high in omega 6 fat) and melanoma. They also found 40% less melanoma among those who regularly eat fish, which is high in omega 3.

A recent Italian study of 300,000 melanoma surgeries (excisions) in 13 countries, found that 90% of them were unnecessary – the suspected melanomas were merely benign moles. It may pay to get a second medical opinion before submitting to expensive and disfiguring surgery.

Non-melanoma skin cancers

The most common skin cancers in NZ are three non-melanoma types – squamous cell, basal cell and solar keratosis They can be unsightly but are rarely life threatening. Two out of three of us will develop at least one of these skin cancers.

The sun is clearly the cause of these three skin cancers, as they occur exactly where you would expect them to – on the face, hands and arms, especially those with sun-sensitive Scottish or Irish ancestry.

Medical treatment of these cancers is normally by freezing with liquid nitrogen or surgery. They can however be treated with less pain and scarring by carefully applying a small blob of paste made from salicylic acid powder and olive oil, waiting at least two hours and then washing it off – repeat for one to three days depending on results.

For more resistant, or deeper-seated cancers, a paste of bloodroot, zinc ammonium chloride and olive oil, thickly applied and covered with a sticking plaster for at least three hours (or overnight), once a day for three days, will nearly always work. However, it's best done under the supervision of an experienced practitioner. Repeat treatments of both these methods can sometimes be necessary a week later.

Going bare headed in the high summer sun for about half an hour is not generally a problem, even if we do get slightly pink. However unless we have dark skin, it is sensible to avoid exposure longer than this, especially on noses, ears and bald heads, by the protection of a hat, plus some sunscreen on our nose. (We burn much quicker here in NZ than other parts of the world.) Skin damage to fair skin can be almost inevitable in later life without protection.

Prostate cancer

Prostate cancer rates in NZ, Australia, Western Europe and the US are the highest in the world. This is probably due to our high sausage, hamburger and processed meat consumption (for the reasons discussed under the heading **Avoid processed meats,** page 208.)

Up to 70% of men in their 70's have some degree of prostate cancer, but most die of something else before the cancer becomes a problem. 'Watchful waiting' is generally the medical recommendation (unless it is an aggressive form of prostate cancer) as surgery to remove the prostate gland is expensive and often results in impotence and urinary leaks.

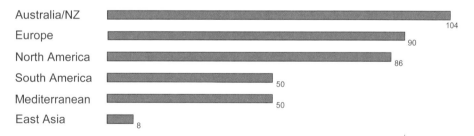

Prostate cancer – world rates per 100,000 men

One role of the prostate gland is to produce a clear fluid which makes up about 30% of semen. A study of 30,000 American men by cancer researcher Dr Michael Leitzman revealed that men who ejaculated three times a week during most of their adult life, had a 33% less risk of developing non-aggressive prostate cancer than those who ejaculated less than twice week. Regular ejaculation is believed to help clear accumulating toxins and reduce prostate enlargement.

Work related stress – Japanese researchers have found that workers on rotating shifts are four times more likely to develop prostate cancer than those working regular hours.

A 14-year study of 48,000 men found that older men who exercised vigorously for three hours or more a week, had a 68% lower risk of advanced prostate cancer. Exercise is an excellent tool to reduce work stress and promote sound sleep.

Prostate cancer is largely a disease of hard-driving businessmen, entrepreneurs and other type A personalities. More relaxed men suffer much less from both enlarged prostate and prostate cancer.

PSA tests only 2% accurate – Dr Thomas Stamey, a research professor of urology, after a study of 1300 prostate tissue samples in 2004 stated – *"PSA no longer has any relationship to the cancer except for 2% of men. The test now indicates nothing more than the size of the prostate gland. Men need to recognize that a PSA between 2 and 10, and in a lot of cases between 2 and 20, is now unrelated to the cancer, but is related to the size of the prostate. If you biopsy men's prostates you're going to find cancer, because we all have age-related prostate cancer. It begins in 8% of men in their 20s ... until 70% of men have prostate cancer in their 70s. Instead of scaring the hell out of the man, you follow it with the fact that the death rate of 226 per 100,000 men over the age of 65 is a pretty small death rate. When men get to be 60 the competing causes of death are huge."*

Progesterone cream – Men with a swollen prostate, known as BPH (benign prostatic hyperplasia) having difficulty urinating can get relief with progesterone cream (prescription only in NZ). Rub 10 mg on the inner thighs daily. Progesterone balances harmful estrogens that can build up in a man's body. A selenium intake of 200 mcg a day can also improve BPH.

Breast cancer

Breast cancer is the leading cause of cancer deaths among NZ women – however this risk can be greatly reduced.

In particular, ensure that your vitamin D blood levels are high. A blood test should read between 150 nmol/L (60 ng/mL) and 200 nmol/L (80 ng/mL). Also ensure that your calcium intake is at least 500 mg a day, and your magnesium intake about 50% of this, to ensure proper absorption.

In a Creighton University trial of 1100 women aged 50 or over (with no cancer at the beginning of the trial) one group took vitamin D and calcium (by supplement) and the other a placebo. At the end of four years there was 77% less breast cancer in the group that took the vitamin D and calcium.

Wearing a bra to bed can hinder lymph flow, as the role of the lymph system is to carry toxins out of the breasts. Research has shown that women who never wear a bra are 125 times less likely to develop breast cancer than women who wear a bra 24 hours a day. There is a controversial book written on this matter called '**Dressed to Kill**' by Singer and Grismaijer.

Avoiding alcohol, or limiting it to one drink a day helps maintain safe iron levels in the breast. Try to avoid inorganic (non-heme) iron after menopause which is commonly added to food. (There is more on this in the chapter on **Iron**.)

Synthetic hormones such as HRT and the contraceptive pill more than double the risk of breast cancer. Try also to avoid aluminium, which is found in under arm anti-perspirants and in baking powder.

Are mammograms risky and unreliable? – Dr Samuel Epstein, chairman of the Cancer Prevention Coalition writes – *"Mammography screening is a profit-driven technology posing risks compounded by unreliability. Mammography is not a technique for early diagnosis. In fact, a breast cancer has usually been present for about 8 years before it can finally be detected. Mammograms miss a third or more of all breast cancers. False positives cause women needless stress, anxiety and pain, which can in turn lower resistance to cancer and other diseases."*

Mammography is a highly competitive billion dollar business. Yet large population studies repeatedly find the five-year survival rate from breast cancer to be no better for women who have annual mammograms than for those who have none.

Many serious cancers missed in mammograms – The August 2005 NZ Medical Journal states – *"Up to 25% of all invasive cancers are not detected by mammography in 40 - 49 year olds"* – and on the other hand, over 60% percent of women who get a terrifying summons for a repeat mammogram, turn out not to have breast cancer at all.

A mammogram compresses breasts so tightly and painfully that it is widely believed it can cause the spread of cancerous cells should they exist. Mammograms also deliver a dangerously high level of cancer-causing radiation (the latest 3D type even more so). The NZ Medical Journal article above, also alarmingly states *"If regular screening is begun at age 40, the number of radiation-induced deaths from breast cancer would be 100 to 200 per million regularly screened women."*

Monthly hand examinations are reported to be as effective as mammograms.

Breast Thermography (heat screening) – A detection method that appears to be more effective (but not yet publicly funded in NZ) is breast thermography or thermograms. These measure heat from the breasts without radiation or compression. They are claimed to detect tiny breast cancer cell clusters, eight years earlier than mammography or hand examinations and with an average 83% accuracy rate.

(A professional woman's account of her breast thermography screening can be read on my www.stayhealthybook.co.nz website.)

A suspect mammogram or thermogram is usually followed up with an ultrasound scan.

Ovarian cancer

As from September 2012 the American Congress of Obstetricians and Gynecologists is no longer recommending screening for ovarian cancer in women, not showing symptoms. Dr Virginia Moyer stated – *"There is no existing method of screening for ovarian cancer that is effective in reducing deaths."*

A survey of 78,000 women found that screening was creating more harm than good – the death rate was not improving and a high percentage of women were receiving false positives and suffering needless major surgery to remove healthy ovaries.

Pancreatic cancer

With this deadly form of cancer, only one person in 50 survives more than five years. The principal causes appear to be cell acidity from excess sugar, additives in processed meat, and lack of vitamin D.

80,000 men and women were studied between 1997 and 2005 and by the end of the study 131 had developed pancreatic cancer. Most at risk were the participants who drank soft drink (soda) twice a day. They had a 90% higher risk than those who never drank them at all. People who added sugar to their tea or coffee, five or more times a day, had a 70% greater risk.

Adequate vitamin D cuts the risk of pancreatic cancer on average by 50%.

Colon cancer

Research has shown there is no cause and effect relationship between constipation and colon cancer, nor in the amount of fibre in the diet, as once thought.

A study of 25,000 people for eight years found that those with vitamin D blood levels of around 90 nmol/L (60 ng/mL) had a huge 80% lower incidence of colon cancer. Average vitamin D levels in NZ are only 20 to 25 nmol/L (8 to 10 ng/mL). The ideal is 150 nmol/L (48 ng/mL) or more.

A large similar study found 400 mcg a day of folate reduced the incidence of colon cancer by 75%, and 200 mcg a day of selenium by 58%.

Physically active adults have an average 50% less risk of colon cancer compared to sedentary adults.

Polyps are little growths in the wall of the colon – about 5% of these eventually become cancerous. Periodically checking for and surgically removing these polyps can also greatly reduce the risk of colon cancer.

"Untreated cancer victims tend to live up to four times longer than treated ones."   Dr Joseph Beasley MD

Help with autism

Autism is increasing in leaps and bounds in developed nations (see graph below). Although virtually unheard of a generation ago, about 2.5% of baby boys now have the affliction, and about 1.5% of girls. Symptoms show up in the first two years of a child's life. Identical twins have a 70% chance of both being autistic, whereas non-identical twins have a 35% chance.

An autistic person is emotionally detached and has difficulty forming normal human relationships. Communication and adaptation to change is poor and their stress tolerance low – they tend to view life solely in terms of their own needs and desires.

Autism appears to be due to incomplete 'wiring' of brain neuron connections during early development in the womb. However, failure to breast feed and exposure to mercury in infancy can aggravate the condition.

Autism rates in boys

1 in 40
1 in 67
1 in 100
1 in 300
1 in 3000   1 in 1500

1975   1985   1995   2005   2008 2016

The most convincing cause appears to be glutamate flavour enhancer (MSG) or chemical sweetener damage to the fetal brain during gestation (see the next chapter on **Avoiding Alzheimer's**).

Neurosurgeon Dr Russell Blaylock, in his book **'Excitotoxins – The Taste That Kills'** reports of repeated experiments with pregnant mice exposed to glutamates that exhibited autistic brain damage in their offspring – and humans are five times more sensitive to glutamates than mice! (Glutamates are also found in some vaccines.)

Infant symptoms of autism

- No babbling during their first year.
- No gesturing, pointing or waving during their first year.
- No single words used by 16 months.
- No two word phrases used by age two.

Treatment of autism

Outright cures of autism are rare. However the full RDI of magnesium, vitamin B6 and omega 3 can improve about 50% of autistic children and adults. These three nutrients improve probiotic health and also offer protection against autism during pregnancy.

The most effective autism treatment devised so far, and reported to benefit about 70% of sufferers, is regular injections of the highest quality, methyl-type vitamin B12.

With a little training these injections can be done by parents at home, using a tiny needle in the child's buttocks every three days. For more information about this treatment do an internet search for 'methyl B12 injections autism'.

Also, an 18 week, double-blind test of sulforaphane (an extract from broccoli) reported substantial "… *improvement in social interaction, abnormal behaviour, and verbal communication.*"

www.ncbi.nlm.nih.gov/pubmed/25313065

"If I could snap my fingers and be non-autistic, I would not. Autism is part of what I am." Dr T. Grandin, (doctor of animal science and best-selling author)

"It seems for success in science or art, a dash of autism is essential." Dr Hans Asperger 1906 –1980, (discoverer of autism)

Avoiding Alzheimer's

Dementia is not a disease in itself – rather it's a medical term for the symptom of a decline in short term memory, lasting six months or more. Normally, this deterioration will also affect time/space awareness, word fluency and problem solving ability.

Dementia symptoms are normally the result of destroyed brain neurons. This destruction is usually caused by stroke or excitotoxin damage (more about excitotoxins shortly). However nutritional deficiencies and the side effects of medication can sometimes mimic the symptoms.

If the dementia is caused by stroke damage, medication, or a nutritional deficiency, it can often be cured. The brain can create new neurons to compensate for the stroke damage, and diet and medications can be corrected. However, if the symptoms are steadily progressive, it is nearly always Alzheimer's.

Alzheimer's is the world's most feared disease (after cancer) – it's currently regarded as medically incurable and is always eventually fatal, unless another terminal disorder intervenes, which often happens.

Alzheimer's is increasing rapidly in countries like NZ, where people eat largely processed foods, do little exercise, and commonly suffer from diabetes. The percentage of elderly people suffering from Alzheimer's is doubling every five years. An estimated 47% of over 85's in NZ display Alzheimer's symptoms.

Alzheimer's rare in some countries

However Alzheimer's is almost non-existent in some sunny countries where the people walk outdoors a lot (good Vitamin D levels are believed to help), have a natural, mostly unprocessed food diet, or have diets very high in fish. The World Health Organisation reports less than 1% incidence of Alzheimer deaths in Fiji, Singapore and many Middle Eastern countries.

Countries with the highest Alzheimer's death rates are Finland 35%, Iceland and the US 25%. The Australian/NZ death rate is 15%. However the percentages of the elderly (over 85) with Alzheimer's are much higher than this (over 50% in the US) but they often die of other causes.

Nutritional causes of Alzheimer's symptoms

Both dementia and Alzheimer's symptoms can be caused by deficiencies of vitamin B12, magnesium, iodine, or from low levels of CoQ10 enzyme (often from taking a cholesterol-lowering statin or beta-blocker drug) and less commonly, by low levels of the hormone DHEA or vitamin K2.

Before assuming Alzheimer's or stroke as the cause of dementia symptoms in people under 85, nutritional deficiencies should be investigated first – especially a lack of vitamin B12, iodine or magnesium.

The most reliable test for a lack of B12 is to simply inject the vitamin daily (1000 mcg of cobalamin) for three days, and then weekly for a month to see if there is an improvement.

Likewise, a daily supplement of 400 mg of magnesium and 200 mcg of iodine for a month should be tried. The same method can be followed using 40 mg of DHEA (the 7 Keto form is available without a prescription) and 100 mcg of vitamin K2.

Symptoms of advanced Alzheimer's

Advanced symptoms of Alzheimer's include –

- No longer aware of the year or day of the week
- Inability to count backwards from 20, or to draw a clock face
- No longer able to operate complex electronic appliances
- Getting lost in familiar surroundings

Preventing Alzheimer's

Hereditary aspects do appear to increase our susceptibility to Alzheimer's, however, by adopting the following lifestyle factors, the risk should be greatly reduced, if not eliminated.

Avoid diabetes – Diabetes is a known risk factor for Alzheimer's and increases chances by 65%. Whatever prevents diabetes, or low blood sugar, will also lower the risk of Alzheimer's. (You can check the diabetes references in the index of this book.)

Avoid free glutamate (MSG) and aspartate – The cause of brain neuron death and associated plaques of Alzheimer's still continue to puzzle most of the medical world – however, in experiments which have been duplicated numerous times, injecting moderate amounts of free glutamate (MSG) or aspartate (chemical sweetener) into the brain bloodstream of mice, causes identical brain neuron death and plaques to those seen in Alzheimer's. (More about this shortly.

Avoid aluminium – Aluminium appears to play a sub-role in Alzheimer's, in that it hinders magnesium absorption in parts of the brain, but is not believed to be a principal cause.

Exercise – Aerobic exercise from age 30 is of great value – it is rare to find dementia symptoms among the elderly who exercise regularly. In a study published in the AHA journal 'Stroke', impairment in brain skills were reduced by 60% among those who exercised 90 minutes a week or more.

Stretch your mind – Keeping our minds active with challenging work, crosswords, musical performance and reading, appear to delay the onset of Alzheimer's but not prevent it.

Sleep well – Proper sleep is vital – a five-year University of California study of 1300 elderly people, found that those with sleep problems doubled their chance of developing Alzheimer's.

Neuron death from glutamate and aspartate

Free glutamate (MSG) and to a lesser extent, aspartate (chemical sweetener), are two amino acids our brain uses to transmit signals between its billions of memory and nerve neurons. They are also used as transmitter chemicals by the neurons of our spinal cord.

Glutamate and aspartate are both made naturally by probiotics in our gut and are strictly controlled in each neuron cell in our brain and spinal cord, to operate in very precise amounts. If free glutamate and aspartate in the blood increase beyond a certain point, our neuron receptors become over-excited and the neuron cells die – some immediately, others within a few hours. This happens more easily when the brain is starved of glucose (blood sugar) as can happen with diabetes.

This neuron death is called excito-toxicity – it is seen in Alzheimer's, Parkinson's, autism, multiple sclerosis, cerebral palsy and nerve cell death in the retina of the eyes, known as dry macular degeneration.

With regard to autism, tests with mice clearly show that the fetus is particularly susceptible to glutamate damage in the womb when the mother has high levels of free glutamate in her blood.

This brain and nerve damage is well explained and demonstrated by retired neurosurgeon Dr Russell Blaylock in his respected book **'Excitotoxins – The Taste That Kills'** which can be chilling reading. Evidently the plaques, commonly found in the brains of those with Alzheimer's, is not the cause, but the result of the disease.

What is glutamate?

Glutamate is found naturally in many protein foods, but is always safely combined with other amino acids – ie, it's not found in the free form manufactured by our body to transmit neuron signals.

However in 1908, a Japanese professor discovered a way to produce free glutamate from seaweed protein. This is the same form of glutamate made by the probiotics in our gut and used by our brain and nervous system to transmit signals. The professor was amazed by how well it enhanced the taste of savoury food – it does this by over exciting the tongue's tastebuds and the linked brain neurons. This non-natural, free glutamate is known as mono sodium glutamate or MSG.

MSG, and the very similar hydrolysed vegetable protein and yeast extracts are used nowadays as flavour enhancers in almost every processed savoury food in NZ and Australia.

When these MSG type flavour enhancers over-excite the neuron transmitters in our taste buds, the taste and addictiveness of savoury food is significantly enhanced – even bland food can taste good with MSG added. Whether neurons in our brain and nervous system are destroyed in the process or not, depends largely on our nutritional status. (More about this below.)

The use of MSG glutamate flavour enhancers has doubled every decade since 1950 – this was when savoury food manufacturers began to become aware of the huge taste improvement obtainable from MSG. It started when American soldiers returned home from action in World War II, reporting that Japanese soldier's ration packs tasted much better than their own.

MSG soon began to be used widely, however, because of countless reports of headaches and other harmful symptoms over the years, MSG soon acquired a bad reputation. So savoury food manufacturers began concealing their glutamate containing additives by listing them on their packaging as 'flavour enhancers' (food additive numbers 621 to 635), or just 'flavours', 'yeast extracts', 'spice extracts' or 'hydrolysed vegetable protein'.

Products containing free glutamate typically include sauces, salad dressings, soups, stocks, dips, sausages, hot dogs, hamburger patties, potato crisps, spaghetti, baked beans, etc. Even *No added MSG* on a label usually means that MSG is in one of the base ingredients.

Soups containing MSG, when taken on an empty stomach can be especially damaging – they can quickly spike our blood stream with high levels of free glutamate (just as a sweet drink can quickly spike our blood sugar levels). Processed meat like sausages can contain large amounts of MSG.

What is aspartate?
Aspartate in our diet comes from chemical sweeteners, especially Aspartame (NutraSweet) additive numbers 951 and 962. These low-calorie sweeteners are commonly used in diet drinks. Aspartame is another product like MSG that has generated countless health complaints over the years, including depression.

According to experiments with mice, when aspartate and glutamate are combined in a meal, the harm from both is intensified.

How to protect yourself from these two excitotoxins
The body's main protectors against neuron death from glutamate and aspartate excitotoxicity are the following dietary nutrients:
- Magnesium
- Zinc

220

- Omega 3 fat
- Folate (the RDI of folate lowers Alzheimer's risk 55%)

Unfortunately, these four nutrients are among the most commonly deficient in our modern, refined diet. Dr Russell Blaylock writes – *"Experimentally we know that neurons are many times more sensitive to the lethal effects of excitotoxins when magnesium is absent or low."*

Nutrients such as selenium, CoQ10 and vitamins A, C, D and E also help limit neuron damage.

Low blood sugar greatly increases the risk of glutamate damage in the brain. Our brain requires huge amounts of energy to protect itself – this energy is supplied by glucose. If we are diabetic, or have been deprived of carbs for a long time, our blood sugar can drop dangerously low – below 3.0 mmol/L (55 mg/dl).

In one MSG experiment, 100% of 14 volunteers who had fasted over-night (and therefore had low blood sugar) developed a headache after taking a common amount of MSG – normally only 10% of people would develop a headache.

In summary – how to avoid Alzheimer's

1. Make sure you get the full RDI for magnesium, iodine, zinc, omega 3, folate (vitamin B9) and also the antioxidants – selenium, CoQ10 and vitamins A, C, D and E. Avoid aluminium and if taking a prescribed diuretic, supplement with extra magnesium.
2. Avoid free glutamate from MSG, hydrolysed vegetable protein and other flavour enhancers as much as possible. Also aspartate from chemical sweeteners – especially from diet drinks.
3. Never consume food containing MSG or aspartate on an empty stomach, as your blood sugar levels are likely to be low, increasing the of risk of glutamate damage to brain and nerve neurons.
4. Exercise five days a week for 20 minutes or more.
5. Ensure you get relaxing and refreshing sleep.

"Modern nutritional deficiencies may account for over half of all disease."
Dr Donald Rudin (author of "The Omega 3 Phenomenon")

HEALTH HINT   Migraine headaches and MSG

High levels of the food additive excitotoxins glutamate (MSG 621) and aspartate (Aspartame or NutraSweet 921) are commonly found in the blood of migraine sufferers.

Migraine researchers in the Neurology Department of San Bortolo Hospital, Vicenza, Italy report – *"During headache, glutamate levels further increased in migraine with aura patients."*

Retired neurosurgeon Dr R. Blaylock MD and author of the book **'Excitotoxins – the Taste that Kills'** also writes of his experience in dramatically reducing migraines in his medical practice – *"Once patients eliminate all forms of excitotoxic food additives from their diet, most find they have a dramatic reduction in the number and severity of attacks. I also instruct them to take 500 g of magnesium lactate or gluconate daily for one week and then switch to a maintenance dose of 250 mg a day."*

(For more on excitotoxins, see chapter on **Avoiding Alzheimer's**.)

HEALTH HINT   Avoiding macular degeneration

Dry macular degeneration (MD) is the destruction of macula neurons in the back of our eyes, which seriously reduces our detailed central vision. It's reaching alarming proportions in those over 80 and is currently the leading cause of blindness in New Zealand. It was virtually unheard of just a few decades ago, and is still rare in undeveloped countries where people eat mostly unprocessed food.

Macular degeneration is regarded medically as a puzzling, mostly incurable disease. Nevertheless, in experiments which have been duplicated numerous times, injecting moderate amounts of glutamate MSG flavour enhancer into the bloodstream of mice, damages the eye's macular nerves in the same way as seen in dry macular degeneration. It would therefore strongly appear that the cause of macular degeneration is the same as that of Alzheimer's. (See chapter on **Avoiding Alzheimer's**.)

So to avoid macular degeneration, or to arrest or even mildly reverse it, take the steps outlined in the **Avoiding Alzheimer's** chapter and avoid as much as possible, MSG (621), hydrolysed vegetable protein and other savoury food flavour enhancers. Also ensure that you get the full RDI of magnesium, zinc, omega 3 and folate, the antioxidants selenium, CoQ10 and vitamins A, C, D and E, and eat plenty of reddish-purple skinned fruit such as blueberries.

Lively exercise for a total of 90 minutes a week also helps greatly.

Nutritional healing

In some parts of the world, especially Japan, France and America, common disorders are being treated successfully, without side effects, by medical doctors who have specialised training in nutritional healing.

Mineral and vitamin supplements, often in high doses are used in skilled combinations, and sometimes with herbs for heightened effect.

All of the following disorders are on record as having been successfully treated with optimum nutrition.

- Acne
- Ageing
- Allergies
- Anemia
- Angina
- Ankylosing spondylitis
- Appendicitis
- Atherosclerosis
- Arthritis (all types)
- Asthma
- Athlete's foot
- Back pain
- Bad breath
- Balance problems
- Bells palsy
- Blood clots
- Body odour
- Boils
- Brain tumour
- Breast cancer
- Bronchial asthma
- Bronchitis
- Bruises
- Bulimia nervosa
- Bursitis
- Cancer – bone
- Cancer – colon
- Cancer – organ
- Cancer – skin
- Candida
- Cardiovascular disease
- Cataracts
- Cerebral palsy
- Chronic fatigue (CFS)
- Circulation disorders
- Clogged arteries
- Coeliac disease
- Cold hands and feet
- Cold sores
- Colic
- Colitis
- Constipation
- Convulsions
- Cot death (or SIDS)
- Cramps
- Crohn's disease
- Cystitis
- Dermatitis
- Diabetes (all types)
- Diarrhea
- Diverticulitis
- Dizziness
- Dry skin
- Eclampsia
- Eczema
- Edema
- Emphysema
- Endometriosis
- Fibrocystic breast
- Gallstones
- Gastritis
- Glaucoma
- Glue ear
- Goitre
- Gout
- Gum disease

223

- Hemorrhoids
- Hair loss (women)
- Halitosis
- Hay fever
- Headaches
- Heart disease
- Hepatitis
- Herpes
- High blood pressure
- Huntington's disease
- Hypertension
- Hyperthyroidism
- Hypoglycemia
- Hypothyroidism
- Immune disorders
- Impotence
- Infections
- Infertility
- Inflammation disorders
- Insomnia
- Irregular heartbeat
- Irritable bowel syndrome (IBS)
- Jaundice
- Kidney stones
- Lead poisoning
- Leukemia
- Liver disease
- Low energy
- Lupus
- M.E (myalgic encephalomyelitis)
- Mastitis
- Meningitis
- Menopausal problems
- Menstrual difficulties
- Migraine
- Miscarriages
- Muscle cramps
- Nausea
- Neck pain
- Numbness in fingers or toes
- Obesity
- Osteoarthritis
- Osteoporosis
- Pancreatitis
- Perotinitis
- Pneumonia
- Pre-eclampsia
- PMT (Premenstrual syndrome)
- Prostate swelling
- Psoriasis
- Reflux
- Rheumatoid arthritis
- Rhinitis
- Ringworm
- Rosacea
- Sciatica
- Shingles
- Sinusitis
- Skin infections
- Stomach disorders
- Stomach pain
- Stunted growth
- Sunburn
- Swollen legs or ankles
- Tendonitis
- Thrush
- Tinnitus
- Tonsillitis
- Tooth decay
- Toxemia (pre-eclampsia)
- Ulcers
- Vertigo
- Warts
- Weak muscles
- Wind

Also the following (mostly) psychiatric disorders:

- ADHD
- Addictions
- Alcoholism
- Anorexia nervosa
- Anxiety
- Bed wetting

- Dementia (non-Alzheimer's)
- Depression
- Eye twitches
- Irritability
- Memory (weak short-term)
- Mood swings
- Nervous breakdowns

- Panic attacks
- Paranoia
- Senility
- Schizophrenia
- Stress
- Tension

Vitamin and mineral supplements have also been used successfully with pregnant women where there's been a history of the following disorders in infants of previous births.

- Autism
- Crooked teeth
- Deformities
- Dwarfism

- Cleft lip and palate
- Malformed bones and spine
- Mental impairment
- Down's syndrome

Orthodox medical treatments

Medical advances in the fields of injury treatment and non-invasive surgical procedures are impressive and continue to improve.

However, the prescribing of pharmaceutical drugs with their inevitable side effects to treat only the symptoms of disease, can do more harm than good, as well as incurring high ongoing costs. Admittedly, there are times when health problems are left too late, and there are no natural alternatives other than medical drugs to relieve intolerable discomfort.

The practice of treating symptoms rather than causes can be compared to a motor mechanic treating an overheating car engine by snipping the wire to the water temperature warning light, and then pronouncing the problem 'fixed'.

For genuine healing, our body needs skilled investigation to address the cause of the problem and then, where possible, correcting the nutritional errors and/or lifestyle that brought it about. This can then allow the body to gradually repair itself.

But we must accept much of the blame ourselves, for the emphasis of orthodox medicine on treating symptoms only, and not the causes of disease. Most people (especially men) are reluctant to discipline themselves and make the changes necessary to maintain good health naturally. We often leave things too late and then become desperate to try anything to lessen our suffering – grasping at the first quick drug or surgical fix for our unpleasant symptoms.

Common sense tells us we should address the causes of our health problems – not the symptoms, and earlier rather than later.

Effective health care is therefore up to us individually – we should avoid smoking and obesity and follow the five simple rules listed in the **Conclusions** chapter (page 243). Also, by insisting that our medical practitioner deal with the causes of our problems, not the symptoms and as naturally as possible.

Dr Ulric Williams – natural healer

Back in the 1930's, a Wanganui GP and hospital surgeon named Ulric Williams became a NZ pioneer in using nutrition as the first approach, instead of resorting to drugs.

He originally had the reputation of being a 'playboy doctor' more interested in sports and golf than his patients. As one of his golfing buddies put it, he would *"rush them through his surgery, filling them up with sedatives and drugs just as quickly as he could, so that he might have more time for his pleasures."*

One night, at age 42, mid-way through his career, when he had pushed through his last patient for the day and was alone in his surgery, he heard a clear voice speak to him saying, *"Are you not ashamed of yourself?"* He believed the voice to be from God and it became a turning point in his life. He rejected what he saw as the hypocrisy of 'the system' and began a career of natural healing. He opened a Health Home in the Wanganui area and began treating chronically ill people who came to him, from all over New Zealand.

He fed them wholesome food, (sometimes just apples and raw farm milk for many days at a time), taught them correct thinking patterns and bullied them into exercising. The results were impressive – almost everyone went home healed after a few weeks, including 'terminally ill' cancer patients.

Dr Ulric Williams died in 1971 at the age of 81. There is an interesting book on his life and treatments written by ex-patient, Brenda Sampson of Wellington called *"New Zealand's Greatest Doctor – Ulric Williams'*. It's available from Health House, Tauranga, www.healthhouse.co.nz.

Alternative health treatments

Alternative health treatments such as herbalism, osteopathy, naturopathy, acupuncture, Bach flowers, homeopathy, etc, are safer and more gentle than orthodox drug treatment. All appear to have similar average success rates (40%) provided treatment is not left too late.

Bach flowers and homeopathy are often ridiculed by those with scientific minds, as having no rational basis. That may be true, but empirical evidence for their effectiveness is certainly not lacking. I once asked a dignified elderly woman, who had run a health shop most of her life, *"What have you found to be the most effective remedy you sell?"*

She replied very emphatically, *"Bach flower remedies!"*

There are numerous testimonials on the Bach flower 'Rescue Remedy' which has a calming effect on both humans and animals.

As with doctors, there are considerable variations in skill levels among alternative practitioners. Also, as with doctors, a caring 'bedside manner' can be hugely beneficial, along with the placebo effect of any remedy. It can be useful to enquire at a nearby health shop as to a practitioner's experience and reputation.

HEALTH HINT   How fit are you?

Research has found that adults who are fit tend to be more alert, healthy, positive and productive than their unfit peers. Our typical resting pulse is usually a good indicator of our fitness.

An approximate guide is as follows:

	Men	Women	
	35	40	Dedicated athlete
Resting	45	50	Very fit
pulse	55	60	Fit
rate	65	70	Average (ie unfit)
	75	80	Very unfit
Over	80	85	See a doctor if it persists

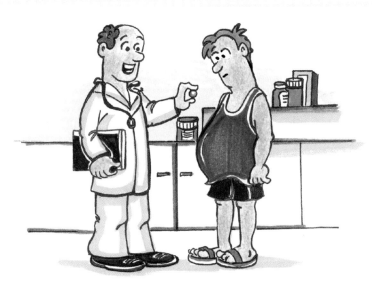

"You're seriously overweight – take this pill every day. Take it for a long walk. Then take it to the gym. Then walk it home again."

Are all vaccines effective?

There are many worrying articles and books (both from inside and outside the medical profession) critical of the dangers and lack of effectiveness of many vaccines.

There is also a surprising absence of convincing responses by the pharmaceutical industry.

Some vaccines are given credit for healing diseases that were in steep decline long before the vaccine was introduced.

Parents of young children might wish to consider the following strong words from Dr Robert Mendelsohn (former president of the National Health Federation and self-confessed 'medical heretic') and investigate further:

"I advise mothers to carefully study the known risks of immunisation – arthritis from German measles shots, encephalitis from measles shots, SID (cot death) following DPT (diphtheria) immunisations, convulsions from whooping cough vaccine and a host of others. There has never been a single vaccine in this country (US) that has ever been submitted to a controlled scientific study. If you want to be kind, you will call vaccines an unproven remedy. If you want to be accurate, you'll call people who give vaccines quacks."

Other concerned doctors have also spoken out strongly.

"Two thirds of the polio cases of this decade (1990's) have been caused by the vaccine itself." **Dr Jonas Salk, developer of the polio vaccine.**

"In 2011, there were an extra 47,500 new cases of NPAFP. Clinically indistinguishable from polio paralysis, but twice as deadly, the incidence of NPAFP was directly proportional to doses of oral polio vaccine received."
Indian Journal of Medical Ethics, 2012.

"In 40 years, I've never healed a single patient. They heal themselves."
Dr Jonathan Wright MD

Do we need supplements?

Are nutritional supplements worthwhile?

If we are having a house built or renovated, and there are insufficient building materials provided to the builder – bricks, nails, paint, etc, our house will be sub-standard.

Supplying twice the amount of some materials, or the wrong materials won't help either – we need to provide the right materials and in the precise amounts to finish the house to a high standard.

So it is with our body – it needs correct nutrients and in specific amounts.

This book can help you identify which nutrients you may be lacking. Almost invariably you will be lacking some dietary minerals (in NZ these are usually the minerals boron, iodine, magnesium, selenium and zinc).

Minerals are critical for our health and all tend to work in groups – ie, being short of one can restrict the activity of a whole group.

Obtaining the RDI of all the minerals we need from our food is difficult, if not impossible nowadays because of nutrient-barren processed foods and mineral-exhausted soils. The only two options we have open to us are going to diet extremes, or simply taking a good mineral supplement.

Vitamins

Vitamins are relatively easy to obtain from our food. In fact, vitamins are best obtained from food whenever possible. The food charts in this book should indicate which vitamins you may be lacking and which foods can supply them. Natural foods should be our first port of call for vitamins – in one large study, synthetic vitamin E was found totally ineffective as a supplement, whereas natural vitamin E from food achieved a massive 62% reduction in heart disease.

Minerals

With the low mineral content of our foods nowadays, mineral supplementation seems almost inescapable. I personally feel confident in obtaining adequate vitamins from my food, but I take a multi-mineral supplement to achieve a balanced mineral intake. I also take omega 3 fish oil, DHEA 7-Keto and CoQ10.

Generally avoid cheap supplements – there are huge variations in quality. Quality ingredients with sufficient levels of absorbable minerals are not cheap. Choose a reputable supplier and check the labels carefully.

Also check the net amount of minerals on a supplement label. Nearly all minerals are combined or chelated with carrier minerals, sugars or proteins and only a percentage of the ingredient is active. For example, boron in most supplements is supplied as a chelate (ie, mixed with another substance to improve absorption). Typically only 5% is boron – the rest is the chelate substance. So 50 mg of boron chelate would only give you 2.5 mg of boron, not 50 mg.

HEALTH HINT **Colloidal silver – a natural antibiotic**

In recent years, the natural antibiotic and antiviral properties of colloidal silver have been rediscovered (colloidal means able to be permanently dissolved in water).

When taken internally (normally two teaspoons a day and/or sprayed in the nose and throat as required) colloidal silver has proven effective in killing many stubborn bacterial infections (including cold viruses) without the side effects of a pharmaceutical antibiotic.

There is no evidence that a normal dose of colloidal silver harms friendly gut probiotics.

It has also proven effective in healing eye infections (as a spray) and for treating skin infections, especially when used as a gel.

Colloidal silver is made by passing a 28-volt electric current through two pure, silver wire electrodes that are suspended apart in distilled water. This can be done at home and there are generator kits available online for home use around the $100 mark that make the process easy.

"You can trace almost every sickness, almost every disease to a mineral deficiency." Dr Linus Pauling, (Nobel prize winner)

Slim for the rest of your life

We clearly have a huge and increasing weight problem in New Zealand. Height and reported daily calorie intake has remained the same for the last three nutrition surveys, so that would indicate that lack of exercise is the problem – increased car ownership also points in this direction.

A few years ago my wife and I visited central New York city, where it's impractical to own a car. I was impressed with the slimness of the native New Yorkers, who tend to live in apartments and walk a lot, especially up and down subway steps. Their slim figures contrasted strikingly with the obese tourists in the central city and the car driving Americans we saw in other parts of America.

My search for painless weight control

I've personally tried many methods for controlling my weight throughout my life – I once fasted for 12 days when I first researched this book back in the 1980's. That worked dramatically. (I had intended fasting longer, but was shocked when I saw how gaunt I looked in a photo, so I began eating again.)

However, since then I've discovered two reliable methods that appear to me to be the best, fastest and most pleasant way to lose weight, and to keep it off permanently. Some discipline is still required however.

The first method I call **Rapid Weight Loss.** This is an effective and relatively painless way to get you down to your ideal weight and can be done quickly as you can easily lose 3 kg (7 lb) a week.

The second method I call **Weight Control.** This allows you to correct the almost inevitable 'weight creep' and retain your slimness for the rest of your life. Use the **Rapid Weight Loss** method first, to drop to your ideal weight, and then the **Weight Control** method to maintain it for the rest of your life.

I'm currently 70 years old and weigh 68 kg (150 lbs), which is about right for my 176 cm (5' 8") height, although my mother always thought I was too skinny. I've never been an athlete but can still run a mile around the seven minute mark. At age 25 my weight was a paunchy and lazy 95 kg (210 lb).

Rapid Weight Loss (lose up to 3 kg (7 lb) per week)

This **Rapid Weight Loss** method can remove all your excess fat, no matter how many years you've carried it around. It works 100% of the time and is probably the most pleasant way possible to seriously lose weight. But only use the full 3 kg (7 lb) **Rapid Weight Loss** method for a maximum of two weeks a month to ensure adequate nutrition.

First prepare yourself mentally a week before beginning. <u>This is most important.</u> Where appropriate, let your household know that you won't be eating normal meals for the following week.

Then using the calorie charts on pages 22-23, or a more detailed source from a booklet or online. (I currently offer a free **Analyse Your Diet** service on my web page www.stayhealthybook.co.nz that may help.) Type up, or write down a list of your favourite daily foods and drinks. Keep these to little servings of between 20 to 100 calories each.

Here's an example of a list you might make –

Half an egg sandwich = 80 cals
Half a glass of fruit juice = 40 cals
1 chocolate biscuit = 60 cals
1 scoop ice cream = 60 cals
1 cob sweet corn = 70 cals
2 med carrots = 30 cals
Half a small can of salmon = 60 cals
2 rye crispbreads = 40 cals – and so on.

Include your favourite foods, but try to aim for sound nutrition. High-fibre vegetable foods provide a full feeling. Carrots, which are very low in calories but high in fibre are excellent for this purpose. Whole grains and beans are also excellent. Include some protein. Try and minimise high glycemic load foods (see chart on page 26) such as white flour, sugar and especially sweet drinks of any kind. You can use stevia as an almost zero-calorie sweetener and drink as much water as you like.

When your chosen week begins, each day eat just three small meals, choosing from among any of the food servings on your list – whichever you most feel like eating at meal time.

Your maximum total calories for each day will be –

  400 calories to lose 3 kg a week
  800 calories to lose 2 kg a week (alternative)
1200   calories to lose 1 kg a week (alternative)

These calories are spread over your three small meals and are likely to be the most enjoyable little meals you'll ever eat.

So to lose 3 kg, you would choose something like 150 + 150 + 100 calories a meal – totalling 400 calories for the day.

Or for a 2 kg loss 250 +300 +250 – total for day = 800 calories.
Or for a 1 kg loss 400 + 400 + 400 – total for day = 1200 calories.

Let's assume you'll be brave and choose the 3 kg a week option – it's easier than you think, especially from the second day forward.

How to do it

When each meal time comes around, decide then and there what you most feel like eating from your list, within the 100 to 150 calories allowed. This makes your little meals enjoyable to look forward to, unlike other weight loss diets where you eat food you don't really like. Try and keep extra busy the first day to keep your mind off food – the rest of the week will be much easier.

Now comes the second part, and this is vital – every evening of this week you are to exercise off most of the 400 calories eaten that day.

Here again, do what you most feel like doing, either outdoors, or indoors at home, or at a gym, or a mix of locations for variety. You might choose:

Running	Brisk walking	Cycling	Skipping	Squash
Tennis	Sit-ups	Skipping	Treadmill	Rowing
Exercycle	Cross trainer	Callanetics	DVD exercise programs	

I suggest doing your exercise to lively music, or while watching TV or a DVD – entertainment helps the time speed by quickly.

The main thing is to get your heart rate up over 100 beats a minute for at least 30 minutes in total – ideally 45 minutes. This generates enough heat to burn lots of calories. More importantly, it keeps your metabolism high, otherwise your body will go into conservation mode to avoid burning calories. This exercise is a key part of the **Rapid Weight Loss** method and the secret to its 100% success rate.

The exercise will also increase your overall fitness – science has found that long term fitness changes begin about the 20 minute mark, so 45 minutes of vigorous exercise is excellent. Elliptical cross-trainers are particularly effective, and also quiet, so that you can better enjoy your chosen entertainment.

You can cut back to 30 minutes if desired for the 2 kg and 1 kg weekly weight loss options, but still get your pulse rate up over 100 for most, if not all the time.

You can do half the exercise in the mornings, but it can create ravenous hunger and sometimes coldness during the day, and you miss out on the valuable fitness effect that only kicks in after 20 minutes.

You must begin this exercise the first evening of the week you begin the method. This is in order to raise your metabolic rate, so that even although you are in effect fasting, you still remain warm, burn off fat and have plenty of energy.

Without this exercise, your body will go into low metabolic 'conservation mode' and restrict heat generation – this can drastically slow down your fat burning, and you're more likely to feel the cold.

One advantage about this weight loss method is that you really do feel like exercising, far more so than when eating full meals.

Your first day will be challenging, but the days that follow are normally a breeze – you'll find that exercise becomes more effortless as the week progresses and your weight drops and your fitness improves.

Other benefits

You will generally find you have increased mental energy and often enhanced spiritual sensitivity. People tend to get much more done than during a typical week and also catch up on postponed tasks. You'll probably find old aches and pains quietly vanishing, your sleep is sounder and you awake earlier, feeling more refreshed.

Your stomach capacity will also shrink significantly over the week and when you begin eating normally again, you'll be satisfied with smaller meals. This effect can easily last for six weeks, or even years if you can avoid overfilling your stomach in the future.

The weeks ahead

Dramatic early weight loss will be largely fluid, which will be regained when your calorie intake is increased. However genuine fat loss should be at least 3 kg (7 lb) a week.

Continue the **Rapid Weight Loss** method for a second week if you feel strong, or eat regular meals for a week and then start again.

Carry on at fortnightly or monthly intervals until you have dropped to your optimum weight – ie, no rolls or flab around your waistline and firm upper arms.

If you have a serious amount of fat to get rid of, approach the task as if you were achieving a university degree – mentally accept that it will take a period of months, and there will need to be serious discipline throughout, but stimulation also. Look forward to a reward that will last a lifetime, and you will never have to do it again. The **Weight Control** method that follows will keep you slim for the rest of your life.

It helps to picture yourself in your mind daily at your ideal weight. Write your ideal weight down, along with the date you should achieve it by. A written goal is immensely powerful when you read it every day – so place it where you'll see it every morning and every evening.

You won't forget your **Rapid Weight Loss** weeks – they become almost a mystical affair. Your senses grow more vivid, your mind becomes clearer and more focused. Minor aches and pains gradually vanish, and when you eventually become fit and slim, you regain the lively 'full of energy' feeling that healthy children enjoy.

Now we move on to the **Weight Control** method.

Weight Control method (to maintain slimness)

After you've achieved your ideal size, using the **Rapid Weight Loss** method – and losing 6 kg (13 lb) a month is achievable – monitor your size weekly by using a tape measure around your waist. (A tape measure is more reliable than relying on weight.) Do this in the morning, on the same day each week.

If your waist measurement increases by ½ cm (or ¼ inch) immediately plan to do this **Weight Control** method. (I find this necessary once or twice a year, especially after Christmas and New Year.)

Here again, psych yourself up the day before – then, for the next two days, eat a medium-size nutritious breakfast and lunch, including some protein. Don't overeat during these two meals, or eat during the afternoon. Drinking water is fine anytime.

Now skip your evening meal entirely and go to bed early. Lying down normally suppresses your appetite within minutes, and without the spike in blood sugar from a meal, you'll generally feel pleasantly sleepy and relaxed in the early evening.

Skipping your evening meal allows your body time to bring itself into better nutritional balance, also to catch up on lost sleep and shed excess fluid. (Calorie restriction is also a scientifically proven method of extending life for all mammals.) If you're a disciplined person, you can omit the early to bed part, however it can be very pleasant.

By following this method for two days, you will normally drop your weight ½ kg (1 lb) or more and reduce your waist size accordingly. I've found this to be the simplest and easiest way to fine-tune my weight. It's not difficult when you psych yourself up the day before and decide firmly to do it. Tell your other household members in advance too.

Initial loss can be as high as 1 kg (2 lb) the following day, but this is largely due to the weight of food not being consumed. Permanent fat loss is nearly always in the region of at least a ¼ kg (½ lb) a day.

It's important of course not to overeat the following day, but this is not normally a problem – the stomach appears to shrink slightly over the two nights and a feeling of fullness is achieved sooner. Besides, it's always a healthy practice at all times to stop eating when 80% full.

I've managed to maintain my ideal weight for years now, even with my sedentary career. When my normal 34 inch waist measurement creeps up to 34¼ inches, I use this **Weight Control** method and I'm back to normal again within two days.

I believe skipping the evening meal is the quickest, most painless way to lose a moderate amount of fat quickly.

Why we get fat

Sitting for hours at a time is without doubt a major cause of fat gain – taxi drivers, truck drivers and deskbound office workers almost inevitably develop a paunch.

My own occupation as a health researcher previously involved mostly sitting, but now I use a stand up desk. Nevertheless, I too can gain weight rapidly if I overeat for even a few days. During the trip to America I mentioned at the beginning of this chapter, I gained 6 kg (13 lb) in just two weeks, sitting for hours in a luxury tour coach and eating high-calorie American meals at hotels and restaurants.

Sitting burns little energy, only about 70 calories an hour – standing can almost double this to around 125 calories an hour, as our large leg and back muscles are brought into play.

Weight gain can also be caused by fluid retention, due to heart defects, food allergies, or nutritional deficiencies, but this is relatively uncommon. When this is the case, the upper body fat usually feels soft and spongy.

Why carb foods fatten us more than fats or protein

The energy value of our three basic food groups – carbs, fats and proteins are mostly converted to glucose by our body, which is the preferred fuel of every body cell.

Although a calorie is a fixed measure of energy, in reality, calories from fats and especially from proteins, are usually less fattening than calories from carb foods. The reason is that fat and protein foods take much longer (often hours) for our body to digest and extract their energy. As a result, glucose enters our blood in a slow and safe manner, without any spikes. This also extends the time it takes for our blood sugar level to drop to the point where hunger is again triggered. Therefore we're not as hungry when the next meal time comes around and we will normally eat less calories. This is the reason low-carb, high protein/high fat diets work.

Carb foods on the other hand, are rapidly converted by our body to glucose (often within minutes of being consumed) especially beverages containing sugar. As a result, our blood supply is quickly spiked with a surge of glucose.

However, if we're not engaged in vigorous physical activity at the time, and our energy reserves (in our muscles and liver) are already full of glucose, we can't use this great surge of extra blood glucose. Therefore, the excess glucose has to be quickly withdrawn from our blood (by insulin) and converted to fat. This is done to protect our brain from high blood sugar levels which cause serious diabetic type problems.

The newly converted fat from the glucose (now called triglycerides) is transported in our blood and deposited around our waistline (and other familiar places) for future energy use, or a famine, which nowadays generally never comes – and so we carry kilos (or pounds) of stored body fat around with us everywhere we go – often for decades.

Just 1 kg (2.2 lb) of body fat stores about 9000 calories, or 4 days of energy. Two soft drinks (sodas) or fruit juices a day can easily load this much stored fat on our body every two weeks.

After a few hours, when our blood glucose level drops below normal, our brain again triggers hunger pangs, usually for fast-digesting carbs – for even though our body has weeks or months of energy stored as fat, it's still quicker (and more pleasurable to the body) to get its glucose from food. This is because it's very time consuming for our liver to convert stored body fat back into usable energy, and so the glucose-to-fat cycle continues.

So, it's not fat or protein foods that normally make us fat, but high glycemic load carb foods, particularly sugary beverages and flour products like bread, cakes and biscuits, all of which quickly spike our blood glucose level.

Eating excess calories from fats can also eventually make us fat, but it's rare for excess protein to turn into fat.

Why our evening meal can be the most fattening

When we come to the close of each day, and sit down to a large, high-calorie evening meal, conditions become ideal for the storing of surplus glucose as fat. This is because –

1. Our daily energy needs have been met by breakfast and lunch.

2. Evenings are generally a time of only light energy use – ie, merely maintaining our body heat as we sit watching TV, or dozing in a chair in a warm room, or lying asleep in bed.

This is why skipping our evening meal using the **Weight Control** method is an astonishingly rapid way to lose weight, and an ideal way to halt weight creep.

Why exercise is a slow way to burn off fat

As every 1 kg (2.2 lb) of body fat is 9000 calories of stored energy, even if we walk briskly for a whole hour, we'd only burn off about 300 calories – about 3% of 1 kg of fat – or the equivalent calories of one slice of cake with icing, three cans of beer, or a small bar of chocolate.

However, if we omit a typical evening meal and go to bed early, we save about 1000 calories from food, and at the same time burn off approx 700 calories in maintaining body heat and other functions. In addition we tend to sleep more deeply, which also helps regulate our weight.

Testing yourself for excess fat

If you are a male, a simple test for excess fat is to stand up and see if you can grab a handful of fat in the centre of your stomach, around the belly button area. If you can, you're overweight, no matter what the scales, tape measure or recommended weight charts might say.

For women, this hand-grab stomach test might be too severe, but the same test can normally be applied to the back of the upper arms.

Ignoring a little age flab, a slender upper arm, consistent in diameter from the elbow upwards to just below the shoulder, is a gold standard of ideal weight for a woman, just as a six pack is for a man.

Why low-carb diets only work short term

If we ever need confirmation that most diets don't work long term, we just need to look at those around us. People on low-carb diets do lose weight, sometimes dramatically, but there is a price to pay. Our brain needs and craves glucose from carbs. Glucose is our brain's energy food, and a slow digesting, high-protein diet with hardly any carbs, typically puts our brain into a glucose deficient state. Without enough glucose feeding our brain, we easily get cranky and depressed and relationships can suffer badly. You will often see stress lines on the faces of people on these diets. Sooner or later the body surrenders to the brain's incessant craving for carbs and the weight goes back on again.

Overcoming comfort eating

Even being aware of all the above, we'll still be defeated if we allow ourselves to become depressed and use food as a comforter. However, good nutrition helps our minds remain cheerful. Most important are the B vitamins and the relaxing minerals magnesium, selenium and calcium.

Equally good is daily exercise, especially brisk walking outdoors and the sound sleep it promotes.

If we have longstanding serious anxieties, perhaps from childhood rejection or abuse, competent help may be necessary. However, self-help is possible – I know a senior, psychiatric nurse who firmly tells me that nearly all his patients could go off their medication and regain normal mental health, if they were to stop blaming others for their problems and forgive the person whose actions have hurt them. In other words – to adopt an attitude such as *"I will leave that person who has hurt me to a just and loving God to deal with, and move on with my life."* Writing a forgiving letter can also greatly help, even if it's never sent.

How to eat 40% less

Research has found that we can normally eat 40% less of a fattening or addictive food, if before eating it, we close our eyes for two to three minutes and just pretend we are already eating and enjoying that food.

It sounds improbable, but has proved true in study after study. The imaginary eating beforehand appears to satisfy the brain's craving to such an extent, that people eat on average 40% less once they start actually eating the food.

"Fewer than 5% of (American) adults meet the minimum guidelines for physical activity."
Dr Joseph Mercola

Slim for the rest of your life

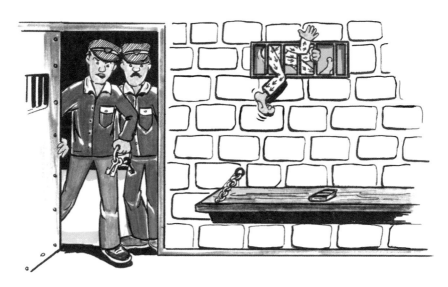

"This one's been on a fast for three weeks now... "

HEALTH HINT   'Super 8' exercise method

A daily one-hour brisk walk can do wonders for our health and mental outlook, and an hourly, cat-like stretch is also excellent for the body. More vigorous, aerobic-type exercise (puffing and perspiration) but without excessive jarring of our bones, can benefit us even more.

However, sports researchers now claim a breakthrough that will give results equal to about two hours of vigorous aerobic exercise, in just 16 minutes. They claim it will improve our health more than ordinary aerobic exercise, and for two hours afterwards, no matter what our age, our body will produce youthful growth hormones, provided we avoid sugar during the recovery period. Growth hormones, they say, should help us lose fat and gain muscle.

I've been using this **'Super 8'** exercise method, five times a week for four years now, using my recumbent exercycle, cross trainer, lifting weights and other heart-rate increasing exercises.

It's not as easy as it sounds – here is what you have to do –

1. Choose an exercise that uses the major muscles of your body and will increase your heart rate rapidly, such as sprinting, hill running, hill cycling, treadmill running, using a cross trainer, recumbent or stationary bike, lifting weights, or crouching down and kicking out both legs then standing again (burpees), etc.

2. After a short warm-up, do your chosen exercise to the maximum of your capacity for 30 seconds, then rest for a minute and a half. If you can do the exercise for 45 seconds you are not working hard enough. You must exhaust yourself, tire your muscles and be puffed out in 30 seconds. Time yourself with a clock, a watch with a second sweep hand or the stopwatch on a cellphone.

3. Repeat the same exercise pattern a further seven times. That is – maximum effort for 30 seconds, rest for 90 seconds, then repeat. Eight times in total (this is where the name **'Super 8'** comes from.)

4. Using your timing device, begin each 30 second exercise on the dot of every second minute. After eight repeats, your time should show that 16 minutes have expired.

You'll have now completed your exercise for the day and should be perspiring.

"Those who have no time for exercise will sooner or later have to find time for illness."   Anonymous

Health and religious beliefs

Throughout my ongoing health research, multiple sources have remarked on the superior health of three religious groups – the Amish, the Seventh Day Adventist Church and the Church of Jesus Christ of Latter Day Saints (Mormons).

The Amish generally reject vaccinations, birth control and consume a largely pre-World War II diet. The rate of autism reported among them is only 1 in 271, whereas non-Amish US rates for boys are 1 in 40. Cancer incidence is 40% less than average, and the mostly HPV virus sexually transmitted cervical cancer is practically non-existent.

The Seventh Day Adventists promote a vegetarian lifestyle that excludes alcohol, tobacco and stimulants. Much of this is based on the writings and teachings of their prophetess Ellen White (1827-1915). Vegetarian Adventists live seven years longer on average than non-Adventists.

The similar Mormon lifestyle does permit sparing amounts of meat, but there is no smoking, no alcohol, no caffeine drinks, and a monthly 24-hour fast from all food and liquids. The diet is based on a revelation said to have been given by Jesus Christ to the prophet Joseph Smith in 1833 and known as the 'Word of Wisdom' – it is reproduced on the next page.

A 1989 study by the University of California of 6000 practising middle-aged Mormon men, found an impressive 65% less cancer and 58% less heart disease than non-Mormons, plus an astonishing 11-year longer average life span.

HEALTH HINT Fasting and health

One age-old health practice that may partially explain superior Mormon health is that of fasting (devout Mormons fast for 24 hours each month).

Specialist German doctors swear by the health benefits of fasting – they treat disease by supervising food fasts of one to three weeks in length, or even up to eight weeks for difficult disorders, such as some venereal diseases.

One elderly German doctor made this statement – *"There is no disease known to man that cannot be healed by fasting, provided the organs are intact."*

"And God said, 'Behold, I have given you every plant, bearing seed... and every... fruit of a tree, yielding seed, to you it shall be for food."

Genesis 1:29

THE WORD OF WISDOM

Behold, verily, thus saith the Lord unto you – in consequence of evils and designs which do and will exist in the hearts of conspiring men in the last days, I have warned you and forewarn you, by giving unto you this word of wisdom, by revelation.

That inasmuch as any man drink wine or strong drink among you, behold it is not good, neither meet in the sight of your Father, only in assembling yourselves together to offer up your sacraments before him, and behold, this should be wine, yea pure wine of the grape of the vine, of your own make. And again, strong drinks are not for the belly but for the washing of your bodies.

And again, tobacco is not for the body, neither for the belly, and is not good for man, but is a herb for bruises and all sick cattle, to be used with judgement and skill.

And again, hot drinks are not for the body or belly.

And again, verily I say unto you, all wholesome herbs God has ordained for the constitution, nature, and use of man. Every herb in the season thereof, and every fruit in the season thereof, all these to be used with prudence and thanksgiving.

Yea, flesh also, of beasts and of the fowls of the air I the Lord have ordained for the use of man with thanksgiving. Nevertheless they are to be used sparingly, and it is pleasing unto me that they should not be used, only in times of winter, or of cold, or famine.

All grain is ordained for the use of man and of beasts, to be the staff of life. Not only for man but for the beasts of the field, and the fowls of heaven, and all wild animals that run or creep on the earth, and these has God made for the use of man only in times of famine and excess of hunger.

All grain is good for the food of man, as also the fruit of the vine, that which yields fruit whether in the ground or above the ground. Nevertheless, wheat for man, and corn for the ox, and oats for the horse, and rye for the fowls and for swine and for all beasts of the field, and barley for all useful animals and for mild drinks, as also other grain.

And all saints who remember to keep and do these sayings, walking in obedience to the commandments, shall receive health in their navel and marrow to their bones, and shall find wisdom and great treasures of knowledge, even hidden treasures, and shall run and not be weary and shall walk and not faint. And I the Lord give unto them a promise, that the destroying angel shall pass by them, as the children of Israel and not slay them. Amen.

Book of Doctrine and Covenants (Section 89)

Conclusions

Updating and revising this latest 10th edition has been a stimulating experience for me. I love this work and have always enjoyed updating and clarifying information from past editions as new and better research becomes available. Future editions of the book will no doubt need to be updated again as even better understanding comes to hand.

Health fads come and go

The media love to report 'new health findings' but all too often when I look more deeply into the research reported on, the news reports have been misleading, and sometimes just plain wrong.

Sorting fact from opinion is a major challenge in the health field. I find the best sources of factual information are mature health practitioners (I like to see grey hair) who have worked for years at the health 'coal-face' so to speak. Men and women who are not afraid to speak out, and like to experiment and see first-hand what actually works, particularly those who write considered books of their findings and experiences in the mature years of their career or life.

Fads such as 'low-fat diets' and claims like 'cholesterol is dangerous' or 'dairy and grains are not good for you' come and go. These fads ignore the obvious fact that millions of people have enjoyed freedom from modern health disorders for centuries while eating these very same foods, and still do.

I also try and apply common sense when some widely held health opinions do not fit into the whole picture. For example, many health practitioners maintain that cow's milk is for calves only, and that calcium in cow's milk can't be absorbed by humans. Then I observe my lively, intelligent 8 year old granddaughter Bella-Chanel, bottle fed with cow's milk almost from birth, growing taller and stronger every week. Yes, 'breast is best' for babies, but observation and common sense also need to be applied, not just theory and opinion. (Nevertheless there are many empirical reports that A2 milk is healthier than the common A1 type.)

I believe that we as a nation, could half empty our hospitals if the majority of New Zealanders understood and practised the laws of good nutrition. I also believe our children would largely avoid the modern plagues of autism, learning difficulties, obesity, addictions, ADHD, anti-social behaviour and drug and alcohol abuse.

So the following are some conclusions that seem relevant to this edition.

243

'Wheat for man?'

Wheat products appear in nearly every food chart in this book – yet rice, which is eaten in greater quantities than wheat worldwide, seldom appears in any food chart (only food servings that provide at least 10% of our RDI are included). You may not accept as God-given revelation, the Mormon *'Word of Wisdom'* (in the previous chapter on **Health and religious beliefs**) nevertheless, the words *"…wheat for man…"* in the eighth paragraph would certainly appear to be true. Wheat-eating nations tend to be invariably taller than rice-eating nations.

Yet there is a growing trend in the Western world to avoid wheat, but we may be poorer nutritionally if we do so. The trend is largely due to wheat flour being fattening, which is certainly true if we eat too much, as wheat is a highly efficient energy food. This is especially so with the new, high-yielding, high-gluten varieties introduced around 1980 (see the Health Hint on page 28, **Overcoming Wheat Allergy**).

Dairy foods

Dairy foods are also widely attacked as promoting cardiovascular disease, cancer, osteoporosis, obesity, etc. However, modern Scandinavian research is finding the opposite – that full cream dairy foods actually protect against these very diseases (the cream in milk helps our body absorb calcium). Dairy, of course, is not exactly a new food and was a staple long before the above diseases became common.

Modifying of natural foods

Misinformation on nutrition and health is rife. It soon becomes obvious to a nutritional researcher like myself, that the real problem is not the natural foods that have sustained humans for thousands of years, but our human interference with those natural foods, to increase shelf life and convenience.

Manufactured margarines and heat-processed vegetable oils are probably the worst examples – it's horrific to contemplate the number of lives cut short over the last 60 years, plus the unnecessary suffering caused (and still being caused) by these cheap but deadly foods.

Sunshine for wellbeing

Sunshine is another excellent source of health that has received bad press for two decades now, especially with regard to melanoma. The surprising truth is that in moderation, sunshine actually protects against this sometimes fatal disease. Vitamin D is now recognised as one of the most essential nutrients of all for cancer avoidance and health.

Excitotoxins

Alarming research findings in recent years are revealing the nerve and brain damage caused by the widespread use of excitotoxins in our foods. Excitotoxins are glutamate-based flavour enhancers like MSG, added to almost every savoury food and processed meat in our supermarkets today. These include soups, sauces, baked beans, sausages and takeaway food. Aspartate chemical sweeteners found in diet drinks are also excitotoxins.

There's overwhelming evidence that we can now avoid progressive and incurable brain and nerve diseases connected with these glutamate and aspartate food additives. These diseases include multiple sclerosis, macular degeneration, Parkinsons, ALS and Alzheimer's. Depression also seems firmly linked with aspartate (see also the chapter on **Avoiding Alzheimer's**). Magnesium, zinc, omega 3, and folate help protect us against these harmful excitotoxins.

Five simple rules for ongoing good health

The bottom line is that we are only as healthy as the probiotics in our gut. We possess a marvellous and complex digestive system that can work reliably non-stop for 80 or 90 years. We just need to abide by five simple rules:

Rule 1 Eat varied and natural foods, to provide close to the RDI (RDA).

Rule 2 Avoid anxiety while our digesting food.

Rule 3 Only eat when hungry, ie, wait until our appetite informs us it has digested our last intake of food before giving it more, and stop eating when we are about 80% full.

Rule 4 Do exercise that makes you sweat, on five or six days of the week.

Rule 5 Avoid antibiotics (by mouth) and other pharmaceutical drugs unless there is no natural alternative. The renowned doctor Robert Willner MD, PhD has stated *"(herbs) are superior 95% of the time to any pharmaceutical drug."*

Rule 1: Eat varied and natural foods – Natural food is vastly superior to processed food. During a three week Middle Eastern trip some years ago (mostly through Muslim countries), I was impressed with the general health, vigour and well-formed teeth of the vast majority of people I saw – even though smoking was common. I saw virtually no obesity (except among the tourists), no walking sticks, and no limping or hobbling due to arthritis.

One reason for this soon became apparent – whenever I walked into a typical Middle Eastern 'supermarket' I would see vast arrays of open sacks on the floor. These sacks contained chickpeas, corn, wheat, barley, or beans, along with large crates of all kinds of raw vegetables and fruit.

Obtaining a variety of natural foods is comparatively easy in NZ – the food charts in this book will help you choose. Select the full colour spectrum of vegetables, fruit and grain over the course of a week – yellow, orange, red, green, brown, purple and white.

Fats, sugars and salt in raw unprocessed foods are not a problem. – the problem foods are the processed ones, high in refined sugar, refined salt, heat damaged fats, flavour enhancing additives, and preservatives for longer shelf life. For superior health we must keep these to a minimum. There's a quip that contains much truth – *'Any food with a bar code is no good for you'*.

Nevertheless, many natural NZ foods are low in important minerals. Until we can persuade our growers to correctly fertilise their soils and not pick produce too early, we will need to supplement our diet with some minerals. The food tables in this book should help you discover which minerals you lack – zinc, magnesium, selenium and boron are common ones.

There appears to be little, or no evidence that food pollutants in NZ foods are responsible for much ill health – a well-nourished body is highly efficient at expelling toxins.

Rule 2: Avoiding anxiety – Mental relaxation, while our food is digesting is more important than we might think. A mind filled with anxiety is a huge contributor to poor health – it seriously affects our digestion by hindering production of stomach acid, digestive enzymes and probiotics, and consequently the uptake of nutrients (excess tummy rumbling can be a symptom of this common problem). Perhaps we should follow the example of animals and rest after eating, or not eat at all when we are emotionally stressed. Fasting has a powerful calming effect and can help overcome food and other addictions.

Hope, love and forgiveness are keys to the nourishment of our body and mind, and to trigger our body's healing powers.

Rule 3: Only eat when hungry – Eating more calories than we need is a massive problem in NZ and the main cause of obesity, diabetes and cardiovascular disorders – diseases virtually unheard of in societies that eat natural foods, walk a lot and have a lower calorie intake. The first law of health is 'Never eat when not hungry'.

Nevertheless, waiting too long between meals and then coming to the table with a ravenous appetite can cause us to seriously over-eat. Japanese sumo wrestlers fatten themselves by fasting during the daytime and then wolfing down an enormous meal at night.

The Muslim city of Cairo in Egypt, generates more food-related garbage during the daylight fasting month of Ramadan than at any other time, because of additional eating and drinking at night.

We should stop eating when we are 80% full. This principle is not easy to follow at first (smaller portions on our plate can help) but the rewards are worthwhile – it protects us against obesity, arthritis, anxiety, loss of energy and poor sleep. The 80% rule also prevents us against stomach capacity stretching, which is a huge factor in overeating.

Rule 4: Exercise has worthwhile benefits – Exercise, both indoors and outdoors that raises a sweat, results in superior blood circulation, which in turn helps nourish our body and rid cells of waste. It also does wonders for our figure, mental outlook, enjoyment of life and inner peace. If we wait until we feel like exercising, or until we have the time, it probably won't happen. We must plan, and work our plan. We can exercise indoors and watch TV at the same time with suitable equipment like a stepper, cross-trainer, exercycle or treadmill. The World Health Organisation recommends an hour of moderate activity every day. (My own exercise regime is outlined in the next section.) A rest and relaxation day is also important – for me it is Sunday.

Healing advice from Dr Ulric Williams

Dr Williams was a well known NZ surgeon and GP who practised between the 1920's and the 1960's. During the 1930's he became a naturopath and began healing patients without drugs or surgery.

"Hardly anyone would be ill if they hadn't made themselves ill, or been made ill by parents or guardians. The life force within, or Spirit of God is the only power that can make us well. It is always striving to restore us to health and keep us well. It will almost always succeed if we give it a chance and withdraw the physical barriers of over-eating the wrong kinds of food, under-eating the right kinds, insufficient outdoor exercise, and indulging in poisons like tobacco and alcohol. "

"And also the psychological barriers, such as fear, resentment, worrying, self pity, jealousy, pride, avarice (greed), gluttony, lust, together with all negative thoughts, beliefs, suggestions, impressions or ideas. Of all the causes of disease, these psychological barriers are far and away the worst. They'll be taken away if you let their cause go."

HEALTH HINT   **Eggs a rich source of nutrients**

Eggs are a rich source of readily available nutrients – superior to any meat. This is not surprising when we take into account that a fully formed, live chicken can be created from the nutrients of one egg.

"I saw a few die of hunger; of eating, a hundred thousand."
Benjamin Franklin

247

My own health

Years of research have gone into the various editions of this book. Day after day – studying medical and health books, cross referencing, checking, discussing, pondering, praying for understanding, attending the occasional lecture, searching the internet, experimenting on myself and testing supplements. It's time consuming but I find it stimulating.

I receive helpful letters, emails and calls from readers. I also enjoy and learn from discussions with health conscious friends and colleagues.

All of this, I feel, has paid off richly for me as I apply (with occasional lapses) the knowledge gained to improve my own health.

I am now 70, and feel that my energy and fitness level is almost as good as it was in my 30s. I sleep right through the night and enjoy complete freedom from the regular and miserable bouts of flu and hay fever that plagued me in my early years.

I rarely catch a cold

I rarely, if ever get a cold, from one year to the next (unless I brag about it) and have not had the flu for over 25 years. I used to get about four colds and two bouts of flu each year. I take a teaspoon of colostrum powder most mornings to help in this area and also a little colloidal silver most days. I have found colloidal silver very effective. If I feel exposed to a cold virus, I'll use a spray bottle and breathe a few puffs of colloidal silver spray in through my nose and mouth and gargle with salty water.

Food and supplements

I'm able to obtain the RDI of all necessary nutrients from wholesome food, apart from zinc, boron, calcium, iodine and omega 3. For these more difficult to obtain minerals, I take four daily supplements, a multi-mineral-vitamin capsule, a coral calcium/magnesium capsule, a fish oil/cod liver oil omega 3 and CoQ10 capsule and DHEA 7-Keto capsule.

I grind organically-grown, whole wheat (spelt) that I first sprout then dry (and sometimes barley) for my home-made bread and my raw porridge recipe (see recipe section).

My six adult children and my wife are not as health-conscious as I am (they would probably say *'not as fanatical'*) but their health has also been above average.

My daily routine

I'm sometimes asked about my daily health routine, so here it is:

Morning exercise – Six mornings a week (about 7.30 am) I do some moderately heavy muscle exercise for about 30–45 minutes. This is done in my home gym (a converted bedroom) while watching pre-recorded TV programs or downloaded documentaries to avoid boredom. Also, to avoid boredom (the enemy of exercise) I vary these morning exercises each day. These variations are – lifting weights, sit-ups, pull-ups, exercycle (recumbent type), cross-trainer, rubber cord leg exercises and a hydraulic rower. About half these exercises are done using the 'Super 8' method described on page 240.

Breakfast – After exercising I have a whey protein milkshake (raw milk from a farm or coconut cream), blended with an egg, a teaspoon of colostrum and some malt powder – I take this protein to try and avert 'old-age' muscle wasting – so far so good. For years I skipped breakfast, in order to have a clearer mind for research and writing, but I find that this protein breakfast doesn't cause me mid-morning drowsiness as a carb breakfast did.

Fruit and supplements – Mid-morning I have a piece of fruit (normally half a banana, a kiwifruit or orange) and a glass of water with apple cider vinegar, honey (or molasses) and a sprinkle of ginger and cinnamon stirred in. With this drink I take my daily omega 3 fish oil and CoQ10 capsule and a DHEA 7-Keto capsule. (I take DHEA to maintain body levels of this important youth hormone.)

Lunch – For lunch I usually have a plate of pre-cooked, mixed vegetables and beans. Once a week I like to fill a slow cooker with a variety of vegetables of all colours, including either navy beans, black eyed peas or chickpeas, then store them in the fridge and warm a plateful each day in the microwave. Following the veges, I usually have a mug of my instant porridge made from ground wholemeal wheat and/or my home-made bread (see recipe section page 259). Sometimes, instead of this I'll have a tin of canned salmon and avocado mixed together, sprinkled with unrefined salt.

I finish lunch with two brazil nuts eaten together with a date (a tasty combination), a home-made healthy afghan and about four teaspoons of roast pumpkin seeds.

I try and resist (not always successfully) the tempting supermarket chocolate biscuits and similar treats that my wife Marie stores in the pantry. Also, my younger daughter Harmony loves to come by and bake for us (and herself) from time to time. So on Sundays I usually fast until evening to atone for my 'diet sins' of the week.

Evening meal – My evening meal nowadays is light and usually just a dessert (unsweetened yoghurt, fruit, and cream) and another of my homemade wheat afghans or a similar treat. Then I'll have a raw fruit, perhaps an apple, or a pear. Soon after I take my daily multi and coral calcium/magnesium capsule with a glass of water, mixed with a sprinkle of ginger, cinnamon and stevia.

Evening and weekend exercise – I also try and exercise every evening. Some evenings I'll go for a brisk walk or run outdoors for 30–40 minutes, or a ride on my mountain bike. If I'm out alone I'll listen to music or talks on an iPod or small belt radio and ear-bud headphones. Saturdays I mow the lawns, do a little gardening or general home maintenance. Sometimes I'll go for a bush tramp or mountain bike with one of my brothers or my brother-in-law.

Future plans – I have no desire to retire – I work from my outside, home office and enjoy it. I believe that stimulating work keeps a person healthy. I plan to continue researching and writing books and being involved in service work within my local church.

It's a true maxim – **'Health is the best wealth.'** I hope this book will also help you to achieve or maintain it.

Feedback to me and help to others

If you have any suggestions that could make future editions of this book more useful to you (without adding to the overall size) please email them to me – stayhealthybook@zealandpublishing.co.nz.

HEALTH HINT   **Banish bad breath**

Most moderate bad breath comes from stagnant bacteria in the mouth, especially on the tongue. Eating usually replaces this bacteria and gives temporary relief.

A permanent solution is, when brushing your teeth (ideally after every meal) to also vigorously brush your tongue with diluted toothpaste. Do this as far back as you can reach without gagging. Also your gums, roof of your mouth and other internal surfaces which might harbour bacteria.

Severe, continual bad breath is usually caused by rotting teeth, infected gums or by a tonsil infection and requires professional help.

"The first requirement of a good life is to be healthy."
Herbert Spencer 1820–1903, (English philosopher)

Food additive code numbers

Food additives are listed on packaging along with the ingredients in descending order of weight.

Typical food additives include –

Colours – to enhance appearance
Preservatives – to kill bacteria and extend shelf life
Antioxidants – to prevent spoilage and extend shelf life
Emulsifiers – to allow mixing of fat and water
Thickeners – to thicken liquids
Stabilisers – to prevent ingredients separating
Modifiers – ie, baking powder to provide gas for raising dough
Flavour enhancers – to enhance taste
Appearance enhancers – glazes, bleach whiteners, etc.
Starches – to extend or thicken food
Gelling agents – to gel liquids
Solvents – to dissolve flavourings

To identify additives and save printing space on food labels, a code number system is often used – below are the code numbers currently used.

Listed alongside each number is the chemical name of the additive, the main use of the additive, and the source.

An asterisk * after a code number indicates that adverse health reactions have been reported. A double asterisk ** indicates greater seriousness of reaction, or that the additive has been banned in some countries. An E before an additive number on overseas food labels means that the additive has been approved for use in the European Union, but it is otherwise identical to one without an E.

Number Chemical name   Use   Source

FOOD COLOURS
100   *Curcumin from Turmeric*. **Yellow colouring.** Turmeric plant.
101   *Riboflavin*. **Yellow colouring.** Yeast.
102**   *Tartrazine*. **Yellow colouring.** Synthetic.
103**   *Alkanet.* **Red colouring.** Alkanet plant root.
104**   *Quinoline*. **Yellow colouring.** Coal tar.
106   *Riboflavin*. **Yellow colouring.** Yeast.
107**   *Yellow 2G*. **Yellow colouring.** Coal tar.
110**   *Sunset Yellow* FCF. **Yellow colouring.** Coal tar.
120**   *Cochineal*. **Red colouring.** Scale insects.
121   *Orcein or Orchil*. **Red/Brown colouring.** Lichen.
122**   *Carmoisine*. **Red colouring.** Coal tar.
123**   *Amaranth*. **Red colouring.** Amaranth plant.
124**   *Ponceau 4R*. **Red colouring.** Coal tar.
125   *Scarlet GN.* **Red colouring.** Synthetic.

Number	Chemical name	Use	Source

126 *Brilliant Crystal Scarlet.* **Red colouring.** Synthetic.
127** *Erythrosine.* **Red colouring.** Coal tar.
128** *Red 2G.* **Red colouring.** Coal tar.
129** *Allura Red AC.* **Red colouring.** Synthetic.
131** *Patent Blue V.* **Blue colouring.** Coal tar.
132* *Indigo carmine.* **Blue colouring.** Coal tar.
133** *Brilliant Blue FCF.* **Blue colouring.** Coal tar.
140 *Chlorophyll.* **Green colouring.** Green plants.
141 *Copper phaeophytin.* **Olive green colouring.** Green plants.
142** *Green S.* **Green colouring.** Coal tar.
150* *Caramel.* **Brown colouring and flavouring.** Heated carbohydrates.
151** *Brilliant Black BN.* **Black colouring.** Coal tar.
153* *Vegetable carbon.* **Black colouring.** Charcoal from burnt plants.
154** *Brown FK.* **Brown colouring.** Synthetic.
155** *Brown HT.* **Brown colouring.** Synthetic.
160a *Carotene.* **Orange-yellow colouring.** Plants.
160b* *Annatto.* **Red-yellow colouring.** Annatto seeds.
160c* *Capsanthin from paprika.* **Orange colouring.** Paprika.
160d* *Lycopene.* **Red colouring.** Tomatoes.
160e *Carotenal beta-apo-8.* **Red-yellow colouring.** Synthetic.
160f *Carotenoic acid apo-8.* **Orange-yellow colouring.** Synthetic.
161 *Xanthopylls.* **Yellow colouring.** Plants.
161a *Flavoxanthin.* **Yellow colouring.** Plants.
161b *Xanthophylls-Lutein.* **Yellow colouring.** Plants.
161c *Cryptoxanthin.* **Yellow colouring.** Plants.
161d *Rubixanthin.* **Yellow colouring.** Plants.
161e *Violoxanthin.* **Yellow colouring.** Plants.
161f *Rhodoxanthin.* **Yellow colouring.** Plants.
161g *Canthaxanthin.* **Orange colouring.** Plants, shellfish or mushrooms.
161h *Citranaxanthin.* **Yellow colouring.** Plants.
162 *Beet Red.* **Red colouring.** Beetroot.
163 *Anthocyanins.* **Red colouring.** Plants.
170 *Calcium carbonate.* **Firming agent and white colouring.** Limestone.
171 *Titanium dioxide.* **White colouring.** Natural mineral.
172 *Iron oxide.* **Yellow-red or Brown-black colouring.** Natural mineral.
173* *Aluminium.* **Silver colouring cake decoration.** Bauxite.
174* *Silver.* **Silver colouring cake decoration.** Natural mineral.
175 *Gold.* **Gold colouring cake decoration.** Natural mineral.
180** *Rubine.* **Red colouring.** Synthetic.
181 *Tannic acid.* **Clarifying agent in alcoholic drinks.** Plants.

FOOD PRESERVATIVES

200 *Sorbic acid.* **Mould inhibitor.** Plants, but mostly synthetic.
201 *Sodium sorbate.* **Preservative.** Plants, but mostly synthetic.
202 *Potassium sorbate.* **Preservative.** Plants, but mostly synthetic.
203 *Calcium sorbate.* **Preservative.** Plants, but mostly synthetic.
210* *Benzoic acid.* **Preservative.** Plants, but mostly synthetic.
211* *Sodium benzoate.* **Preservative.** Plants, but mostly synthetic.
212* *Potassium benzoate.* **Preservative.** Plants, but mostly synthetic.
213* *Calcium benzoate.* **Preservative.** Plants, but mostly synthetic.
214* *Ethyl p-hydroxybenzoate.* **Preservative.** Plants, but mostly synthetic.
215* *Sodium ethyl para-hydroxybenzoate.* **Preservative.** Plants, but mostly synthetic.
216* *Propyl para-hydroxybenzoate.* **Preservative.** Plants, but mostly synthetic.

| Number | Chemical name | Use | Source |

217*   *Sodium propyl para-hydroxybenzoate.* **Preservative.** Plants, but mostly synthetic.
218*   *Methyl para-hydroxybenzoate.* **Preservative.** Plants, but mostly synthetic.
219*   *Sodium methyl hydroxybenzoate.* **Preservative.** Plants, but mostly synthetic.
220*   *Sulphur dioxide gas.* **Preservative, stabiliser, antioxidant and bleach.** Sulphur.
221*   *Sodium sulphite.* **Preservative and antioxidant.** Sulphurous acid.
222*   *Sodium bisulphite.* **Preservative and bleach.** Sulphurous acid.
223*   *Sodium metabisulphite.* **Preservative and antioxidant.** Sulphurous acid.
224*   *Potassium metabisulphite.* **Preservative.** Sulphurous acid.
225*   *Potassium sulphite.* **Preservative.** Sulphurous acid.
226*   *Calcium sulphite.* **Preservative and firming agent.** Sulphurous acid.
227*   *Calcium hydrogen sulphite.* **Preservative and firming agent.** Sulphurous acid.
228   *Potassium bisulphite.* **Preservative.** Sulphurous acid.
234   *Nisin.* **Preservative.** Bacteria.
235*   *Natamycin.* **Preservative.** Bacteria.
236**   *Formic acid.* **Preservative.** Synthetic.
249**   *Potassium nitrate.* **Meat curer and preservative.** Nitrous acid.
250**   *Sodium nitrate.* **Meat curer and preservative.** Nitrous acid.
251*   *Chile saltpetre.* **Meat curer and preservative.** Natural mineral.
252**   *Potassium nitrate (saltpetre).* **Meat curer and preservative.** Natural mineral.
260   *Acetic acid (vinegar).* **Preservative and colour diluent.** Synthetic.
261*   *Potassium acetate.* **Preservative and acidity regulator.** Vinegar.
262   *Sodium diacetate.* **Preservative and acidity regulator.** Vinegar.
263   *Calcium acetate.* **Preservative, thickener and acidity regulator.** Vinegar.
264*   *Ammonium acetate.* **Preservative.** Vinegar.
270   *Lactic acid.* **Preservative, acidity regulator and flavouring.** Milk and plants.
280*   *Propionic acid.* **Preservative.** Fermentation of plants.
281*   *Sodium propionate.* **Preservative.** Propionic acid.
282*   *Calcium propionate.* **Preservative.** Propionic acid.
283   *Potassium propionate.* **Preservative.** Propionic acid.
290   *Carbon dioxide.* **Preservative gas, freezant and spray can propellant.** Natural gas.
296   *Malic acid.* **Acid flavouring.** Synthetic.
297   *Fumaric acid.* **Acid flavouring.** Fermentation of plants.

ANTIOXIDANTS, EMULSIFIERS AND STABILISERS

300   *Ascorbic acid.* **Vitamin C, antioxidant and flour improver**. Synthetic.
301   *Sodium ascorbate.* **Vitamin C and antioxidant.** Ascorbic acid.
302   *Calcium ascorbate.* **Vitamin C and antioxidant.** Ascorbic acid.
303   *Potassium ascorbate.* **Vitamin C and antioxidant.** Ascorbic acid.
304   *Ascorbyl palmitate.* **Vitamin C and antioxidant.** Ascorbic acid.
306   *Tocopherol.* **Vitamin E and antioxidant.** Seeds.
307   *a-Tocopherol.* **Vitamin E and antioxidant.** Synthetic.
308   *y-Tocopherol.* **Vitamin E and antioxidant.** Synthetic.
309   *Tocopherol.* **Vitamin E and antioxidant.** Synthetic.
310**   *Propyl gallate.* **Antioxidant.** Tannins.
311*   *Octal gallate.* **Antioxidant.** Tannins.
312*   *Dodecyl gallate.* **Antioxidant.** Tannins.
314   *Guaiac gum.* **Antioxidant in cola drinks.** Guaiacum tree resin.
315   *Erythorbic acid.* **Antioxidant.** Sucrose.
316   *Sodium erythorbic.* **Antioxidant**. Sucrose.
318   *Calcium isoascorbate.* **Antioxidant.** Ascorbic acid.
319*   *tert-Butylhydroquinone.* **Antioxidant and synthetic vitamin E.** Petroleum**.**
320**   *Butylated hydroxyanisole.* **Antioxidant and synthetic vitamin E.** Petroleum.
321   *Butylated hydroxytoluene (BHT).* **Antioxidant and synthetic vitamin E.** Petroleum.

Food additive code numbers

322 *Lecithin.* **Stabiliser, antioxidant, thickener and emulsifier.** Mostly Soy beans.
325 *Sodium lactate.* **Antioxidant, acidity regulator and moistener.** Lactic acid.
326 *Potassium lactate.* **Antioxidant and acidity regulator.** Lactic acid.
327 *Calcium lactate.* **Antioxidant, acidity regulator and firmer.** Lactic acid.
328 *Ammonium lactate.* **Stabiliser.** Lactic acid.
329 *Magnesium lactate.* **Stabiliser and magnesium supplement.** Lactic acid.
330 *Citric acid.* **Stabiliser, preservative, gelling agent and flavouring.** Corn or molasses.
331 *Sodium citrate.* **Antioxidant, acidity regulator and emulsifier.** Citric acid.
332 *Potassium citrate.* **Food acid, antioxidant and emulsifier.** Citric acid.
333 *Calcium citrate.* **Emulsifier, firming agent and acidity regulator.** Citric acid.
334 *Tartaric acid.* **Antioxidant, diluent and food acid.** Grapes.
335 *Sodium tartrate.* **Antioxidant, emulsifier and stabiliser.** Tartaric acid.
336 *Cream of tartar.* **Antioxidant, emulsifier and stabiliser.** Tartaric acid.
337 *Potassium sodium tartrate.* **Antioxidant, emulsifier and stabiliser**. Tartaric acid.
338 * *Phosphoric acid.* **Food acid and antioxidant.** Phosphate ore.
339 *Sodium phosphate.* **Stabiliser and antioxidant.** Phosphoric acid.
339b *Di-sodium phosphate.* **Stabiliser, nutrient and gelling agent.** Phosphoric acid.
340 *Potassium phosphate.* **Stabiliser, antioxidant and emulsifier.** Phosphoric acid.
341 *Calcium phosphate.* **Raising agent, alkaliser, firming agent, anti-caking, antioxidant, toothpaste abrasive, nutrient and emulsifier**. Natural mineral.
343 *Magnesium phosphate.* **Magnesium supplement and anti-caking.** Natural mineral.
350 *Sodium malate.* **Stabiliser and seasoning.** Malic acid.
351 *Potassium malate.* **Stabiliser.** Malic acid.
352 *Calcium malate.* **Stabiliser, seasoning and firming agent**. Malic acid.
353 *Metatartaric acid.* **Removing calcium from wine.** Tartaric acid.
354 *Calcium tartrate.* **Food acid and preservative**. Tartaric acid.
355 *Adipic acid.* **Food acid, salt substitute and raising agent.** Synthetic.
357 *Potassium adipate.* **Firming and raising agent.** Adipic acid.
363* *Succinic acid.* **Food acid and gelling agent.** Vinegar.
365 *Sodium fumarate.* **Bread dough volume increaser.** Fumaric acid.
366 *Potassium fumarate.* **Food acid and gelling agent.** Fumaric acid.
367 *Calcium fumarate.* **Food acid and gelling agent.** Fumaric acid.
370* *1,4-Heptonolactone.* **Food acid and gelling agent.** Synthetic.
375 *Niacin (or nicotinamide).* **Vitamin B3 and colour stabiliser.** Nicotinic acid.
380 *Ammonium citrate.* **Food acid, emulsifier and stabiliser.** Citric acid.
381 *Ammonium ferric citrate.* **Iron supplement**. Citric acid.
385** *Calcium disodium EDTA.* **Flavourer, emulsifier and stabiliser.** Synthetic.
387 *Oxystearin.* **Food fat stabiliser.** Vegetable oil.

EMULSIFIERS AND THICKENING AGENTS

400 *Alginic acid.* **Stabiliser and thickening agent.** Seaweed (carrageenan).
401 *Sodium alginate.* **Thickening and gelling agent.** Alginic acid.
402 *Potassium alginate.* **Thickening and gelling agent.** Alginic acid.
403 *Ammonium alginate.* **Thickening and gelling agent.** Alginic acid.
404 *Calcium alginate.* **Thickening and gelling agent.** Alginic acid.
405* *Propylene glycol alginate.* **Emulsifier, thickener and solvent.** Petroleum.
406 *Agar.* **Thickening and gelling agent.** Seaweed.
407* *Irish moss (carrageenan).* **Thickening and gelling agent.** Seaweed.
409 *Larch gum.* **Chewing gum.** Plant gum.
410 *Carob gum.* **Thickening and gelling agent.** Carob (locust) beans.
411 *Oat gum.* **Thickening agent.** Oats.
412* *Guar gum.* **Thickening agent.** Guar beans.
413* *Tragacanth gum.* **Emulsifier and thickener.** Tree resin.

254

| Number | Chemical name | Use | Source |

414   *Acacia gum*. **Stabiliser, emulsifier, glazing agent and thickener.** Acacia tree resin.
415   *Xanthan gum*. **Emulsifier and thickener.** Corn sugar.
416   *Karaya gum*. **Stabiliser, emulsifier and thickener**. Tree resin.
417   *Tara gum*. **Stabiliser.** Tree resin.
418   *Gellan gum*. **Gelling agent.** Fermentation of bacteria.
420*   *Sorbitol*. **Sweetening agent and stabiliser.** Glucose.
421*   *Mannitol*. **Sweetener and anti-caking agent.** Seaweed or plants.
422   *Glycerol*. **Solvent, moistener, sweetener and lubricant**. Fats and oils.
430   *Polyoxyethylene*. **Emulsifier and stabiliser.** Synthetic.
431   *Polyoxyethylene 40*. **Emulsifier.** Synthetic.
432**   *Polysorbate 20*. **Emulsifier and stabiliser.** Synthetic.
433**   *Polysorbate 80*. **Stabiliser and moistener.** Sorbitol.
434**   *Polysorbate 40*. **Stabiliser and moistener.** Sorbitol.
435   *Polysorbate 60*. **Stabiliser, foaming agent, emulsifier and moistener.** Sorbitol.
436   *Polysorbate 65*. **Stabiliser, defoaming agent, emulsifier and moistener,** Sorbitol.
440   *Pectin*, **Emulsifier and gelling agent,** Apples and citrus.
440a   *Ammonium Pectin*, **Stabiliser, gelling agent and thickener.** Pectin.
441   *Gelatine*. **Gelling agent and thickener.** Collagen from animal bones or skin.
442   *Ammonium phosphatidic acid*. **Stabiliser and emulsifier.** Ammonia and plant oils.
444   *Surcrose acetate isobutyrate*. **Stabiliser.** Synthetic.
445*   *Glycerol ester*. **Stabiliser.** Glycerol and wood resin.
450*   *Sodium pyrophosphate*. **Stabiliser, emulsifier and raising agent.** Phosphoric acid.
450a   *Ammonium phosphate*. **Food acid and yeast activator.** Phosphoric acid.
451   *Potassium tripolyphosphate*. **Moisturiser and stabiliser.** Phosphoric acid.
452   *Sodium polyphosphate*. **Stabiliser**. Phosphoric acid.
460   *Cellulose*. **Fibrous thickener, tablet binder and anti-caking agent.** Plants.
461*   *Methyl cellulose*. **Fibrous thickener, binder and emulsifier.** Wood pulp.
463**   *Hydroxypropyl cellulose*. **Gelling agent.** Cellulose.
464   *Hydropropyl methyl cellulose*. **Gelling agent.** Cellulose.
465   *Methyl ethyl cellulose*. **Emulsifier and thickener.** Cellulose.
466   *Sodium carboxymethyl cellulose*. **Emulsifier, gelling agent and thickener.** Cellulose.
469   *Sodium caseinate*. **Whitener and emulsifier.** Milk casein.
470   *Magnesium stearate*. **Emulsifier, thickener and flow agent.** Magnesium and sodium.
470a   *Mineral salts from fats*. **Emulsifier and stabiliser.** Seed oils.
471   *Processed fat*. **Emulsifier, solvent, stabiliser, lubricant and thickener**. Seed oils.
472   *Glycerol acids*. **Emulsifier, solvent and lubricant.** Glycerol.
472a   *Acetic acid ester*. **Emulsifier, solvent and lubricant.** Vinegar.
472b   *Lactic acid ester*. **Emulsifier and stabiliser.** Lactic acid.
472c   *Citric acid ester*. **Emulsifier and stabiliser.** Citric acid.
472d   *Tartaric acid ester*. **Emulsifier and stabiliser.** Tartaric acid.
472e   *Diacetyltartaric acid ester*. **Emulsifier and stabiliser.** Tartaric acid.
473   *Sucrose esters*. **Emulsifier and stabiliser.** Glycerol and sugar.
474*   *Sucroglyceride*. **Emulsifier and stabiliser.** Glycerol and sugar.
475   *Polyglycerol acids*. **Emulsifier and stabiliser.** Synthetic.
476   *Polyglycerol polyricinoleate*. **Emulsifier and fat substitute.** Castor oil and glycerol.
477*   *Propane-1. 2 ester*. **Emulsifier and stabiliser.** Propylene glycol.
478*   *Fatty acid ester*. **Emulsifier and stabiliser.** Lactic acid.
480   *Dioctyl sodium sulphosuccinate DSS*. **Emulsifier and dissolving agent.** Synthetic.
481   *Sodium stearoyl lactylate*. **Flour processing stabiliser and emulsifier.** Lactic acid.
482   *Calcium stearoyl lactylate*. **Flour processing stabiliser and emulsifier.** Lactic acid.
483**   *Stearyl tartrate*. **Emulsifier and stabiliser.** Stearic and tartaric acid.
491   *Sorbitan monostearate*. **Emulsifier, stabiliser and glazing agent.** Stearic acid.
492*   *Sorbitan tristearate*. **Emulsifier and stabiliser.** Stearic acid.

Number	Chemical name	Use	Source

493** *Sorbitan monolaurate.* **Emulsifier, stabiliser and anti-foaming agent.** Lauric acid.
494** *Sorbitan mono-oleate.* **Emulsifier and stabiliser.** Oleic acid.
495** *Sorbitan monopalmitate.* **Emulsifier and stabiliser.** Synthetic.

FOOD MODIFIERS

500 *Bicarbonate of soda.* **Food alkali, diluent and raising agent.** Seawater.
501 *Potassium carbonate or bicarbonate.* **Food alkali.** Potassium and carbon.
503 *Ammonium bicarbonate.* **Stabiliser, alkali and raising agent.** Natural minerals.
504 *Magnesium carbonate.* **Alkali, anti-caking, anti-bleaching agent.** Natural mineral.
507 *Hydrochloric acid.* **Food acid.** Synthetic.
508 *Potassium chloride.* **Salt substitute, nutrient and gelling agent.** Natural minerals.
509 *Calcium chloride.* **Stabiliser and firming agent.** Natural minerals.
510 *Ammonium chloride.* **Yeast activator and flavourer.** Hydrochloric acid and ammonia.
511 *Magnesium chloride.* **Yeast activator.** Natural minerals.
512 *Stannous chloride.* **Colour retention agent and antioxidant.** Synthetic.
513** *Sulphuric acid.* **Food acid.** Sulphur dioxide.
514 *Sodium sulphate.* **Diluent for colour powders.** Natural mineral.
515 *Potassium sulphate.* **Low sodium salt substitute.** Natural mineral.
516 *Calcium sulphate.* **Firming agent, nutrient, stabiliser, yeast activator.** Limestone.
518 *Epsom salts (magnesium sulphate).* **Nutrient, laxative and firming agent.** Salt water.
519 *Copper sulphate.* **Firming agent, and anti-caking agent.** Natural mineral.
520 *Aluminium sulphate.* **Brewing and vegetable processing additive.** Natural mineral.
521 *Aluminium sodium sulphate.* **Bleaching of flour.** Natural mineral.
522 *Aluminium potassium sulphate.* **Acidifying of baking powder.** Natural mineral.
524** *Sodium hydroxide.* **Acid neutraliser and colour solvent.** Synthetic.
525* *Potassium hydroxide.* **Food alkali.** Synthetic.
526 *Calcium hydroxide.* **Food alkali, firming and neutralising agent.** Limestone.
527** *Ammonium hydroxide.* **Food alkali.** Diluted ammonia.
528** *Magnesium hydroxide (milk of magnesia).* **Food alkali.** Natural mineral.
529 *Calcium oxide.* **Food alkali, stabiliser and nutrient.** Limestone.
530 *Magnesium oxide.* **Food alkali, anti-caking agent and nutrient.** Natural mineral.
535 *Sodium ferrocyanide.* **Anti-caking agent.** Synthetic.
536** *Potassium ferrocyanide gas.* **Anti-caking agent, removes metals from wine.** Synthetic.
537 *Ferrohexacyano manganate.* **Anti-caking agent.** Synthetic.
538 *Calcium ferrocyanide.* **Anti-caking agent in table salt.** Synthetic.
539 *Sodium thiosulphate.* **Antioxidant to inhibit browning of potato.** Synthetic.
540 *Dicalcium diphosphate.* **Nutrient and raising agent.** Synthetic.
541* *Sodium aluminium sulphate.* **Raising agent, emulsifier and food acid.** Synthetic.
542 *Bone phosphate.* **Anti-caking agent, nutrient and tablet base.** Animal bones.
543 *Calcium sodium polyphosphate.* **Cheese stabiliser.** Synthetic.
544* *Calcium polyphosphate.* **Cheese stabiliser.** Calcium phosphate.
545 *Ammonium polyphosphate.* **Emulsifier and water binder in meat.** Synthetic.
550 *Sodium silicate.* **Flavour carrier, anti-caking agent and thickener.** Quartz sand.
551 *Silicon dioxide.* **Suspender, anti-caking agent and thickener.** Quartz sand.
552 *Calcium silicate.* **Anti-caking and non-stick agent.** Limestone.
553a *Magnesium silicate.* **Antacid, anti-caking and non-stick agent.** Natural minerals.
553b *Talc (French chalk).* **Non-stick agent.** Natural mineral.
554* *Aluminium sodium silicate.* **Anti-caking agent.** Natural mineral.
556* *Aluminium calcium silicate.* **Anti-caking agent.** Natural mineral.
558 *Bentonite.* **Filler, emulsifier, clarifier and anti-caking agent.** Clay.
559 *Kaolin (aluminium silicate).* **Anti-caking agent.** Clay.
570 *Stearic acid.* **Anti-caking agent.** Fats.
572 *Magnesium stearate.* **Emulsifier, anti-caking and non-stick agent.** Staeric acid.

Number	Chemical name	Use	Source

574   *Gluconic acid.* **Food acid, chelater and stabiliser.** Glucose.
575   *Glucono delta-lactone.* **Food acid and stabiliser.** Glucose.
576*   *Sodium gluconate.* **Neutraliser of adverse minerals, diet supplement.** Gluconic acid.
577   *Potassium gluconate.* **Neutraliser of adverse minerals.** Gluconic acid.
578   *Calcium gluconate.* **Stabiliser, firming agent, neutraliser.** Gluconic acid.
579*   *Ferrous gluconate.* **Colour stabiliser, iron supplement.** Gluconic acid.
585   *Ferrous lactate.* **Iron supplement in infant formula.** Gluconic acid.

FLAVOUR ENHANCERS

620   *Glutamic acid.* **Flavour enhancer and salt substitute.** Fermentation of molasses.
621**   *Monosodium glutamate* (MSG). **Protein flavour enhancer.** Hydrolysed protein.
622**   *Monopotassium glutamate.* **Flavour enhancer, salt substitute.** Hydrolysed protein.
623*   *Calcium glutamate.* **Flavour enhancer and salt substitute.** Hydrolysed protein.
624*   *Monoammonium glutamate.* **Flavour enhancer, salt substitute.** Hydrolysed protein.
626*   *Guanylic acid.* **Flavour enhancer.** Yeast extract.
627*   *Disodium guanylate.* **Flavour enhancer.** Yeast extract.
628*   *Dipotassium guanylate.* **Flavour enhancer.** Yeast extract.
629*   *Calcium guanylate.* **Flavour enhancer.** Yeast extract.
630*   *Inosinic acid.* **Flavour enhancer.** Meat or fish protein.
631*   *Disodium inosinate.* **Flavour enhancer.** Meat or fish protein.
632*   *Dipotassium inosinate.* **Flavour enhancer.** Meat or fish protein.
633*   *Calcium inosinate.* **Flavour enhancer.** Meat or fish protein.
634*   *Calcium ribonucleotides.* **Flavour enhancer.** Made from 626 and 630.
635*   *Disodium ribonucleotides.* **Flavour enhancer.** Made from 627 and 631.
636   *Maltol.* **Flavour and aroma enhancer.** Plants and synthetic.
637   *Ethyl maltol.* **Sweetener and flavour enhancer.** Maltol.
640   *Glycine.* **Sweetener and flavour enhancer.** Gelatine.
641   *L-leucine (amino acid).* **Flavour enhancer.** Animal collagen.

FOOD APPEARANCE ENHANCERS

900   *Dimethylpolysiloxane.* **Anti-foaming agent and water repellent.** Synthetic.
901   *Beeswax.* **Glazing and non-stick agent.** Honeycomb.
902   *Candelilla wax.* **Glazing agent for confectionery.** Candelilla plant leaves.
903*   *Carnuba wax.* **Glazing agent for confectionery.** Carnuba Palm leaves.
904   *Shellac.* **Glazing agent for confectionery.** Lac insects.
905a*   *Mineral oil.* **Glazing, non-stick agent and lubricant.** Synthetic.
905b*   *Petroleum jelly (Vaseline).* **Non-stick agent, medication and lubricant.** Synthetic.
905c   *Paraffin wax.* **Non-stick agent.** Synthetic.
906   *Benzoic gum.* **Ingredient of flavours, essences and perfumes.** Styrax tree.
907*   *Microcrystalline wax.* **Non-stick agent.** Synthetic.
908   *Rice bran wax.* **Non-stick agent and chewing gum ingredient.** Rice bran.
910   *L-cysteine (Amino acid).* **Flavour, white flour improver.** Animal collagen.
912*   *Montanic acid wax.* **Coating for citrus fruit.** Brown coal.
913   *Lanolin (sheep wool fat).* **Chewing gum and ointment ingredient.** Sheep wool.
914*   *Polyethylene wax.* **Coating for fruit and vegetables.** Synthetic.
915   *Colophane resin.* **Citrus flavour and stabiliser.** Pine tree.
920   *L-cysteine hydrochloride.* **Flour improver and flavour enhancer.** Animal collagen.
922   *Potassium persulphate.* **Bread enhancer.** Synthetic.
922   *Ammonium persulphate.* **Bread enhancer.** Synthetic.
924*   *Potassium bromate.* **Oxidiser and flour bleaching agent.** Synthetic.
925*   *Chlorine.* **Disinfectant and flour bleaching agent.** Synthetic.
926*   *Chlorine dioxide.* **Antibacterial agent, oxidiser and bleach.** Synthetic.
927a*   *Azodicarbonamide.* **Bread dough fermentation improver.** Synthetic.
927   *Carbamide.* **Fermentation improver, teeth bleaching.** Synthetic.
928*   *Benzoyl peroxide.* **Food bleaching agent.** Synthetic.
930*   *Calcium peroxide.* **Flour bleaching and bread enhancer.** Synthetic.

Number	Chemical name	Use	Source

Number   Chemical name   Use   Source

940   *Dichlorodifluoromethane.* **Anti-freeze and spray can propellant.** Synthetic gas.
941   *Nitrogen.* **Antioxidant and spray can propellant.** Natural gas.
942   *Nitrous oxide (laughing gas).* **Flour bleaching and whipping agent.** Natural gas.
943   *Butane.* **Spray can propellant.** Natural gas.
944   *Propane.* **Spray can propellant.** Natural gas.
950**   *Acesulphame potassium.* **Intense synthetic sweetener.** Synthetic.
951**   *Aspartame.* **Intense synthetic sweetener.** Synthetic.
952*   *Cyclamic acid.* **Synthetic sweetener.** Synthetic.
953*   *Isomalt.* **Sweetener.** Glucose and mannitol.
954**   *Saccharin.* **Intense synthetic sweetener.** Synthetic (from toluene).
955**   *Sucralose (Splenda).* **Intense synthetic sweetener.** Synthetic.
956   *Alitame (Aclame).* **Intense synthetic sweetener.** Synthetic.
957   *Thaumatin.* **Intense sweetening agent.** Plant.
959*   *Neohesperidine DC.* **Intense sweetening agent.** Citrus.
960   *Stevia.* **Intense sweetener.** Plant.
961   *Neotame.* **Intense synthetic sweetener.** Synthetic (improved Aspartame).
962**   *Aspartame-Acesulphame ('Twinsweet').* **Intense synthetic sweetener.** Synthetic.
965   *Maltitol glucose syrup.* **Sweetening and bulking agent.** Plants.
966   *Lactitol.* **Sweetening and bulking agent.** Milk.
967   *Xylitol.* **Sweetener.** Wood pulp.
968   *Erythritol.* **Sweetener.** Yeast and glucose.

MISCELLANEOUS ADDITIVES
1000   *Cholic acid.* **Emulsifier used in egg powder.** Cow bile.
1100   *Amylase.* **Bread flour treatment agent.** Natural enzyme.
1101   *Protease,* **Flour treatment agent, stabiliser and flavour enhancer.** Natural enzyme.
1102   *Glucose oxidase.* **Antioxidant.** Natural enzyme.
1104   *Lipase.* **Flavour enhancer.** Animal sources.
1105   *Lysozyme.* **Beer preservative.** Egg white.
1200   *Polydextrose.* **Bulking agent, anti-freeze and texture regulator.** Synthetic.
1201   *Polyvinylpolypyrrolidone (PVP).* **Stabiliser and tablet binder.** Synthetic.
1202   *Insoluble Polyvinylpolypyrrolidone (PVP).* **Clarifying agent, tablet binder.** Synthetic.

MODIFIED STARCHES
1400-1500   *Modified plant starches.* **Food thickening agents.** Plants.

FLAVOUR SOLVENTS
1501   *Benzylated hydrocarbons,* **Flavour and fragrance compound.** Synthetic.
1502   *Butane-1,3-diol,* **Flavour solvent for tobacco products.** Synthetic.
1503   *Castor oil,* **Flavour solvent and mould inhibitor.** Castor bean.
1504   *Ethyl acetate,* **Flavour solvent.** Vinegar.
1505   *Triethyl citrate,* **Flavour solvent.** Citric Acid.
1510   *Alcohol,* **Ingredient and flavour solvent.** Fermented sugars.
1516   *Glycerol monoacetate,* **Flavour solvent.** Vinegar.
1517*   *Glycerol diacetate,* **Flavour solvent, humectant and fruit coating.** Vinegar.
1518   *Glycerol triacetate,* **Flavour solvent.** Glycerol and vinegar.
1520   *Propylene glycol,* **Anti-freeze and solvent for antioxidants.** Synthetic.
1521*   *Polyethylene glycerol 8000,* **Artificial sweetener and anti-foam agent.** Synthetic.

Recipes

Below are three of my own recipes that I've developed over the years.

I previously used my own ground wholemeal wheat flour, however, during an extensive health check up at age 70, a naturopath found that I was low in the minerals zinc, magnesium, manganese and iron. This surprised me, as my intake should have been adequate.

However, unsoaked, unleavened or unsprouted grains, retain their naturally high levels of phosphorus in a form called phytate. This phytate has a binding effect on the above four minerals and typically blocks the absorption of about 40% of them in the gut. I had come across this fact many times before, but assumed a healthy digestive system and a good probiotic supplement should overcome this problem – evidently not.

So I now sprout my wheat before drying the sprouts and grinding them into flour – this overcomes the phytate problem and greatly enhances the nutritional value (and taste) of a grain. Malt is made by the same process, but mostly with barley.

My quick method of sprouting grains

As I normally grind about 7 cups of whole wheat (spelt) grains at a time (and sometimes barley) I now soak this same amount in a bowl overnight in water. Next morning, I tip the grain into a pillowcase and tie the top around my bathroom shower bracket. For the next two days, morning and night I briefly water the grain using my detachable shower head and allow it to drain – takes only a few seconds. (I cut a hole in the upper part of the pillowcase to provide air circulation and give access for the shower head.)

By the morning of the third day the grains have white sprouts about as long as the grain. (If the sprouts grow any longer they tangle and make the grain difficult to pass through the wheat mill.)

I then spread the sprouted grain on two oven trays and dry them in a lukewarm oven – about 55°C (130°F) for approx 5 hours or overnight. Later I grind them to flour in my wheat mill. The flour is finer, and sweeter than regular flour but otherwise can be treated as normal flour.

Delicious instant raw porridge

Ingredients (stir together in a mug then eat immediately)

4 tsps (heaped)	Freshly ground, sprouted wholemeal flour
1 tsp	Brown sugar (or liquid malt extract, or molasses)
6 tsp	Cream
4 tsp (approx)	Milk or coconut cream (to regulate consistency)

---

10 Minute wholemeal bread
Makes two tasty, healthy loaves with a crisp crust
Ingredients

7 cups	Freshly ground, sprouted wholemeal flour
2 tsp (raised)	Baking soda (mixed in ½ cup of milk)
1½ cups	Ground flaxseed (available from health stores)
¾ cup	Brown sugar or treacle (light molasses)
5½ cups (approx)	Water

Stir all the ingredients together in a large bowl with a sturdy wooden spoon, altering the water content until you have an elastic dough that will hold its shape without slumping (approx 2 minutes mixing). Kneading is not required.

Put into two, baking paper lined or non-stick, full-size loaf tins and leave to rise for 35 minutes in an oven that has been pre-heated to 160°C (320 °F) and then switched off.

Then turn the oven back on, set to 200°C (390 °F) and bake for 60 minutes. For a crisp, all-over crust, remove the loaves from the tins while they are still warm.

Healthy wholemeal Afghan biscuits (cookies)
Ingredients

4½ cups	Freshly ground, sprouted wholemeal flour
600 g	Butter
1¼ cups	Cocoa
1 cup	Brown sugar
2 tsps (level)	Stevia 100 natural sweetener (vary amount to taste)
2½ cups	Cornflakes (or cacao nibs)

Semi-melt butter then mix all ingredients together. Place tablespoon size amounts on non-stick trays and flatten with a fork.

Bake at 180°C (360 °F) for 25 minutes.

Icing (optional): 1 part cocoa, 1 part butter and 2 parts treacle (light molasses). Experiment with amount according to desired thickness.

Index

(See also **Calcium growths; Osteoporosis) 90 day cure 181;** Australian doctor reports 90% of his patients improve with boron 118; excess non-heme iron 146; lack of boron 118; lack of manganese 155; lack of molybdenum 159; lack of niacin (factor) 73; lack of selenium 171; lack of sodium 175; lack of vitamin C 97; lack of vitamin K2 115; the lower the level of boron in soil, higher the incidence of osteoarthritis 118;

Aspartame (See also **Aspartate**) chemical sweetener 200 times sweeter than sugar 36; numerous adverse reactions reported 34;

Aspartate (See also **Glutamate (MSG)** amino acid used by brain and nerve neurons to transmit signals 219; an excitotoxin found in diet drinks sweetened with aspartame 220, 245; has generated countless health complaints over the years, including depression 220; magnesium, zinc, omega 3 fat and folate protect against 220; multiple sclerosis, macular degeneration, Parkinsons, ALS, Alzheimer's and depression linked with aspartate sweeteners 245; selenium, CoQ10 and vitamins A, C, D and E limit the neuron damage 221;

Aspirin delays the clotting of blood 114; can cause stomach bleeding 114;

Asthma drinking more water can help avoid 57; excess LA omega 6 fat 42; phosphorus exceeding calcium intake 162; excess sugar increases sensitivity to 31; excess vitamin B6 80; how to avoid 139; lack of fibre 37; lack of magnesium 150; lack of omega 3 fat 41; lack of selenium 171; lack of vitamin C (factor) 97; lack of vitamin E 107; lack of zinc 186; magnesium can stop attacks instantly when administered intravenously 149; NZ'ers with low selenium five times more likely to suffer from 169; sulphite preservative in processed meats can trigger 139; main indoor causes - wool dust mites and dry saliva from cat fur 139; pet dog exposure reduces incidence 139; overcleanliness with children increases incidence 139;

Athletes perform better short term on carbs 59; can have a heartbeat low as 35 227;

Attention disorder See **ADHD**

Autism section on 215; lack of vitamin B6 and magnesium in pregnancy 80, 150; excess copper 134; lack of zinc in pregnancy 186; symptoms appear by age two 215; main cause appears to be glutamate flavour enhancer (MSG) or aspartate chemical sweetener damage to fetal brain neurons in pregnancy 215, 218-221; mercury can aggravate symptoms of 215; graph of incidence in boys 215; incomplete 'wiring' of brain neurons while in womb 215; increasing in leaps and bounds 215; infant symptoms of 216; most effective treatment - regular injections of methyl-type vitamin B12 216; treatment can improve symptoms 50% 216; sulforaphane – an extract of broccoli substantially improves 215: Amish have about six times less incidence than US average 241;

Auto-immune disorders (See also **Immune system suppressed**) lack of vitamin B12 89; role of oxidised cholesterol 193; lack of omega 3 fat 47, 148;

Avocado oil (Also see **Fats**) good source of omega 9 fat 40; one of best oils for cooking 40;

B

Baby in womb See **Birth defects**

Bach Flowers (See also **Nutritional healing**) 'Rescue Remedy' has calming effect on both humans and animals 227; often ridiculed but reported success rate similar to orthodox medicine 226;

Back pain, lower drinking more water can help 57; lack of magnesium 150; lack of vitamin C 97; stress can cause 58; excellent exercise 58;

Bacteria vitamin C able to destroy 94;

Bacteria, friendly gut See **Probiotics**

Bad breath excess selenium 171; how to banish 250; lack of vitamin C 96;

Baking powder contains aluminium 117; recipe for home made 117;

Baking soda can destroy riboflavin on contact 70; can neutralise pantothenic acid 76; contains sodium 173; used to raise pH in cancer cure 204;

Balance problems lack of vitamin B12 88; lack of manganese 155;

Baldness See **Hair loss men**

Bed rest need to minimise long term125;

Bed sores lack of vitamin C 96; lack of vitamin E from food 107; lack of zinc 186;

Biotin (vitamin H) chapter on 112; diabetic nerve damage halted or reversed with injections of 112; lack can cause cradle cap in infants 112; made by our bodies in intestines 112; male baldness improved and female baldness cured with 10 mg a day 112;

Birth control pill can lower vitamin B6 and B12 levels79, 87; can double copper levels in women 133; nutrients needed for pregnancy after pill 131; require extra folate and riboflavin 69, 83;

Birth defects (See also **Cleft palate; Malformities; Autism**) excess retinol form of vitamin A 63; lack of folate in pregnancy 85; lack of iodine in pregnancy can reduce infant's IQ 10 to 15 points 140; lack of lecithin 91; lack of manganese 155; lack of selenium 171; lack of vitamin B6 80; lack of vitamin B6 80; lack of vitamin E from food in pregnancy 107;

Bladder stones lack of magnesium 150;

Bleeding, internal lack of vitamin C 96; lack of vitamin K1 115; taking aspirin or warfarin 114;

Bleeding, excessive menstrual lack of iron 146; lack of vitamin E from food 107; lack of vitamin K1 114;

265

all processed meats such as sausages, hot dogs, hamburger, luncheon, etc 208; avoid burning protein food 208; avoiding diabetes reduces risk 40% 208; maintain 1 part acidic phosphorus to 2 parts calcium in diet 160, 206; stale air and dampness suppress immune system 208; reduce sugar intake 207; eat mainly alkaline foods 209; exercise half an hour a day, five days a week 208; keep ratio of omega 6 to omega 3 below 9 to 1 (optimum 3 to 1) 206; maintain saliva pH to 6.8 or higher 207; list of alkaline foods found in author's free booklet 'Is Your pH healthy?' 209; relax, minimise stress and sleep well 209; much truth in traditional saying 'happy people rarely get cancer'209; older men who exercise vigorously have a 68% lower risk of prostate cancer 211; practising Mormon men have 65% less cancer 241; 200 mcg of selenium daily reduces risk of cancer 42% 209; books on phosphorus and cancer 207; vitamin D blood level should average 150 nmol/L 100, 121, 207; women need 900 mg and men 1500 mg daily of omega 3 206; workers on rotating shifts at higher risk 211;

Cancer, breast section on 212; 77% less risk when vitamin D and calcium levels high 212; thermography can detect cancer eight years earlier than mammography 213; lack of vitamin E from food 107; excess iron 146, 212; HRT and pill more than double risk 213; calcium intake should be 500 mg a day or higher 212; lack of iodine 141; lack of vitamin D (blood level should be 150 nmol/L or higher) 101 103, 212; mammograms miss 25% of cancers and 5-year survival rate no better 213; trans fat increases risk 75% 44; risk five times higher when vitamin E intake from food low 106; women who never wear a bra 125 times less likely to get 212;

Cancer, colon section on 214; 200 mcg daily of selenium reduced by 58% 214; 400 mcg daily of folate reduced by 75% 209; 5% of polyps become cancerous 214; drinking more water can help avoid 57; fibre does not protect from 36; lack of folate 85; lack of molybdenum 159; physically active adults have 50% less risk 214;

Cancer, cervical lack of folate 85; almost non-existent among Amish 241; sexually transmitted 241;

Cancer cures See **Cancer, alternative treatments**

Cancer, leukemia lack of vitamin K2 115;

Cancer, liver lack of vitamin K2 115;

Cancer, lung deaths 60 times higher since change to polyunsaturated LA omega 6 fats 42; 40% less with 67% increase in selenium 168; lack of vitamin K2 115;

Cancer, melanoma section on 209; yearly increase 11% worldwide 209; 40% lower risk among those who regularly eat fish 210; 90% of melanoma surgeries unnecessary 210; Australian beach lifeguards have far lower

incidence than office workers 103, 209; Australian outdoor workers have less than indoor workers 210; strong link between margarine eating and melanoma 210; excess LA omega 6 believed responsible for alarming increase 43; higher levels of vitamin D protect against 203, 210; Iceland with weak sunshine has much higher rate than sunny tropical regions of world 210; lack of vitamin D 101, 103; moderate sun exposure protects against 209; occurs more frequently on areas not exposed to the sun 43; office workers under fluorescent lights have highest incidence 210; over-use of sunscreen believed to increase risk 210; Swedish researchers found no link to childhood sunburn, but three bouts of adult sunburn each year can double risk 210; sunbeds linked with melanoma 103, 202;

Cancer, ovarian section on 214; high percent of false positives and needless surgery 214; screening no longer recommended unless symptoms present 214;

Cancer, pancreatic section on 214; deadly form of cancer 214; principal causes – acidity from excess sugar, additives in processed meats and lack of vitamin D 214, 208; adequate vitamin D cuts risk 50% 214;

Cancer, prostate section on 211; Aust/NZ rate highest in world 211; lack of boron – 62% lower incidence on 2 mg a day 118; lack of iodine 141; lack of selenium 168; lack of vitamin E from food 107; lack of vitamin K2 115; largely disease of hard-driving businessmen, entrepreneurs and type-A personalities 212; older men who exercise vigorously have 68% lower risk 211; over 200 mg of a vitamin E supplement can increase risk by inhibiting selenium 107; major cause – processed meat and charring when cooking, 208, 211; PSA tests only 2% accurate 212; regular ejaculation reduces risk 33% 211; four times higher risk for workers on rotating shifts (stress factor) 211;

Cancer, skin (See also **Cancer, melanoma**) **section on 210;** common, non-melanoma types are squamous cell, basal cell and solar keratosis 210; home remedies to treat 212; lack of vitamin A 62; sun clearly the cause of non-melanoma skin cancers 210;

Candida See **Yeast infections**

Canola oil See **Fats**

Carbohydrates (carbs) chapter on 25; glycemic load chart 26; athletes perform better on 59; carb calories can be more fattening than protein or fat calories 20; cancer cells can be starved to death by eliminating all carbs (new finding) 206; only 25% of calories from carbs recommended daily 27; why low-carb diets work only short term 238;

Cardiovascular disease (See also **Arteries, hardened; Artery, inflammation; Arteries, narrowed; Arteries, weak walls; Blood clots;**

Cholesterol; Heart attack; Blood pressure high; Chapter on avoiding heart attack and stroke 189; 62% reduction when adequate vitamin E taken in food form 143; became major problem when animal fat intake fell in 1970's and processed vegetable oils greatly increased 195; blood tests for risk of 196; cardiologist never saw a heart attack before 1928 46; causes of a blood clot 190; causes of angina pain 193; conclusions on cardiovascular disease 198; death rates five-fold higher since use of margarine and vegetable oils/fats 43; eight steps to avoid a heart attack or stroke 195; exercise of major importance for cardiovascular health 196; excess calcium 124; excess non-heme iron 146; excess LA omega 6 fat 42; excess sugar (major cause) 33; five most common disorders are clot, aneurysm, arrhythmia, leaky valve, inflammation 189; smoking and heart disease 199; the higher our HDL cholesterol the safer we are 52; lack of vitamin B12; lack of CoQ10 111; lack of folate 84; lack of iodine 141; lack of magnesium 150; lack of omega 3 fat 41; lack of selenium 171; lack of vitamin B6 79; minimise stress – learn to relax and sleep well 209; practising Mormon men have 58% less heart disease 241; proven heart medications 197; reducing ratio of omega 6 to omega 3 decreased cardiovascular disease 70% 44; require full RDI of all vitamins and minerals to avoid 55; risks of smoking 195; stress a major cause of heart attacks and stroke 194; triglyceride reading above 2 mmol/L (175 mg/dl) a greater risk than high LDL cholesterol 55, 193; workers with jobs at risk had 50% increased risk 194;

Cardiovascular medications (See also **Statin drugs**) ACE inhibitors, angiotension and beta-blockers, calcium channel blockers, vaso-dilators, diuretics, digitalis, statins 198; anti-coagulants warfarin (coumadin) and aspirin lower risk of blood clots 197; more cost-effective and free means to reduce heart attacks 54; list of proven heart medications 197, 198; nitroglycerin angina reliever has saved countless lives 197; statins have only minor effect on cardiovascular deaths 54;

Carotene See **Vitamin A**

Carpal Tunnel Syndrome See **Repetitive Strain Injury (RSI)**

Cataract See **Eyes cataract**

CFS See **Chronic fatigue**

Chelated minerals absorption satisfactory at approx 50% 181; bound with a substance to improve absorption 230;

Chemotherapy Sydney hospital 5-year survival rate of adults treated with chemotherapy only 2.3% 204;

Chest infection See **Cystic fibrosis**

Chest pressure or tightness See **Heart attack; Anxiety; Asthma**

Childbirth See **Pregnancy**

Children, slow growth lack of copper 133; lack of iron 145; lack of protein 60; lack of ribo-flavin 69; lack of thiamine 67; lack of iodine 141; lack of zinc 186;

Chocolate avoiding tooth decay from 139; exercise required to burn off four squares or 125 cals 21; major cause of tooth decay 32;

Chloride/Chlorine **chapter on 126; food table 127;** chloride amply supplied by salt in diet 126; chloride found in every cell of body 126; chlorine a necessary evil in domestic water supplies 126; how to rid drinking water of chlorine 128; no evidence chlorinated water kills useful gut bacteria 126; part of hydro-chloric acid in our stomach 126; required to maintain body electrolyte balance 164;

Cholesterol **chapter on 51;** 80% made by our body, 20% supplied by protein foods 51; anxiety has profound effect on levels 55; artificially lowering not effective at preventing heart disease 55; half all heart attack victims have normal cholesterol levels 51; HDL carries repair debris from body cells for recycling 52; high overall cholesterol over age 75 protective of health 51; the higher our HDL the lower our risk of cardiovascular disease 52; LDL essential for every cell in our body 52; LDL only blocks arteries when oxidised and hardened 52; LDL oxidises when not cleared fast enough by HDL 52; LDL repairs artery inflammation and other damage 52; cholesterol required for countless functions in every cell of body 51; niacin helps maintains healthy levels 73; omega 3 helps maintain healthy HDL/LDL levels 46; only one kind of cholesterol but takes on different characteristics 52; its negative image 51;

Cholesterol blood test anxiety can have profound effect on readings 55; HDL should be 40% or more of total cholesterol 55; optimum readings to look for 52; the important TC/HDL ratio 52; total cholesterol level almost worthless in determining risk 55;

Cholesterol, HDL too low anger and anxiety can have profound effect on levels 54; role of HDL to clear away debris of LDL artery repairs 196; causes of low HDL 53; below 2.0 mmol/l (80 mg/dl) can be dangerous 53; excess sugar 31; lack of lecithin 91; lack of magnesium 150; lack of manganese 155; lack of niacin 72; lack of omega 3 fat 47; lack of vitamin C 97; panto-thenic acid *'best substance on planet for establishing optimal levels'* Dr Atkins 75; should be 2.0 mmol/l (80 mg/dl) or higher 197; think H for healthy 52; total cholesterol to HDL ratio should be 2.5 or lower 197;

Cholesterol, LDL too high anger and anxiety has profound effect on level 54; blocks arteries only when oxidised 52; causes of high LDL 54; how to read blood test results 197; lack of chromium 130; lack of inositol 92; lack of iodine 141; lack of magnesium 150; lack of niacin 73;

133; preserves elasticity of skin, arteries and veins 132; turkeys died suddenly from ruptured arteries due to lack of 132;

CoQ10 chapter on 109; food table 111; 74% of heart attack patients recovered fully when given 109; author takes daily 249; blood pressure readings dropped from 141/97 to 126/90 with 60 mg daily 109; body gradually loses ability to make after age 30 109; can increase desire to exercise 110; can rebuild aged skin collagen 110; CoQ enzymes have other numbers besides CoQ10 109; disease and mental deterioration inevitable when CoQ10 drops to 25% of normal levels 109; helps generate over 90% of body's energy 109; can sometimes dramatically increases energy 110; low levels can cause Alzheimer's symptoms 111; patients awaiting heart transplants no longer needed them 110; statin drugs and beta-blockers reduce body's manufacture of 109; ubiquinol four times cost of ubiquinone to make and has shorter shelf life 110;

Corn syrup liquid sugar extracted from maize, contains 65% fructose 34;

Cortisol increases blood sugar for more energy 194, 201; long term high levels increase risk of heart attack or stroke 50%194;

Cot death lack of thiamine 67; lack of selenium 171;

Cracks in skin/mouth See **Mouth, cracks/sores at corners; Skin, dry/cracked**

Cradle cap lack of biotin 112;

Cramp, leg (See also **Muscle cramp)** excess sodium (after high salt meal)175; how to avoid 177; lack of calcium 124; lack of magnesium 150; lack of potassium 166; lack of sodium (after heavy sweating) 175;

Cravings See **Salt craving; Sugar cravings**

Crohn's disease lack of omega 3 fat 41, 84; lack of pantothenic acid 76, 84; lack of folate, 84; lack of vitamin D 102; lack of magnesium 150; lack of zinc 186;

Cystic fibrosis lack of selenium 171;

D

Dairy dairy fat linked with a lower risk of coronary heart disease 195; requires correct probiotics in gut to be digested well 195; was thought to cause heart disease, cancer and obesity but Scandinavian research finding opposite 244;

Dandruff lack of selenium 171; lack of zinc 186;

Daniel in Babylon health tested with pulse vegetables for 10 days 60;

Deafness See **Hearing loss**

Deformities See **Birth defects**

Delirium lack of water 57;

Dementia See **Alzheimer's; Alzheimer's-like symptoms**

Depression (See also **Apathy; Anxiety; Post natal depression)** 80% of depressed people lacked vitamin B6 78; excess folate 85; excess trans fat 44; lack of carbs 60; lack of copper 134; low HDL cholesterol 53; lack of magnesium 150; lack of manganese 155; lack of omega 3 fat 41; lack of pantothenic acid 76; lack of potassium 166; lack of selenium 171; lack of thiamine 67; lack of vitamin B6 80; lack of vitamin B12 88; lack of vitamin C 97; lack of zinc 186; linked with aspartame sweetener 220; long term high levels of adrenalin and cortisol increase risk of 194; vigorous exercise in open air an antidote to mild depression 68;

DHEA (youth hormone) bone-building hormone 160; boron helps maintain levels of 118; low levels linked with Alzheimer's symptoms 217; author takes 7-Keto type 249;

Diabetes type 1 lack of vitamin D 101; lack of niacin, which can cut incidence more than 50% 72, 73; has been reversed by taking 600 mcg of chromium a day for two months 129;

Diabetes type 2 400% greater risk when vitamin E intake low 105; deaths quadrupled in 20 years due to 400% increase in sugar intake 33; diabetic nerve damage halted or reversed with injections of biotin 112; dramatic fall-off during World War II due to starvation19; excess blood sugar (triglycerides) 193; excess carb calories 47, 247; excess fructose 30; excess LA omega 6 fat 43; can easily test your own blood sugar at home 131; fasting insulin level test above 15 µIU/mL a sign of 208; lack of chromium 129; lack of CoQ10 111; lack of magnesium 150; lack of fibre 37; lack of manganese 155; lack of potassium 166; lack of vitamin B6 79; lack of vitamin D 101; lack of vitamin E 107; lack of zinc 186; often found with heart disease 154; modern, high-yield wheat strains linked with 28; raises Alzheimer's risk 65% 218; raises cancer risk 25% 208;

Diarrhea can occur when changing to higher fibre diet 36; excess magnesium 151; excess non-heme iron 146; excess vitamin C 97;

Diet (See also **Slimming, permanent)** free **Analyse Your Diet** service on web page www.stayhealthybook.co.nz 232; how to eat 40% less 239; major changes should be phased in gradually 65; our bodies thrive on regularity 65; overcoming comfort eating 238; why low-carb diets only work short term 238;

Digestion poor (See also **Appetite, loss of)** anxiety hinders 13, 246; drugs such as Losec suppress strength of stomach acid 124; lack of magnesium 151; lack of pantothenic acid 76; lack of vitamin B6 79; lack of vitamin C 96; low strength of stomach acid 126;

Dirt eating lack of zinc 186;

Diuretic drugs (See also **Fluid retention)** drugs like frusemide can dangerously deplete potassium, magnesium, sodium and thiamine

arrest or mildly reverse 222; 90 minutes of exercise a week helps greatly 222; excess LA type omega 6 47; excitotoxins glutamate and aspartate in food destroy macular nerve neurons 218-221; lack of copper 133; lack of folate 85; lack of iodine (factor) 141; lack of magnesium 150; lack of selenium (factor) 171; lack of zinc 186; loss of central vision 222;

Eyes, over-sensitive to light lack of magnesium 150; lack of riboflavin 69;

Eyes, poor night vision lack of vitamin A 63; lack of zinc 186;

Eyes, red eyelids lack of niacin 73; lack of riboflavin 69; lack of vitamin B6 79;

Eyes, twitchy lids lack of calcium124; lack of lecithin 91; lack of magnesium 150; lack of vitamin B6 80;

Eyes, weak sight in elderly See **Eyes, macular degeneration**

F

Face, eczema on (See also **Eczema; Skin rashes**) lack of biotin 112; lack of riboflavin 69;

Face, haggard (See also **Skin, premature ageing/wrinkling**) smoking a cause 96;

Face, red and inflamed (rosacea) lack of GLA type omega 6; lack of niacin 73; lack of riboflavin 69;

Facial twitches See **Nervous twitches**

Fainting (See also **Light headedness; Blood pressure low**) heart fibrillation 191; lack of sodium 175; lack of water 57;

Fasting health benefits of 241; Mormons fast 24-hours monthly from all food and liquids 241; no disease that cannot be healed by fasting provided organs intact 241;

Fatigue See **Low energy**

Fat, losing See **Slimming, permanent**

Fats (See also **Trigliceridies**) **chapter on 39**; food tables 48-50; high fat foods (table) 48-49; percent of fat types in common oils (table) 49; 30% of calories recommended daily 27; currently 37% of total calories in NZ diet 39; author's daily fat choices 46; can suppress hunger for long periods 46; four families of - saturated, poly-unsaturated, monounsaturated and trans 38; go rancid in presence of light 47; help body absorb vitamins A, E, D and K 46; maintain body warmth by insulation 46; required for healthy skin, hair and bones 46; niacin helps lower in blood 73; one kg contains 9000 calories 19, 236; wrong fats linked with many modern diseases 38;

Fats, cooking oils become toxic and unhealthy when heated to smoking point 45; dark containers protect against rancidity from light 45; unless cold-pressed, have generally been subject to heat during chemical extraction 45; list of high smoking point oils 45;

olive and avocado oils regarded as best for cooking 45; refined oils better for frying than cold-pressed oils 45;

Fats, omega 3 **section on 41; food tables 48-50;** a polyunsaturated fatty acid 40; 60% deficient intake in surveys 8; one reason for superior health of Mediterranean people 41; helps maintain healthy HDL/LDL cholesterol levels 46; develops and protects brain and nerve cells 46; fish only good animal source nowadays 40; found mostly in fish, nuts, seeds, algae and leafy greens 40; when from fish oil called EPA and DHA 41; helps keep skin moist and supple 46; lack of can harden arteries 47; lowers blood fats (triglycerides) 41; maintains mental clarity and well being 46; modern farming/fertilising methods have almost eliminated omega 3 from animal fats 40; needed for body to absorb vitamins A, D, E and K 40; omega 3 from plant seed oils called ALA 41; pantothenic acid needed to absorb 76; protects against blood clots and fibrillation 41, 46;

Fats, omega 6 **section on 42-44; food tables 48-50;** a polyunsaturated fatty acid 40; 3 types - LA from plant seeds, GLA from evening primrose and borage and CLA from animal fat 41; assists with omega 3 functions 46; CLA form from animal fat has powerful anti-cancer properties 41; excess LA type depresses human immune system when ratio to omega 3 exceeds 9 to 1 42; found mostly in bean, seed and grain oils 40; healthy ratios to omega 3 44; how to avoid excess LA 44; reducing ratio of LA to omega 3, to 4 to 1 can decrease cardiovascular disease 70% 44; regulates brain functions 46; typical NZ diet has six times too much LA 203; LA type high in supermarket oils 44;

Fats, omega 9 **section on 40; food tables 48-50;** a polyunsaturated fatty acid 40; can be made by body from saturated fat 40; helps prevent insulin resistance 40; olive and avocado oils good source 40;

Fats, polyunsaturated See **Fats, Omega 3; Fats omega 6; Fats, omega 9**

Fats, saturated **section on 39; food tables 48-50;** diseases once thought due to excess saturated fat, actually due to a lack of omega 3 40; increases absorption of calcium and magnesium 40; in moderation surprisingly good for body 40; mostly found in animal, nut and coconut products 39; mostly solid at room temperature 39; undeserved reputation for being harmful 40;

Fats, trans **section on 44; 194;** harmful when partly-hydrogenated - higher risk of breast cancer 75%, infertility 73% and depression 48% 44; largely removed from supermarket margarines nowadays 195; natural animal trans fat not harmful 45; partly hydrogenated still found in unlabelled commercial baking and frying fats 39, 44, 195; not tested for in NZ foods 44; risk of heart attack doubles for every

I

Immune system suppressed excess LA type omega 6 fat 42- 47; excess stale air and dampness 208; excess sugar 29, 207, excess trans fat 44; lack of CLA omega 6 (from animal fat) 47; probiotics play major role 113; lack of CoQ10 111; lack of iron 146; lack of omega 3 fat 47; lack of pantothenic acid 76; lack of oxygen 161, 202-208; lack of selenium 171; lack of thiamine 67; lack of vitamin A 63; lack of vitamin B6 82; 63; lack of vitamin C 97; lack of vitamin D 101; lack of vitamin E from food 107; lack of zinc 186; stress hormones adrenalin and cortisol weaken over time 209; smiling can strengthen 74; alkaline food diet boosts 205;

Immunising vaccines See **Vaccines**

Impotency See **Erectile disfunction**

Indigestion lack of pantothenic acid 76;

Infections, repeated (See also **Immune system suppressed**) colloidal silver a natural bacteria killer 230, 248; excess LA omega 6 fat 42; lack of copper 134; lack of iron 146; lack of pantothenic acid 76; lack of selenium 171; lack of vitamin A 63; lack of vitamin C 96; lack of vitamin E from food 107; lack of zinc 186;

Infections, respiratory (See also **Immune system suppressed**) dramatic fall-off at close of World War ll due to starvation 19;

Infertility (See also **Low sperm count**) excess trans fat 44; lack of iodine 141; lack of iron 146; lack of selenium 171; lack of PABA 92; lack of vitamin C 97; lack of zinc 186;

Inflammation (See also **Artery inflammation**) excess LA omega 6 fat 42, 43; lack of copper 133; lack of magnesium 150; lack of pantothenic acid 76; lack of zinc 186;

Inositol chapter on 92; food table 93; 6 g daily for two weeks relieved severe cases of anxiety 92; can reduce blood pressure and LDL cholesterol 92; high levels found in breast milk 92; lack of can aggravate stress disorders 92; Nature's tranquilliser and sleeping pill - can replace medication 92;

Insect bites large dose of thiamine can repel 49

Insomnia See **Sleep**

Insulin converts excess glucose to fat 30;

Insulin resistance lack of chromium 130; lack of manganese 155; major cause of type 2 diabetes and cardiovascular disease 30; omega 9 fat helps prevent 40; too much fructose can cause 30;

Intelligence low See **Brain; Mental impairment**

Iodine chapter on 140; food table 142; increase intake during pregnancy 131; 100% deficient in NZ 2009 survey 140; 96% of a doctor's patients deficient 142; kelp an abundant source 141; lack causes goitre

(swollen throat area of neck) 140; lack in pregnancy can cause birth defects and reduce infant's IQ 140; lack linked with painful breast lumps and breast and prostate cancer 140; lack can increase artery inflammation 141;

Iron chapter on 143; food table 147; 34% NZ teenage girls lacking 143; builds bone and tissues 145; women can lose 10 to 30 mg during menstruation 143; copper helps body absorb 133; excess non-heme iron (from food additives) a serious health problem 144; excess can cause free radicals 155; excess in breast linked to breast cancer 213; how to read hemoglobin blood test readings 145; healthy gut probiotics critical for absorption 143; how to absorb more 143; inorganic non-heme iron absorbed up to 10 times more than organic heme iron 144; iron overload causes LDL cholesterol to oxidise 144; long-distance runners and cyclists can lack 143; low energy caused by both excess and lack of iron 144; low risk of heart disease among child bearing age women due to low iron levels 144; molybdenum needed to absorb 159; mostly enough iron in diet – poor absorption the problem 143; need for triple amount during pregnancy 13; how to read serum ferritin test readings 145; stomach acid lowering drugs can hinder absorption 144; strengthens bones 145; transports energy in blood 143; vitamins B6, D and C needed for absorption 79, 101, 96;

Irritability (See also **Anxiety; Stress**) lack of calcium 124; lack of carbs 60; lack of folate 85; lack of iron 145; lack of magnesium 150; lack of vitamin B6 80; sign of hypoglycemia 32;

Irritable bowel (IBS) lack of folate 85; lack of pantothenic acid 76; lack of probiotics 113:

J

Joint pain or disorders See **Arthritis**

K

Kelp powder rich source of iodine 141

Kidney failure lack of vitamin C 97;

Kidney stones drinking more water can lower risk of 57; excess or lack of calcium 124; lack of boron 119; lack of magnesium 150; lack of vitamin K2 115;

Kilojoules (See also **Energy**) divide by 4.18 to convert to calories 19;

L

LA (linoleic acid) (See also **Fats omega 6**) omega 6 fat from plant seeds 41;

Lactose milk sugar 33;

Lead poisoning excess fluoride allows 137; lack of thiamine 67; lack of vitamin C 97; lack of zinc 186;

Learning difficulties See **ADHD**

M

Manganese chapter on 154; food table 156; assists in sex hormone production 155; asthmatics can have only quarter normal blood level 155; deficiencies firmly linked with modern health disorders 154; diabetic levels half those of healthy people 155; helps create enzymes for thousands of body processes 154; helps maintain healthy collagen in bones, joints, arteries and skin 155; high levels can turn bore water blackish and stain toilets and clothes 155; MS and epilepsy reported cured by manganese and zinc supplements 155; how to read normal blood test levels 155;

Manic-depressive disorder See **Mental disorders**

Margarine section on margarine vs butter 45; nearly all nutritive value destroyed in processing 45; a source of heat-damaged LA omega 6 fat 42;

ME See **Chronic Fatigue**

Measures and abbreviations explanation of those in this book 15;

Meat NZ unprocessed meats high in nutrients 8;

Meat, processed (See also **Cancer, avoiding**) **section on avoiding 208;** 67% increase in risk of pancreatic cancer 208 contain nitrites which are known carcinogens 208; contain sulphite preservatives that can trigger asthma 139; often have acidic phosphorus added 161; can contain huge amounts of salt 173; cancer researchers strongly recommend avoiding 208; often contain MSG-type flavour enhancers 208; one sausage a day raises risk of colon cancer 20% 208;

Medical treatment, orthodox See **Orthodox medical treatment; Nutritional healing**

Melanoma See **Cancer, melanoma**

Memory, poor long term lack of niacin 73; lack of thiamine 67; lack of zinc 186;

Memory, poor short-term (See also **Alzheimer's- like symptoms**) 10 g of lecithin a day can considerably improve 91; excess aluminium (but can be removed by optimising magnesium, zinc and vitamin C levels) 117; lack of vitamin B12 89; lack of boron 118; lack of lecithin 91; lack of thiamine 67; lack of vitamin B6 80; lack of zinc 186;

Menstrual discomfort See **PMT**

Menopausal discomfort 10 mg of boron daily can substitute for hormone replacement therapy 118; imbalance of estrogen to progesterone (estrogen drops much less than progesterone after menopause due to estrogen in diet) 122; lack of boron 119; lack of folate (can be cause of hot flushes) 85; lack of magnesium 150; raising of progesterone to match estrogen level can avoid menopausal problems 122;

Mental disorders 50% incidence of hypoglycemia among psychiatric patients 32;

excess copper 132; excess vitamin B6 79; lack of calcium 124; lack of chromium 129; lack of CoQ10 109; lack of folate 85; lack of iodine 140; lack of inositol 92; lack of manganese 155; lack of omega 3 41, 47; lack of niacin 72; lack of sleep 90; lack of thiamine 67; lack of vitamin B12; lack of vitamin C (nearly all psychiatric hospital patients lack this vitamin) 96; lack of zinc 185; mental affirmations can help 71; negative thinking major cause of 67;

Mental impairment lack of folate in pregnancy 85; lack of iodine in pregnancy 141; lack of iron 145; lack of lecithin in pregnancy 91;

Mercury can aggravate symptoms of autism 215; little trace of in NZ grown foods 71; selenium helps neutralise effects of 169; vitamin C helps body expel 94;

Metals, toxic See **Toxins in body**

Migraine See **Headache, migraine**

Microflora See **Probiotics**

Milk (See also **Dairy**) allergies to if lacking correct gut probiotics 33, 113; author drinks unpasteurised whole 249; can supply vitamin B12 needs 88, 93; cow's milk a nutritious food despite criticisms 243; A1 type reported better than A2 195, 243; cows milk three times higher in protein than human 59; cream helps body absorb minerals of better 40; difficult to digest for many adult Maori and Pacific Islanders 123; Dr Ulric Williams fed his patients unpasteurised 226; false theory that calcium not absorbed from cow's milk 243; has a sleep-inducing effect on the body due to tryptophan content 152; largest source of calcium in NZ diet 123; lower risk of cardiovascular disease with high milk consumption 195; pasteurising destroys vitamin C 95; good source of riboflavin 70; unpasteurised milk now able to be bought direct from NZ dairy farmers 250; yoghurt more easily digested than milk 123; yoghurt nutrients virtually identical to milk 16;

Milk, human contains 1 part magnesium to 10 parts calcium 121; has vitamin C in useful amounts 95; has six times more selenium and twice as much vitamin E as cow's milk 169;

Minerals in food soil mineral depletion chart 157; every major update of this book has had to drop plant foods off food charts due to reduced mineral content 154; phosphorus a major acidic mineral - most others alkaline 160, 206; phosphorus and potassium content remain high as they are part of common crop fertilisers 154; steady decline of minerals in crop-growing soils 154; top five macro (bulk) minerals are potassium, sodium, chloride, calcium and phosphorus 206;

Miscarriage See **Pregnancy, miscarriage**

Molasses author of book takes daily 249; final by-product of sugar refining and therefore rich in trace minerals 34;

Nutritional healing chapter on and list of ailments healed by 223 Bach flower 'Rescue Remedy' has calming effect on both humans and animals 226; Bach flowers and homeopathy often ridiculed by science but empirical evidence for effectiveness not lacking 226; can be useful to enquire at a nearby health shop as to a practitioner's experience and reputation 227; caring bedside manner can play a huge role 227; cause of problem should be treated, not symptoms 225; considerable variations in skill among alternative practitioners 227; herbalism, osteopathy, naturopathy, acupuncture, Bach flowers, homeopathy, etc, safer and more gentle than orthodox drug treatment 226; similar success rate to orthodox medicine 226; Wanganui hospital surgeon Dr Ulric Williams a NZ pioneer in using nutritional healing 226;

Nutrition Survey NZ 2009 list of typical NZ mineral and vitamin deficiencies 8;

O

Obesity (See also **Slimming - permanent**) **chapter on permanent slimming 231;** calories from carbs the most fattening 20, 59; lack of chromium 129; lack of fat and protein in diet 47; lack of fibre in diet 37; lack of iodine 141; lack of walking 231; modern high-yield wheat strains linked to 28;

Oestrogen See **Estrogen**

Oils See **Fats**

Old age spots See **Skin, age spots**

Olive oil (See also **Fats}** good source of omega 9 40; one of best oils for cooking 40;

Omega 3 See **Fats omega 3**

Omega 6 See **Fats omega 6**

Omega 9 See **Fats omega 9**

OOS See **Repetitive Strain Injury**

Organically grown food average 60% higher zinc content in food from certified organic growers 183; emphasis on avoidance of toxic chemicals rather than optimum mineral content 183;

Orthodox medical treatment section on 225; chapter on doctors training 10; emphasis on treating symptoms rather than causes 225; skills of injury treatment and non-invasive surgical procedures impressive 225; patients show little interest in changing eating habits or exercising 10;

Osteoarthritis See **Arthritis, osteo**

Osteopathy (See also **Healing, nutritional**) similar success rate to orthodox medicine 226;

Osteoporosis section on avoiding 121; bones become like a dead branch of a tree 120; caused by collagen and calcium migrating from bones 120; full fat dairy foods can protect against 244; excess aluminium from antacids

117; excess fluoride 137; excess retinol vitamin A (hinders vitamin D) 63; healthy levels of estrogen, progesterone and testosterone protect against 118, 122; lack of boron 118; lack of calcium 124; lack of copper 133; lack of magnesium 150; lack of zinc 186; lack of vitamin B12 89; lack of vitamin D 101; lack of vitamin K2 115; phosphorus exceeding calcium intake 160-162; race horses can develop 123; sex hormones play big role in bone formation and maintenance 121; weight exercise helps retain calcium in bones 122; women in poor countries suffer less from 120;

Overeating excess fructose can interfere with appetite regulator leptin 30; how to eat 40% less 239; lack of fibre (which provides a sense of fullness) 37; stretching of stomach a factor 246;

Ovarian cysts lack of iodine 141;

Oxygen cancer cells die in presence of high levels of oxygen 161, 203; ensure constant change of fresh air in home 208; helps avoid colds and flu 202; low cell pH seriously lessens amount of oxygen that can enter body cells 161; most important nutrient of body 202; vital for immune system 202;

P

Pale skin See **Anemia**

Palpitations See **Heartbeat, rapid or irregular**

Pancreatitis lack of selenium 171;

Panic attacks (See also **Anxiety, Fearfulness**) lack of inositol 92; lack of magnesium 150; lack of niacin 73; lack of thiamine 67; sign of hypoglycemia (low blood sugar) 32;

Pantothenic acid (vitamin B5) chapter on 75; food table 77; baking soda can neutralise 76; Dr Atkins claimed it the best substance on the planet for establishing optimal levels of cholesterol and triglycerides in the blood 75; can be made in intestines but smoking hinders 75; found in most foods 75; helps prevent inflammation in body 75; important for healthy digestive system 75, 76; increases average life span of mice to human equivalent of 90 years 76; can lower LDL cholesterol by 21% and blood triglycerides by 32%. 75; number one nutrient used in Dr Atkin's practice 75; protects against acne and burning feet 75;

Paralysed arms or legs lack of potassium 166;

Paranoia See **Mental disorders**

Parasites, intestinal lack of zinc 186;

Parkinson's disease excess glutamate and aspartate 219; excess manganese 156; excess non-heme iron 146; lack of CoQ10 111; lack of magnesium 150;

Peace inner exercise can produce 247;

Period discomfort See **PMT**

Pesticides section on 71; low in NZ foods 71; organic food emphasis is on avoiding 183;

meal normally the most fattening 237; exercise necessary to raise metabolism rate otherwise body conserves calories 233; exercise to lively music or while watching TV/video 233; first day challenging but following days a breeze 234; fluid retention can be cause of weight problem 236; high glycemic-load carb foods the most fattening 237; how to eat 40% less 239; new 'Super 8' exercise method 240; one kg of fat stores 9000 calories 236; optimum weight is no rolls or flab around waistline and firm upper arms 234; overcoming comfort eating 238; skipping evening meal a rapid way to lose weight 237; stomach capacity shrinks 234; stop eating when 80% full 246; testing yourself for excess fat 237; use stevia as an almost zero-calorie sweetener 232; why exercise is a slow way to burn off fat 237; why low-carb diets only work short term 238;

Slow growth See **Children, slow growth**

Slow learning See **ADHD**

Slow healing or illness recovery lack of iron 146; lack of vitamin A 63; lack of vitamin C 97; lack of zinc 186;

Smell, poor sense of lack of copper 134; lack of zinc 186,

Smoking (See also **Addictions**) after quitting 10 years, cardiovascular risk drops to normal 199; a sign of stress 199; can drain body of folate 83; can lower vitamin B12 87; cause of low HDL cholesterol 53; depletes vitamin E 106; destroys 27% of vitamin C in blood 96, 193; destroys skin collagen 110; hinders manufacture of pantothenic acid in intestines 76; increases risk of cardiovascular disease 196, 199; increases tendency of blood to clot 190; lowers vitamin B6 79; 'tobacco not for the body' Mormon 'Word of Wisdom' 242;

Sodium (See also **Chloride/Chlorine; Salt**) chapter on 173; food table 176; diuretic drugs can severely deplete body of 174; should not increase blood pressure if potassium intake matched 173; essential for every cell 173; helps regulate heartbeat and blood pressure 175; a litre of perspiration causes loss of 950 mg 173; long living Japanese consume 11,000 mg a day 173; maintains body's electrolyte balance along with potassium and chloride 174; natural foods low in sodium 173; normal RDI 700 mg (a fifth of a teaspoon) 173; obtained from common salt which is 40% sodium, 60% chloride 173;

Soil mineral depletion chart of drop in 157; NZ soils mostly deficient in selenium 169;

Soy bean oil See **Fats, cooking oils**

Sperm count low See **Low sperm count; Infertility**

Spina bifida lack of folate in pregnancy 83;

Spinal disorders (See also **Glutamate; Aspartate**) lack of manganese 155; lack of vitamin D 101;

Spinal malformities lack of vitamin D in pregnancy 101;

Statin drugs 70% of people give up within a few months 55; artificially lowers liver production of cholesterol 54; can hinder formation of vitamin D 99; more cost-effective or free means to reduce heart attacks 54; have only minor effect on cardiovascular deaths 54; high dose of niacin far superior to 72; Lipex, Lipitor, etc statins 54; reduce body's manu-facture of CoQ10 52% 109; side effects include sore, weak muscles, dementia-like symptoms, liver damage 54;

Stevia a plant sugar 250 times sweeter than table sugar 34; has virtually zero calories 194, 232; author drinks water with sprinkle of ginger, cinnamon and stevia 250;

Stillbirth See **Birth defects**

Stomach acid, deficient anxiety hinders production of 246;

Stomach acid reducing drugs can hinder iron absorption 144; dangers of 124;

Stomach, rumbling sign of anxiety 246;

Stomach, ulcers excess aspirin 114; lack of vitamin A 63;

Stools grey or black excess non-heme iron

Stress (See also **Anxiety**) major cause of chronic fatigue 153; arteries squeezed narrow by stress hormone adrenaline 193-194, 201; benefits of smiling and cheerfulness 74; best antidote is vigorous exercise in fresh air 68, 212; can cause lower back pain 58; cause of acid reflux 76; excess or lack of vitamin B6 80; greatest need of nutrients during times of 13; hinders absorption of nutrients 13; how to lower 82; lack of calcium 124; lack of inositol 92; lack of magnesium 150; lack of manganese 155; lack of niacin 72; lack of selenium 171; lack of sunshine 99; lack of thiamine 66; lack of vitamin C 97; lack of zinc 186; LDL cholesterol of shift workers high 54; linked to numerous health disorders 152; stress main cause of high blood pressure 200; major cause of heart attacks, stroke and nearly all diseases 194, 209; major factor in artery plaques during active war service 33; stress arises mostly from family, finances or fellow workers 82; pets can help you avoid 209; smoking a sign of 199; stress hormones adrenalin and cortisol linked with inflamed joints 152,181; test of Confronters and Avoiders 201; three rules to minimise 82; workers with jobs at risk had 50% increase in cardiovascular disease 194;

Stretch marks lack of zinc 186;

Stroke (See also **Cardiovascular disease**) chapter on avoiding 189; 90% of caused by blood clots 190; why blood clots occur 190; eight steps to avoid 193; excess calcium 124; excess sodium (indirect factor) 175; high homocysteine a risk factor for clots 196; how to lower your stroke risk 166; lack of chromium 130; lack of CoQ10 111; lack of folate 85; lack of iodine 141; lack of magnesium 150; lack of manganese 155; lack of omega 3 fat 47; lack of potassium 166; lack of selenium 171; lack of vitamin B6 79; lack of vitamin D 101; lack of vitamin E 107; lack of zinc 186; long term high levels of adrenalin and cortisol can increase risk by 50%194; require full RDI of all vitamins and minerals to avoid 55; risk from smoking drops to normal after quitting smoking ten years 199; stress a major cause of 194; medical tests for risk of 196; women who ate 225 g of fish each week cut risk by 47% 194;

Sucralose chemical sweetener 600 times sweeter than sugar 36;

Sucrose term for table sugar 33;

Sugar (See also **Sweeteners**) **chapter on 29; different types of sugars listed 33;** best to use unrefined 131; blood triglycerides (fats) formed from excess 31; body requires chromium to process 129; contains few if any nutrients 29; cravings for 175; excess can cause cardio-vascular disease 29; excess can lower vitamin B12 87; excess surest way to create disease 31; fattens faster than other foods 29; feeds yeast infections and cancer cells 29; highly addictive and suppressive to immune system 29; levels in processed foods 29; major cause of cardio-vascular disease 33; only 10% to 15% of calories from recommended daily 27; sources of unrefined 131; tame that sweet tooth 24; use stevia as an almost zero-calorie sweetener 232; white sugar one of three deadly white foods 174; WHO now recommends only 10% of our calories be from sugar29;

Sugar, fructose (fruit sugar) 70% sweeter than sugar 33; can interfere with leptin our appetite regulator 30; man collapsed into a diabetic coma after living on oranges 31; more fattening than regular glucose sugar 30; one third converted directly to fat by liver 30; too much can cause insulin resistance, diabetes, cardiovascular disease and gout 30;

Sugar, craving why sugar cravings 175; lack of chromium 130; lack of magnesium 151;

Sulphur chapter on 179; food table 180; nature's beauty mineral 179; necessary for health of joints and nervous system 179; eggs a high quality source but rheumatoid arthritis sufferers seem to dislike 179; found in every cell of body 179; helps multiply useful bacteria in intestines 179; MSM a safer organic form of sulphur 179; required to make collagen 179; RDI normally met with sufficient protein intake 179;

Summary See **Conclusions**

Sunburn Swedish researchers found no link between childhood sunburn and melanoma 210; three bouts of adult sunburn every year doubles risk of melanoma 210; sunbeds linked with melanoma 103, 202;

Sunbathing helps avoid cancer 103; NZ sunshine chart to obtain vitamin D 103; UVA

and UVB rays explained 99; vitamin D from the sun one of most essential nutrients for cancer avoidance and health 244; sunbeds linked with melanoma 103, 202;

Supplements chapter on 229; check net amount of minerals on a supplement label as it is often only a small percent of main listing 230; difficult to obtain full RDI of all minerals nowa-days because of nutrient-barren processed foods and mineral-exhausted soils 157, 229; huge variations in supplement quality 229; mineral supplementation seems almost inescapable nowadays 229; minerals critical for good health 229; most common lacking minerals in NZ – boron, iodine, magnesium, selenium and zinc 229; most vitamins relatively easy to obtain from food 229; nutrients tend to work in groups - being short of one can restrict activity of whole group 229; supplements author takes 248, 249; vitamin E ineffective in supplement form but achieved 62% reduction in heart disease when obtained from food 105, 229;

Surgery See **Orthodox medical treatment**

Swallowing, painful or difficult lack of iron 146;

Sweeteners See **Sugar**

Swelling of tissue See **Fluid retention**

T

Tantrums See **Irritability**

Taste, poor sense of lack of copper 134; lack of zinc 186,

Teeth (See also **Fluoride**) calcium maintains health of 123; molybdenum strengthens enamel 158; phosphorus maintains health of 162; tooth enamel largely magnesium 149; vitamin A regulates spacing and straightness of 63; vitamin C assists body in forming and main-taining 96; vitamin D maintains health of 101;

Teeth, brittle excess fluoride 136;

Teeth, crooked lack of vitamin A 63;

Teeth, decayed acidity of sticky sweets and chocolate a major cause 32; high blood sugar can also cause 32; how to avoid decay 139; lack of calcium 124; lack of magnesium 150; lack of molybdenum 159; lack of phosphorus 162; lack of vitamin A 63; lack of vitamin C 96; lack of vitamin D 101; should remove chocolate residue from molars by eating dry bread or apple afterwards 139; sugar-acid decay takes place during 30 minutes after eating 139;

Teeth, loose lack of vitamin C 96;

Teeth, malformed lack of phosphorus 162; lack of vitamin A 63;

Teeth, mottled excess fluoride 136

Teeth, weak lack of vitamin A 63; lack of vitamin C 96; wrong phosphorus-calcium balance 162;

Tendonitis See **Arthritis**

284

Voice thick lack of iodine 141;

Vomiting (See also **Nausea**) lack of sodium 175;

W

Walking brisk walking burns 300 calories hour - four times that of sitting 19, 237; calorie use table 21; excellent for improving health and mental outlook 240; helps avoid headaches 116; improves sleep 90; helps prevent constipation and varicose veins 37, 86; linked with longevity 172; mid-city New York dwellers without cars much slimmer than car-using Americans 231; obesity and Alzheimer's rare in societies that walk a lot 217, 246;

Warfarin anticoagulant (See **Cardiovascular medications**)

Water (See also **Fluoride**) **chapter on 56**; can increase muscle power 58; dehydration can raise blood pressure 56; excess can flush out potassium and sodium 57; food supplies about 25% of daily need 56; helps prevent consti-pation 57; high natural manganese levels can turn bore water blackish and stain toilets and clothes 155; lack of reduces physical and mental performance 57; lack of thirst in elderly regarded as side effect of dementia 56; loss of just under one litre can cause health problems 56; should you drink eight glasses a day? 56; nutritionists consider four glasses of water a day adequate during winter 57;

Water retention See **Fluid retention**

Weak red blood cells See **Anemia**

Weight averages 75% of NZ men and 63% of women overweight 14;

Weight loss See **Slimming, permanent**

Weight, difficult to lose (See also **Thyroid underactive**) lack of calcium (if after menopause) 124; can be fluid retention due to heart defect 236; lack of progesterone 121;

Wellbeing, sense of inositol and vitamin B6 promote 79, 92; words can have marked effect on 77;

Wheat better provider of nutrition than rice 243; stone ground flour from health shops retains wheat germ 106; wheat germ absent from supermarket flour products 106; modern high-yield strains can be faster digesting and higher in gluten 28; older strains of wheat may be more healthy - Einkorn, Spelt, etc 28; over-coming allergy to 28; NZ should be grateful for wholegrain weetbix 158;

Williams Dr Ulric See **Doctor Ulric Williams**

Wind can be an allergic reaction to milk 123; digestive probiotics for a type of food lacking 113; excess vitamin C 97;

Words power of affirmations 71; power on health 77;

Wound healing slow See **Slow healing or illness recovery**

Wrinkled skin See **Skin, premature ageing/-wrinkling**

X

Xylitol plant sugar - does not decay teeth 34;

Y

Yeast infections can eventually lead to cancer 205; excess sugar 29, 31; lack of iron 146; lack of molybdenum 158; lack of pantothenic acid 75; lack of probiotics 113; lack of vitamin B6 79; lack of zinc 186; over-acidic body cells 205;

Yoghurt can help body re-establish some hardy probiotics following antibiotics 113; more easily digested than milk 123; nutrients virtually identical to milk so not included in food tables 16;

Z

Zinc chapter on 183; food table 187; 52% to 90% deficient in NZ, depending on age 8; 60% higher content in food from certified organic growers 183; 66% lost from wheat during milling 183; assists in healing wounds and surgery 185; blondes have become brown-haired taking zinc supplements 185; can double testosterone in men over 60 185; cancer and inflammation quickly exhaust body's supply 185; critically important in protecting brain and eyes from MSG/aspartate excitotoxin damage 183; deficiencies common among children and elderly 185; excess phosphorus can cause deficiency of 162; has limited storage in body so deficiencies can develop quickly 184; helps body eliminate toxins along with vitamin C 186; helps body repair DNA genes 185; helps maintain bone density and muscle bulk 186; helps maintain sexual fertility and libido 185; how to make a cheap zinc sulphate heptahydrate liquid to test for deficiency 184; home-made zinc spray can knock out a developing cold virus 185; more known roles in body for zinc than any other nutrient 183; nearly all NZ men aged over 70 deficient 183; necessary to maintain sense of taste and smell 185; not included in commonly used fertilisers 183; rock oysters only natural rich source 183; vitamin B6 needed for absorption 79; zinc and magnesium deficiencies tend to go together 183;

Bibliography

As this book is intended for the lay person I have not taken up valuable space with numerous pages of references – in most cases there should be sufficient detail in the text for readers to do further research online.

Key Findings of the 2008/09 New Zealand Adult Nutrition Survey
Ministry of Health, 2011

Nutrient Reference Values for Australia and New Zealand
Ministry of Health, 2010

Dr Atkins Vita-Nutrient Solution – Nature's Answer to Drugs
Dr Robert C. Atkins MD 1998

NZ Food Composition Database 2010
Ministry of Health and NZ Institute for Plant & Food Research Ltd

Weston A. Price Foundation 2011
www.westonaprice.org

Vitamins, Herbs, Minerals & Supplements – The Complete Guide
Dr H. Winter Griffith MD 1998

BioBalance
Rudolf A. Wiley, Ph.D.

Natural Remedies That Really Work – A NZ Guide
Dr Shaun Holt, MD. 2008

A Physician's Guide to Natural Health Products That Work
Dr James A. Howenstine, MD. 2008

Excitotoxins – The Taste That Kills
Dr George R. Schwartz MD. 1996

Healing Through Nutrition
Dr Melvyn R. Werbach MD. Thorsons, 1995

Nutritional Medicine
Dr Stephen Davies & Dr Alan Stewart, Pan.

The Vitamin Bible
Earl Mindell, Ph.B.,R.Ph, Arlington Books, 1999

The Miracle Nutrient CoQ10
Dr E.G. Bliznakov, MD, & G.L. Hunt, Bantam, 1987

Mental and Elemental Nutrients
Dr Carl Pfeiffer, Kents Publishing, Conn. US. 1976

Fit For Life
Harvey & Marilyn Diamond, Harper Collins, 2010

NZ's Greatest Doctor – Ulric Williams
Brenda Sampson, 2003. Zealand Publishing House.

Living the Low Carb Life
Jonny Bowden, MA, CNS, 2004

Cancer: Cause and Cure
Percy Weston, 2005